New Insights into Prostate Cancer Diagnosis and Treatment

New Insights into Prostate Cancer Diagnosis and Treatment

Guest Editor

Sazan Rasul

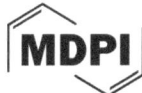

Basel • Beijing • Wuhan • Barcelona • Belgrade • Novi Sad • Cluj • Manchester

Guest Editor
Sazan Rasul
Medical University of Vienna
Vienna
Austria

Editorial Office
MDPI AG
Grosspeteranlage 5
4052 Basel, Switzerland

This is a reprint of the Special Issue, published open access by the journal *Current Oncology* (ISSN 1718-7729), freely accessible at: https://www.mdpi.com/journal/curroncol/topical_collections/New_Frontiers_Prostate_Cancer_Diagnosis_Treatment.

For citation purposes, cite each article independently as indicated on the article page online and as indicated below:

Lastname, A.A.; Lastname, B.B. Article Title. *Journal Name* **Year**, *Volume Number*, Page Range.

ISBN 978-3-7258-2681-0 (Hbk)
ISBN 978-3-7258-2682-7 (PDF)
https://doi.org/10.3390/books978-3-7258-2682-7

© 2025 by the authors. Articles in this book are Open Access and distributed under the Creative Commons Attribution (CC BY) license. The book as a whole is distributed by MDPI under the terms and conditions of the Creative Commons Attribution-NonCommercial-NoDerivs (CC BY-NC-ND) license (https://creativecommons.org/licenses/by-nc-nd/4.0/).

Contents

About the Editor ix

Preface xi

Cristina V. Berenguer, Ferdinando Pereira, José S. Câmara and Jorge A. M. Pereira
Underlying Features of Prostate Cancer—Statistics, Risk Factors, and Emerging Methods for Its Diagnosis
Reprinted from: *Curr. Oncol.* **2023**, *30*, 2300–2321, https://doi.org/10.3390/curroncol30020178 . **1**

Ahmad N. Alzubaidi, Amy Zheng, Mohammad Said, Xuanjia Fan, Michael Maidaa, R. Grant Owens, et al.
Prior Negative Biopsy, PSA Density, and Anatomic Location Impact Cancer Detection Rate of MRI-Targeted PI-RADS Index Lesions
Reprinted from: *Curr. Oncol.* **2024**, *31*, 4406–4413, https://doi.org/10.3390/curroncol31080329 . **23**

Raidizon Mercedes, Dennis Head, Elizabeth Zook, Eric Eidelman, Jeffrey Tomaszewski, Serge Ginzburg, et al.
Appropriateness of Imaging for Low-Risk Prostate Cancer—Real World Data from the Pennsylvania Urologic Regional Collaboration (PURC)
Reprinted from: *Curr. Oncol.* **2024**, *31*, 4746–4752, https://doi.org/10.3390/curroncol31080354 . **31**

Giulia Riccio, Cristina V. Berenguer, Rosa Perestrelo, Ferdinando Pereira, Pedro Berenguer, Cristina P. Ornelas, et al.
Differences in the Volatilomic Urinary Biosignature of Prostate Cancer Patients as a Feasibility Study for the Detection of Potential Biomarkers
Reprinted from: *Curr. Oncol.* **2023**, *30*, 4904–4921, https://doi.org/10.3390/curroncol30050370 . **38**

Bernhard Grubmüller, Nicolai A. Huebner, Sazan Rasul, Paola Clauser, Nina Pötsch, Karl Hermann Grubmüller, et al.
Dual-Tracer PET-MRI-Derived Imaging Biomarkers for Prediction of Clinically Significant Prostate Cancer
Reprinted from: *Curr. Oncol.* **2023**, *30*, 1683–1691, https://doi.org/10.3390/curroncol30020129 . **56**

Takafumi Yanagisawa, Pawel Rajwa, Tatsushi Kawada, Kensuke Bekku, Ekaterina Laukhtina, Markus von Deimling, et al.
An Updated Systematic and Comprehensive Review of Cytoreductive Prostatectomy for Metastatic Prostate Cancer
Reprinted from: *Curr. Oncol.* **2023**, *30*, 2194–2216, https://doi.org/10.3390/curroncol30020170 . **65**

Lewis Wardale, Ryan Cardenas, Vincent J. Gnanapragasam, Colin S. Cooper, Jeremy Clark and Daniel S. Brewer
Combining Molecular Subtypes with Multivariable Clinical Models Has the Potential to Improve Prediction of Treatment Outcomes in Prostate Cancer at Diagnosis
Reprinted from: *Curr. Oncol.* **2023**, *30*, 157–170, https://doi.org/10.3390/curroncol30010013 . . . **88**

Marco Oderda, Giorgio Calleris, Daniele D'Agate, Marco Falcone, Riccardo Faletti, Marco Gatti, et al.
Intraoperative 3D-US-mpMRI Elastic Fusion Imaging-Guided Robotic Radical Prostatectomy: A Pilot Study
Reprinted from: *Curr. Oncol.* **2023**, *30*, 110–117, https://doi.org/10.3390/curroncol30010009 . . . **102**

Ying Hao, Qing Zhang, Junke Hang, Linfeng Xu, Shiwei Zhang and Hongqian Guo
Development of a Prediction Model for Positive Surgical Margin in Robot-Assisted Laparoscopic Radical Prostatectomy
Reprinted from: *Curr. Oncol.* **2022**, *29*, 9560–9571, https://doi.org/10.3390/curroncol29120751 . **110**

Siroos Mirzaei, Rainer Lipp, Shahin Zandieh and Asha Leisser
Single-Center Comparison of [^{64}Cu]-DOTAGA-PSMA and [^{18}F]-PSMA PET–CT for Imaging Prostate Cancer
Reprinted from: *Curr. Oncol.* **2021**, *28*, 4167–4173, https://doi.org/10.3390/curroncol28050353 . **122**

Nikolaos Kalampokis, Nikolaos Grivas, Markos Karavitakis, Ioannis Leotsakos, Ioannis Katafigiotis, Marcio Covas Moschovas, et al.
Nondetectable Prostate Carcinoma (pT0) after Radical Prostatectomy: A Narrative Review
Reprinted from: *Curr. Oncol.* **2022**, *29*, 1309–1315, https://doi.org/10.3390/curroncol29030111 . **129**

Benedikt Hoeh, Felix Preisser, Mike Wenzel, Clara Humke, Clarissa Wittler, Jan L. Hohenhorst, et al.
Correlation of Urine Loss after Catheter Removal and Early Continence in Men Undergoing Radical Prostatectomy
Reprinted from: *Curr. Oncol.* **2021**, *28*, 4738–4747, https://doi.org/10.3390/curroncol28060399 . **136**

Darren M. C. Poon, Daisy Lam, Kenneth Wong, Cheuk Man Chu, Michael Cheung, Frankie Mo, et al.
Prospective Randomized Phase II Study of Stereotactic Body Radiotherapy (SBRT) vs. Conventional Fractionated Radiotherapy (CFRT) for Chinese Patients with Early-Stage Localized Prostate Cancer †
Reprinted from: *Curr. Oncol.* **2022**, *29*, 27–37, https://doi.org/10.3390/curroncol29010003 . . . . **146**

Raffaella Lucchini, Ciro Franzese, Suela Vukcaj, Giorgio Purrello, Denis Panizza, Valeria Faccenda, et al.
Acute Toxicity and Quality of Life in a Post-Prostatectomy Ablative Radiation Therapy (POPART) Multicentric Trial
Reprinted from: *Curr. Oncol.* **2022**, *29*, 9349–9356, https://doi.org/10.3390/curroncol29120733 . **157**

Dalia Ahmad Khalil, Jörg Wulff, Danny Jazmati, Dirk Geismar, Christian Bäumer, Paul-Heinz Kramer, et al.
Is an Endorectal Balloon Beneficial for Rectal Sparing after Spacer Implantation in Prostate Cancer Patients Treated with Hypofractionated Intensity-Modulated Proton Beam Therapy? A Dosimetric and Radiobiological Comparison Study
Reprinted from: *Curr. Oncol.* **2023**, *30*, 758–768, https://doi.org/10.3390/curroncol30010058 . . . **165**

Bernhard Grubmüller, Victoria Jahrreiss, Stephan Brönimann, Fahad Quhal, Keiichiro Mori, Axel Heidenreich, Alberto Briganti, et al.
Salvage Radical Prostatectomy for Radio-Recurrent Prostate Cancer: An Updated Systematic Review of Oncologic, Histopathologic and Functional Outcomes and Predictors of Good Response
Reprinted from: *Curr. Oncol.* **2021**, *28*, 2881–2892, https://doi.org/10.3390/curroncol28040252 . **176**

Jonathan Wallach, Irini Youssef, Andrea Leaf and David Schwartz
Diagnostic and Therapeutic Challenges in a Patient with Synchronous Very High-Risk Prostate Adenocarcinoma and Anal Carcinoma
Reprinted from: *Curr. Oncol.* **2022**, *29*, 377–382, https://doi.org/10.3390/curroncol29010033 . . . **188**

Stefano Salciccia, Marco Frisenda, Giulio Bevilacqua, Pietro Viscuso, Paolo Casale, Ettore De Berardinis, et al.
Comparative Prospective and Longitudinal Analysis on the Platelet-to-Lymphocyte, Neutrophil-to-Lymphocyte, and Albumin-to-Globulin Ratio in Patients with Non-Metastatic and Metastatic Prostate Cancer
Reprinted from: *Curr. Oncol.* **2022**, *29*, 9474–9500, https://doi.org/10.3390/curroncol29120745 . **194**

Tim Wollenweber, Lucia Zisser, Elisabeth Kretschmer-Chott, Michael Weber, Bernhard Grubmüller, Gero Kramer, et al.
Renal and Salivary Gland Functions after Three Cycles of PSMA-617 Therapy Every Four Weeks in Patients with Metastatic Castration-Resistant Prostate Cancer
Reprinted from: *Curr. Oncol.* **2021**, *28*, 3692–3704, https://doi.org/10.3390/curroncol28050315 . **221**

Chetanya Mittal, Hardik Gupta, Chitrakshi Nagpal, Ranjit K. Sahoo, Aparna Sharma, Bharat B. Gangadharaiah, et al.
Quality of Life Determinants in Patients with Metastatic Prostate Cancer: Insights from a Cross-Sectional Questionnaire-Based Study
Reprinted from: *Curr. Oncol.* **2024**, *31*, 4940–4954, https://doi.org/10.3390/curroncol31090366 . **234**

About the Editor

Sazan Rasul

Sazan Rasul (MD, PhD) is the Head of the PET Center (PET/CT and PET/MRI) at the Vienna General Hospital and Deputy Head of the Department of Nuclear Medicine at the Medical University of Vienna, Austria. She studied Medicine at the Salahaddin College of Medicine in Erbil, Iraq, and at the Medical University of Vienna, Austria. Professor Dr. Rasul is a specialist in general medicine and nuclear medicine and holds a PhD in the field of endocrinology and metabolism and a professorship in the field of nuclear medicine, both from the Medical University of Vienna, Austria.

Preface

The incidence of prostate cancer is increasing worldwide as a result of the rising age of the male population and improvements in diagnostic methods for early detection of the disease. However, despite advances in the diagnosis and treatment of this type of cancer, the mortality rate is still high. Prostate cancer remains the second most common cause of cancer-related death in men since the disease has highly complicated genetic and pathological diversity.

Sazan Rasul
Guest Editor

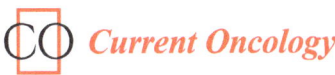

Review

Underlying Features of Prostate Cancer—Statistics, Risk Factors, and Emerging Methods for Its Diagnosis

Cristina V. Berenguer [1], Ferdinando Pereira [2], José S. Câmara [1,3] and Jorge A. M. Pereira [1,*]

[1] CQM—Centro de Química da Madeira, NPRG, Campus da Penteada, Universidade da Madeira, 9020-105 Funchal, Portugal
[2] SESARAM—Serviço de Saúde da Região Autónoma da Madeira, EPERAM, Hospital Dr. Nélio Mendonça, Avenida Luís de Camões 6180, 9000-177 Funchal, Portugal
[3] Departamento de Química, Faculdade de Ciências Exatas e Engenharia, Campus da Penteada, Universidade da Madeira, 9020-105 Funchal, Portugal
* Correspondence: jorge.pereira@staff.uma.pt

Abstract: Prostate cancer (PCa) is the most frequently occurring type of malignant tumor and a leading cause of oncological death in men. PCa is very heterogeneous in terms of grade, phenotypes, and genetics, displaying complex features. This tumor often has indolent growth, not compromising the patient's quality of life, while its more aggressive forms can manifest rapid growth with progression to adjacent organs and spread to lymph nodes and bones. Nevertheless, the overtreatment of PCa patients leads to important physical, mental, and economic burdens, which can be avoided with careful monitoring. Early detection, even in the cases of locally advanced and metastatic tumors, provides a higher chance of cure, and patients can thus go through less aggressive treatments with fewer side effects. Furthermore, it is important to offer knowledge about how modifiable risk factors can be an effective method for reducing cancer risk. Innovations in PCa diagnostics and therapy are still required to overcome some of the limitations of the current screening techniques, in terms of specificity and sensitivity. In this context, this review provides a brief overview of PCa statistics, reporting its incidence and mortality rates worldwide, risk factors, and emerging screening strategies.

Keywords: prostate cancer; incidence; mortality; risk factors; biomarkers

1. Introduction

Prostate cancer (PCa) is the second most frequent type of malignancy cancer among men worldwide [1,2]. PCa burden was very dramatic until the beginning of the 21st century, due to the increased use of the prostate-specific antigen (PSA) tests for screening. From this date onwards, different innovations increasing the efficacy of the therapeutic methods, along with earlier diagnoses, led to a significant reduction in the number of deaths, and a less pronounced downward trend in the incidence of PCa.

Epidemiological studies have shown that the geographical and racial distribution differences in PCa incidence and mortality rates reflect differences in the distribution of populations, with varying degrees of genetic susceptibility [3,4]. Epigenetic factors such as different lifestyles also contribute to these differences, particularly unbalanced diets, and tobacco and alcohol consumption [2,3,5]. Another difference is in the availability and use of, and access to, medical care, especially regional differences in the diagnosis of latent cancers through PSA screening [5,6]. Generally, most men are reluctant to go through PCa screening, since it is based on invasive and unpleasant procedures. For cancer control, it is of the utmost importance to build a sustainable platform for the dissemination of cancer prevention and the provision of cancer care, specifically in low-income and transitioning countries. These results highlight the need to increase health literacy and ensure that opportunistic screening is preceded by a thorough discussion about its potential benefits and risks [7]. Hence, it is crucial to develop more focused diagnostic tools for the early and

Citation: Berenguer, C.V.; Pereira, F.; Câmara, J.S.; Pereira, J.A.M. Underlying Features of Prostate Cancer—Statistics, Risk Factors, and Emerging Methods for Its Diagnosis. *Curr. Oncol.* **2023**, *30*, 2300–2321. https://doi.org/10.3390/curroncol30020178

Received: 5 January 2023
Revised: 9 February 2023
Accepted: 12 February 2023
Published: 15 February 2023

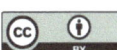

Copyright: © 2023 by the authors. Licensee MDPI, Basel, Switzerland. This article is an open access article distributed under the terms and conditions of the Creative Commons Attribution (CC BY) license (https:// creativecommons.org/licenses/by/ 4.0/).

non-invasive detection of PCa that can classify patients according to the severity of their cancers, and, as a result, guide their treatment decisions. In this review, PCa statistics are briefly summarized, reporting its incidence and mortality rates worldwide, and risk factors and emerging screening strategies are presented and discussed.

2. Incidence and Mortality Rates Worldwide

The prevalence of PCa varies among different racial groups, and the vast disparity has been associated with socioeconomic conditions, as well as environmental and biological factors, which play an important role in the etiology of PCa. Variations in the incidence rates may be due to underdiagnosis, differences in screening methods, and disparities in healthcare access [2]. Requesting PSA tests directly influences the incidence values around the world. In more developed countries, the use of the PSA test has resulted in a reduction in the mortality rates, while in less developed countries, they have shown an increase, reflecting the access to early detection and available therapies yielded by the PSA result [1,8]. For instance, PCa incidence in Europe is high when compared with other geographical areas, such as Africa or Asia, due to the use of PSA for early detection [9]. Regional differences are related to environmental risk factors and differences in healthcare policies across individual countries, such as the access to and availability of costly targeted therapies, in addition to heterogeneity in health and socioeconomic status [9,10]. In 2020, PCa was the most frequently diagnosed cancer among men in 121 of 185 countries around the world [1,2,5] (Figure 1). The world age-standardized incidence rates (wASR) are three times higher in areas with high or very high human development index scores [1,5] when compared with less developed countries (37.5 and 11.3/100,000, respectively), while the mortality rates are almost constant (8.1 and 5.9/100,000, respectively).

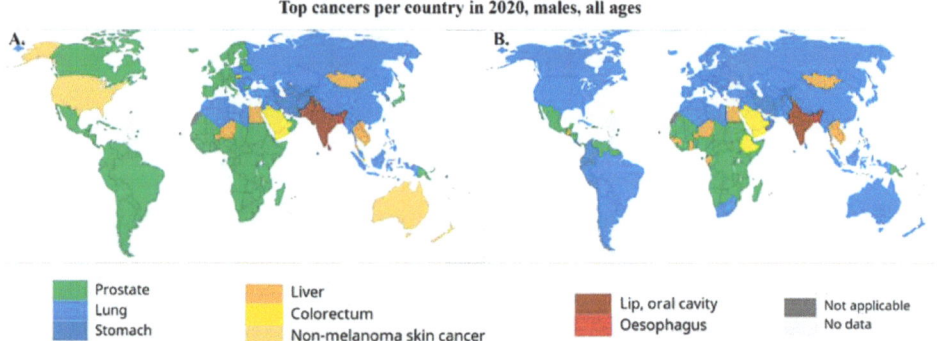

Figure 1. (**A**) Most diagnosed types of cancer among men worldwide, 2020. Nonmelanoma skin cancer was included in calculations of top cancer per country. (**B**) Leading cause of cancer deaths among men worldwide, 2020. Source: GLOBOCAN 2020 [1].

Social determinants, such as poverty, lack of education, lack of social support, and social isolation, play an important role in the PCa stage at diagnosis and survival. A later stage at diagnosis may be due to lower PCa screening rates or population-specific variations in environmental exposures, including diet, physical activity, or occupational exposures. Additionally, men may be persuaded by their partner, other family members, or others within their social network to undergo PCa screening [11]. Social media can be employed in research, advocacy, and awareness campaigns in the PCa community. Evidence suggests that social media initiatives may enhance cancer screening and early detection. Patients and their caregivers can also take advantage of networking and educational opportunities. Nevertheless, a few concerns remain regarding inconsistent information quality [12].

Overall, in the last 5 years, the mortality rates have declined, most probably due to improved access to treatments and dissemination of therapies, such as surgery and hormonotherapy. The projections for the next 5 years show an increasing trend in the estimated number of new cases and deaths (Figure 2), for all continents. Furthermore, in the upcoming years, the number of PCa cases may increase, because the diversion of resources to the COVID-19 pandemic has delayed diagnosis, patient management, treatment, and research. Many cancer patients had their management delayed as PCa care changed and shifted towards patterns that limited the risk of COVID-19 infection, including increased use of transperineal biopsy and hypofractionated radiation therapy regimens, as well as the substitution of docetaxel with enzalutamide [13]. This pandemic will lead to an increasing number of men diagnosed with more advanced diseases, which will have a negative impact on their prognosis. Consequently, treating patients with locally advanced or metastatic diseases is also expected to be more expensive than treating those with less advanced diseases. Therefore, to control the clinical, economical, and welfare costs to society, urgently coordinated action is needed to address the diagnostic and treatment deficiencies in PCa services [13].

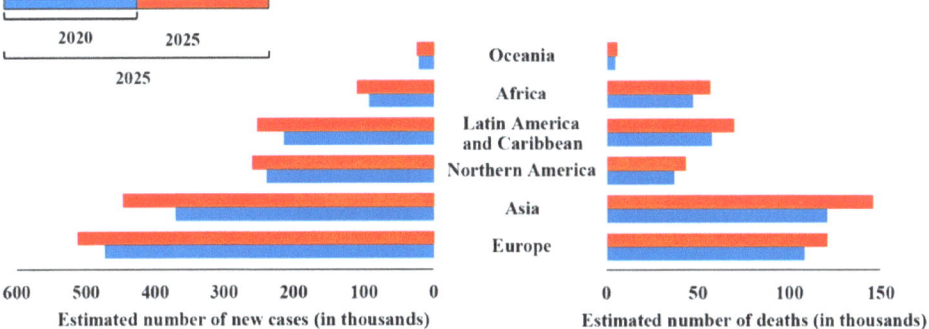

Figure 2. Estimated number of new cases and deaths from prostate cancer from 2020 to 2025. Source: GLOBOCAN 2020 [1,5].

3. Prostate Cancer Risk Factors

The well-established PCa risk factors are advancing age, ethnicity (Black race), certain genetic mutations, insulin-like growth factors (IGF), and family history of this malignancy (Table 1) [5]. Lifestyle, including diet, tobacco and alcohol consumption, obesity and physical inactivity, and environmental factors, such as exposure to chemicals or ionizing radiation, may also increase the risk of advanced PCa (Figure 3) [2,5,14].

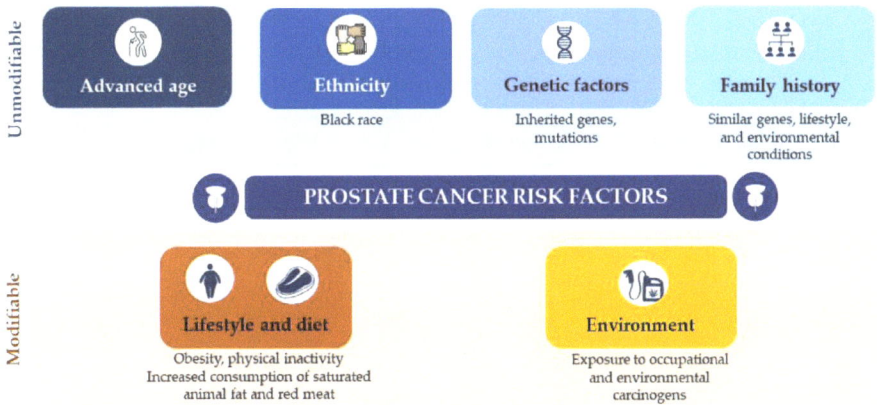

Figure 3. Modifiable and unmodifiable prostate cancer risk factors.

Table 1. Prostate cancer risk factors and their roles in the development of this tumor (articles from the last 5 years).

Risk Factor	Role in PCa	Reference
Ethnicity	PCa incidence, morbidity, and mortality rates vary significantly by race and ethnicity. African-American, Black, and Caribbean men show the highest PCa rates worldwide. These disparities are mostly related to differences in access to screening and treatment, exposure to PCa risk factors, and variations in genomic susceptibility (e.g., risk loci found at chromosome 8q24), among other biological factors.	[15–20]
Family history and genetic factors	According to estimates, around 5 to 15% of PCa cases have been related to hereditary factors. In genome-wide association studies, almost 170 loci of susceptibility for hereditary PCa (about 33% of familial PCa risks) have been identified. Many genes show a strong association with hereditary PCa risk, including *BRCA1*, *BRCA2*, *ATM*, *CHEK2*, and *PALB2*, and Lynch syndrome *MLH1*, *MSH2*, *MSH6*, and *PMS2* genes. Other genes, however, have an unclear cancer risk and unknown clinical importance.	[4,20–26]
Obesity, overweight and physical inactivity	Obesity is implicated in the dysregulation of various hormonal pathways, leading to higher levels of insulin and IGF, oxidative stress, and inflammatory cytokines, and lower levels of adiponectin, testosterone, and sex hormone-binding globulin. Obesity is associated with an increased risk of PCa mortality and recurrence, worsened treatment-related adverse effects, development of obesity-related comorbidities, and the earlier progression and development of metastatic disease. Nevertheless, the physiological mechanisms associated between obesity and poor PCa outcomes remain unknown.	[3,27–33]
Tobacco use	Smoking increases the risk of death from PCa, which increases with obesity, specifically for advanced PCa. Moreover, tobacco smoking increases the risk of biochemical recurrence and metastasis. Nevertheless, the association between tobacco smoking and PCa prognosis needs to be explored.	[3,32,34–38]
Lycopene and tomato-based products	Epidemiologic studies have focused on tomatoes as a specific source of lycopene, with more consistent findings supporting the protective effect of a higher intake of tomatoes on PCa risk. Furthermore, studies have shown a reduced risk of advanced PCa with the consumption of cooked tomatoes, since these products have more available lycopene. Current epidemiologic evidence is not definitive but suggests that a higher intake of tomato-based products is associated with a reduced risk of PCa and a potentially lower risk of progression. Further studies are required to determine whether the effect is because of lycopene or other components of tomatoes.	[3,32,39–44]
Calcium, dairy products, and vitamin D	An intake of dairy products above the daily recommended dose has been positively associated with PCa risk. A potential mechanism underlying the association with calcium is through suppressing circulating levels of dihydroxyvitamin D, which seems to have a protective effect against PCa. The mechanisms behind this association are not yet fully understood, but researchers suggest reducing dairy intake while increasing the consumption of fish and tomato products for PCa prevention.	[3,32,45–48]
Cruciferous, soy, and green tea	Cruciferous, soy, and green tea seem to have a role in decreasing the risk of PCa due to compounds with anticarcinogenic properties in their composition. Asian populations consume soy foods as a part of their regular diet, which might contribute to the lower PCa incidence found in these countries. However, the preventive action of these compounds needs to be further explored.	[32,43,49–54]

3.1. Unmodifiable Risk Factors: Ethnicity, Family History, and Genetic Factors

PCa is infamous for its ethnic disparity, which raises the possibility that inheritance plays an important role in oncogenesis. The highest incidences of this cancer are documented in descendants of Northern Europeans and African-Americans, while native

Africans and Asians are much less susceptible to the disease [55]. For instance, African-American, Caribbean, and Black men in Europe have the highest incidences of PCa and are more likely to develop the disease earlier in life when compared to other racial and ethnic groups [17,56,57]. These individuals possess a common genetic background more prone to the development of cancer, such as specific genes (e.g., chromosome 8q24) that are more susceptible to mutation (Table 1) [2,16,58]. The migration and colonization history of Scandinavians is intimately related to the susceptibility to PCa in Europe. Subsequently, the incidences in other ethnic groups are related to the history of European settlement and the degree of admixture. Some research has suggested that PCa has been transmitted through a hereditary predisposition that resides in the Northern European genome [55]. A proportion of the patients in the European, European American, and African-American populations share two polymorphisms at chromosome 8q24, transmitted by admixture [59–61]. The low frequency of these alleles among native Africans and other ethnic groups, however, suggests transmission by admixture between Europeans and African-Americans. The Caribbean countries have a history of colonization by Europeans, including the Scandinavians. At the same time, the slave trade brought many Africans. Given these reasons, many of the Caribbean countries now show high PCa incidence [55].

The prevalence of family PCa is estimated to be around 20%, while the rate of inherited PCa is about 5% to 15% [10,21]. The presence of similar genes, similar lifestyles, and similar environmental conditions are among the reasons associated with family PCa. Inherited PCa occurs when a gene mutation is transmitted from one generation to the next, when at least three of their first-degree relatives are affected by PCa, or when three or two generations of a family, or more close relatives (such as the father, brother, son, grandfather, uncle, or nephew), are affected by this cancer [21,22]. Some cancer predisposition genes have been identified to affect the risk of PCa, including hereditary mutation of *HOXB13* as well as *BRCA1*, *BRCA2*, *ATM*, *CHEK2*, and *PALB2*, and Lynch syndrome *MLH1*, *MSH2*, *MSH6*, and *PMS2* genes (Table 1) [21]. Other genes have a poorly defined cancer risk with unknown clinical significance. Nevertheless, the genetics behind family and hereditary PCa remains complex [10,21,22].

3.2. Modifiable Risk Factors: Lifestyle, Diet, and Environment

Lifestyle factors are modifiable and may provide an effective method for reducing cancer risk (Figure 3). According to the World Health Organization (WHO), 30 to 50% of cancers are preventable by healthy lifestyle choices, such as avoidance of tobacco and alcohol consumption, and public health measures, such as immunization against cancer-causing infections [3,5,14,32]. Men with PCa have been shown to exhibit upregulated oxidative stress and impaired antioxidant defense systems [62]. Animal studies have reported that nutrients, such as fat, protein, carbohydrates, vitamins (vitamins A, D and E), and polyphenols, are involved in PCa pathogenesis, and progression through several mechanisms, including inflammation, antioxidant effects, and the effects of sex hormones [63]. However, it has been difficult to determine which nutrients have a beneficial or harmful impact on PCa incidence and progression due to divergent results in clinical studies [3,32,64].

Diets involving plant-based foods, such as tomatoes, cruciferous, and soybeans, have been associated with a lower risk of developing PCa [32,43,49]. Cruciferous or Brassica vegetables are known to possess anticancer properties mediated by phenylethyl isothiocyanate, sulforaphane, phytochemicals, and indole-3-carbinol [54]. Similarly, lycopene, a carotenoid mostly found in tomatoes and other red fruits and vegetables, has been shown to have powerful antioxidant properties and cancer-preventive effects by reducing lipid peroxidation and inhibiting cell growth [39–41,65], and is associated with a decreased risk of PCa [41,42,44]. Such effects are certainly correlated with the observation that lycopene acts on the androgen receptors and reverses the effects of dihydrotestosterone [66]. Soy and green tea have also been investigated for their chemo-preventive capacity in relation to PCa (Table 1). Soy isoflavones and their derivatives, genistein and daidzein, reportedly show efficacy in preventing PCa [63]. Genistein acts as a chemotherapeutic agent in various cancer cells, modulating cell angiogenesis, apoptosis, and metastasis [62]. Moreover, soy isoflavones are similar in structure to 17β-estradiol, and thus can bind to the estrogen receptor and act as phytoestrogens. In addition to estrogenic effects, isoflavones reportedly exert antioxidant and inhibitory effects on tyrosine kinase activity [63]. However, the inadequate intake of isoflavones may lead to PCa progression [63]. The catechins found in green tea exhibit anticarcinogenic effects that may prevent various stages of carcinogenesis and metastasis [50–53]. Vitamin D and its analogues seem to protect from PCa, through the inhibition of cell proliferation and invasion, and inflammatory signaling (Table 1). For instance, several epidemiological studies suggest that PCa occurs more frequently in older men with vitamin D deficiency [2,47,67]. Moreover, a high dietary intake of dairy products rich in calcium, higher than the daily recommendation, also increases PCa risk, due to decreased serum levels of vitamin D [45,46,48,68]. Nevertheless, the research about nutrient intake and PCa needs to be further elucidated and extended.

Several epidemiological studies have shown a positive correlation between PCa mortality and per capita consumption of meat, fat, and dairy products [3,32,33,65]. The promotion of prostate carcinogenesis through androgen signaling, increased levels of reactive oxygen species (ROS), leukotrienes, and prostaglandins from lipid metabolism, as well as increased basal metabolism, IGFs levels, and tumor proliferation, are a few biological mechanisms that are thought to connect trans and saturated animal fat and PCa risk. Additionally, aromatic hydrocarbons and mutagenic heterocyclic amines, which are formed while cooking all of the components in meat at high temperatures—including creatine, amino acids, and sugar—can result in lipid peroxidation and DNA damage through the production of free radicals [2,69]. Unsaturated fatty acids such as Omega-3 fats, abundant in fish and vegetable oils, have been reported to reduce the risk of PCa. However, Omega-6 fats seem to have a pro-inflammatory effect through linoleic acid [2,70]. Arachidonic acid, a metabolite of linoleic acid, leads to the formation of pro-inflammatory prostaglandins (PG), such as PGE2, involved in cell proliferation, and 5-hydroxyeicosatetraenoic acid, which is found to be increasingly expressed in malignant PCa [3,32,33].

Changes in the metabolic profile caused by metabolic disorders such as obesity, insulin resistance, and changes in the hormonal profile are often associated with PCa, and some conditions can lead to more aggressive tumors [3,32–34]. Obese men show alterations in circulating levels of metabolic and sex steroid hormones, both known to be involved in prostate development and oncogenesis. Clinical studies have demonstrated that obesity might have clinical implications for disease detection and management [27,28,71]. Additionally, insulin is a risk factor of promoting PCa initiation and/or progression. In aggressive PCa tumors, for instance, elevated circulating insulin concentrations were found, supporting the role of insulin in PCa growth [72]. Tobacco consumption is another PCa risk factor (Table 1) [34,36,37]. The incidence and mortality rates of PCa have increased significantly with the increase in tobacco use, due to exposure to carcinogens and alterations in circulating levels of hormones [73]. Functional polymorphisms in genes involved in the polycyclic aromatic hydrocarbons (PAHs) metabolism, one of the carcinogenic chemicals of cigarette smoke, may affect cancer onset and progression [2]. Researchers found that smoking increases the metabolism of serum estrogen, which is involved in a more aggressive tumor phenotype, resulting in increased PCa-related deaths [74]. Moreover, cigarette smoking has been associated with adverse pathological features and worse oncological control [10].

4. Prostate Cancer Screening

Screening for PCa is based on the PSA biomarker values in blood serum (>4.0 ng/mL) and DRE. After suspicion, a magnetic resonance imaging (MRI) scan is usually performed, which indicates whether a prostate biopsy should be performed, considering the prostate imaging–reporting and data system (PI-RADS) value (PI-RADS > 3). Following the histological confirmation (biopsy) of malignant neoplasia, staging tests are performed, through imaging techniques such as computed tomography (CT) or positron emission tomography

(PET). In turn, the results of these tests dictate the patient's therapy based on a combination of surgical strategies, hormone therapy, radiotherapy, and chemotherapy (Figure 4) [75].

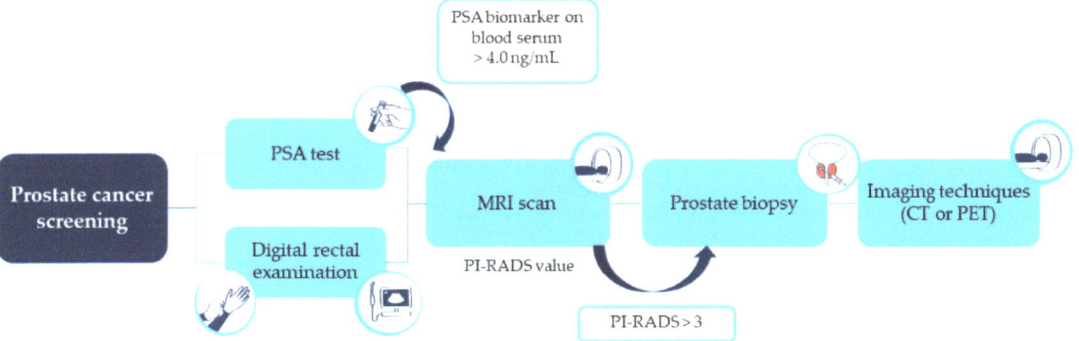

Figure 4. PCa diagnosis pathway.

PSA is a glycoprotein normally expressed by the prostate tissue with a cut-off of 4.0 ng/mL [5]. However, this test shows low selectivity to detect PCa and monitor the disease's progression [76], due to its limited sensitivity (20.5%) [77], accuracy (62–75%) [78], and specificity (51–91%) [79]. PSA screening cannot differentiate patients in terms of the aggressiveness of the tumor [80], and cannot distinguish between benign prostatic hyperplasia and prostatitis [81]. Furthermore, PSA levels may be affected by several other factors, such as age, body mass index (BMI), and urinary tract infection, leading to false-positive results [77,82]. Due to concerns about overdiagnosis and overtreatment, along with the high rate of false-positive results, the United States Preventive Services Task Force made recommendations against PSA testing among men over 70 years old [7,76]. This decision resulted in a decline in the incidence of PCa from 2007 to 2014. Between 2013 and 2017, the mortality rates flattened, most likely because of a decline in the use of PSA, which consequently resulted in the diagnosis of more men with metastatic PCa [76]. Therefore, it has become very important that men are fully informed of the potential benefits and harms of PSA screening [83].

A decisive diagnosis of PCa is based on a prostate biopsy when PSA and DRE show abnormal results [84,85]. Besides being an invasive, unpleasant, and potentially harmful procedure [86], prostate biopsies also show the risk of severe infection, due to the introduction of rectal commensal or other bacteria through a needle into the sterile prostate [87]. Moreover, this procedure can still lead to both false-positive and false-negative results [2,88,89]. False-negative results may occur when the tumor is small, when the cancer cells are distributed heterogeneously, and in early PCa stages when, histologically, the tumor appears benign. Accordingly, the samples obtained during the biopsy may not be representative of cancer. Another issue is the overdiagnosis and overtreatment of relatively indolent tumors with low potential for morbidity or death if left untreated [90,91]. Hence, serum PSA levels and prostate biopsy histology have very limited accuracy in predicting the clinical behavior of individual tumors, especially the ones prone to becoming aggressive at a later stage. Several studies have focused on the development of new methods to overcome these limitations and provide more accurate tools for PCa detection and management (Table 2).

Table 2. Emerging diagnostic methods for prostate cancer detection and management (articles from the last 5 years).

Method	Evidence/Aim	Reference
PSMA radioligand targeted therapy and molecular imaging	Evidence: Molecular imaging techniques detect PCa lesions that are occult on anatomic imaging. PSMA radioligand therapy shows promising response rates with low toxicity in extensively pre-treated patients with PCa. Aim: Theragnostic applications—diagnosis, management, and treatment of metastatic PCa.	[92–100]
EVs	Evidence: EVs can mediate PCa progression and metastasis. EVs have great potential to be used as liquid biopsy biomarkers in the diagnosis of PCa. EVs can be used in risk stratification and to predict the response to hormonal, chemo-, immune- and targeted therapy. Aim: Diagnosis and treatment. Can be used to personalize and guide treatment decisions.	[76,87,89,101–105]
lncRNAs (PCA3, MALAT1, SChLAP1, BDNF-AS, FALEC)	Evidence: lncRNAs provide new insights into cancer signaling networks, along with novel strategies and methods for PCa diagnosis and treatment. lncRNAs analysis has the potential to improve the specificity and sensitivity of existing biomarkers. Aim: Novel biomarkers (predictive, diagnostic, prognostic) and therapeutic targets.	[106–112]

Legend: EVs: extracellular vesicles; lncRNAs: long non-coding RNAs; PSMA: molecular targeting of prostate-specific membrane antigen.

4.1. Prostate-Specific Membrane Antigen: A Theranostic Approach

Imaging methods are used to define the stage of PCa and so guide its management. However, PCa's more aggressive forms can manifest rapid growth with progression to adjacent organs and spread to lymph nodes and bones [2,113,114], and CT, bone scan, and MRI have limited performance abilities in the detection of lymph node metastasis [92]. Patients with castration-resistant PCa (CRPCa) have a 90 to 95% probability of developing bone metastases, which leads to severe morbidity, including bone pain, pathological fractures, spinal cord compression, and hematological consequences of bone marrow infiltration [115–117]. Due to the importance of bone metastases in the overall disease progression, bone-targeted therapy constitutes an essential part of the treatment of CRPCa [118]. A possible therapy may be based on the use of radiopharmaceuticals systemically administered to slow or reverse the bone metastatic progression [117].

Current research is focused on the molecular targeting of prostate-specific membrane antigen (PSMA) as a theragnostic approach, to diagnose, monitor, and treat PCa [92]. PMSA is a transmembrane enzymatic protein found on most PCa cells, and its overexpression correlates to adverse factors, such as androgen independence, metastasis, and progression, making PSMA an antigenic marker for PCa progression [92,93,117,118]. Hence, PMSA can be used for diagnostic and therapeutic purposes, and several clinical trials have been investigating its effectiveness as a diagnostic tool and for direct radioligand therapy (Table 2) [92].

4.1.1. Molecular Imaging

PSMA scans can detect metastatic lesions that are missed by conventional imaging techniques [92], so small molecules, antibodies, and antibody fragments that target PSMA have been created, radiolabeled, and used for molecular imaging [98].

PET is emerging as a highly sensitive molecular imaging technique in the detection and localization of primary PCa. PET uses a positron emitter to label key molecules that are intravenously injected, and their distribution and uptake images provide insights into metabolic changes associated with cancer [119]. This technique has been reported as a valuable tool in the diagnosis of PCa patients with negative MRI and systematic biopsies [98]. Recently, ligands of PSMA were introduced in PET to diagnose and manage PCa (reviewed by Mena et al., 2020 [99]). This approach can improve PCa detection by identifying lesions that are not visible on MRI, providing better estimates of tumor volume [98]. PSMA-PET can be used in the diagnosis, staging, and management of PCa patients [99]. PSMA-PET has an important role in the initial staging of PCa, superior diagnostic performance to anatomical imaging, and enhanced sensitivity to detect node metastasis (reaching 99% [119]), outperforming other molecule imaging techniques, including PET-CT [98,99]. Furthermore, PSMA-PET can be combined with anatomical CT (PET/CT) and MRI (PET/MRI) images for the detection of bone metastases [99,100] (Table 2). PSMA-PET/MRI consistently outperforms multiparametric MRI (mpMRI) in the detection or localization of PCa in intermediate- or high-risk PCa patients (reviewed by Moradi et al., 2021 [98] and Mena et al., 2020 [99]). PSMA-PET/CT has greater sensitivity in the detection of bone metastasis when compared to whole-body bone scans [100], and has shown the most utility in biochemical recurrence [119]. PSMA-PET/CT was first coupled with gallium-68 (^{68}Ga) and is considered the most sensitive and specific method for staging high-risk PCa and imaging recurrent PCa [92,98]. Moreover, ^{68}Ga-labeled ligands have shown higher sensitivity and specificity in the diagnosis of primary and recurrent PCa [100]. In a retrospective analysis, Maurer et al. [120] investigated the diagnostic efficacy of ^{68}Ga-PSMA-PET for lymph node staging in patients with PCa and compared it to CT and MRI imaging. In their analyses, ^{68}Ga-PSMA-11 showed sensitivity, specificity, and accuracy levels of 65.9%, 98.9%, and 88.5%, respectively, in the detection of nodal metastases, compared with the values of 43.9%, 85.4%, and 72.3% achieved by morphological imaging [120]. In another study, Thomas et al. [100] investigated the difference between technetium-99m (^{99m}Tc)-methyl diphosphate (MDP) bone scans and ^{68}Ga-PSMA-PET/CT for the detection of bone metastases in PCa. The authors compared the number of identified lesions and found that the PSMA-PET/CT method detected twice the number of lesions, especially in the thorax and pelvis. Their results suggest that when patients go through ^{68}Ga-PSMA-PET/CT, the bone scan is not mandatory [100].

4.1.2. Radioligand Targeted Therapy

Recent studies suggest that newer molecular theragnostic approaches, based on PSMA radioligands, have the potential to provide even more effective and personalized treatment options for diagnostic, prognostic, and therapeutic applications in patients with CRPCa, with fewer toxicities and adverse effects [92–94]. This approach has been developed to select patients, and delivers irradiation to all tumor sites, including osseous, nodal, and visceral metastases [92]. PSMA radioligand therapy uses small-molecule inhibitors of PSMA, usually labeled with beta and alpha-emitting radionuclides that emit cytotoxic radioactive decay [92,93]. Alpha and beta radionuclides differ in energy, tissue range, linear energy transfer, and the number of DNA hits needed for cell destruction [117]. These radiopharmaceuticals deliver targeted irradiation to the active bone turnover sites, where metastatic infiltration and destruction are happening. This approach can simultaneously treat multiple sites of disease, ease administration, and be integrated or combined with other treatments. Alpha-emitters include actinium-225 (^{225}Ac), thorium-227 (^{227}Th), radium-223 (^{223}Ra), and astatine-211 (^{211}At). Recently, ^{223}Ra was approved to treat bone metastases from PCa. This authorization follows the symptomatic relief and significant improvement in the overall survival of CRPCa with predominant bone metastases that ^{223}Ra was shown to elicit [121]. Beta-emitting radiopharmaceuticals, including lutetium-117 (^{177}Lu), strontium-89 (^{89}Sr), samarium-153 (^{153}Sm), and rhenium-186 (^{186}Re), have been used for bone palliation. ^{177}Lu is the most used beta-emitter, due to its favorable safety profile, short range of emissions, and relatively long half-life, allowing the delivery of a high degree of radiation to specific lesions [92]. For instance, [^{177}Lu] Lu-PSMA-617 shows a favorable safety profile due to reduced kidney uptake, and has demonstrated promising results in prospective trials with high response rates, low toxic effects, and the reduction of pain in men with metastatic CRPCa who progressed after standard treatments [95–97]. In general, radioligand therapy shows promising response rates with low toxicity in extensively pretreated patients with PCa [92]. While most of these studies remain experimental and the effects of this therapy on overall survival and safety are yet to be determined, their clinical observations are very promising [95,118,122–124].

PSMA-targeted imaging and therapy have proven to be excellent diagnostic and therapeutic options for metastatic PCa, but further studies are still required to determine the effect of this approach on overall survival and safety. Moreover, current research is still ongoing regarding the exact role of PSMA in various stages of PCa care [92].

4.2. Tumor Biomarkers

In recent years, new potential biomarkers for PCa screening and management have been developed through advances in molecular medicine, particularly OMICs genomics, proteomics, transcriptomics, and lipidomics. In addition to molecular biomarkers for urine, serum, and tissue samples, extracellular vesicles (EVs), circulating tumor cells (CTCs) and DNA (ctDNA), and cell-free DNA (cfDNA), common liquid biopsy biomarkers [125] and long noncoding ribonucleic acids (lncRNAs) have emerged as promising PCa biomarkers.

4.2.1. Molecular Biomarkers

Based on the combination of imaging techniques with other methodologies such as gene or protein profiling, several molecular biomarkers have been developed for urine, serum, and tissue samples to improve cancer detection, pre-biopsy decision-making, cancer risk assessment, and the therapeutic management of PCa [126]. Additionally, risk calculators (RCs) are used in combination with these tests to help identify each individual's specific cancer risk, hence reducing the number of unnecessary biopsies. The guidelines on PCa treatment are therefore recommending the use of these tests in addition to the current PCa screening methods [77]. These biomarkers include several derivatives of PSA, such as the Prostate Health Index (PHI), approved by the US Food and Drug Administration (FDA), which combines total PSA, free PSA, and [−2] proPSA, and the Four-Kallikrein (4KScore) blood tests, which consist of kallikrein-related peptidase 2 (hK2), intact PSA, free PSA, and total PSA [104]. Transcriptomic methodologies also contributed to the discovery of biomarkers, and Progensa Prostate Cancer Antigen 3 (PCA3) is the first and only urine test approved by the FDA, which detects the PCa gene 3 transcript levels. The MyProstateScore (MPS) assay requires the collection of urine post-DRE and is based on combinations of multiple gene analyses, including total serum PSA, the PCA3 assay, and the expression of the TMPRSS2: ERG fusion gene [127,128]. These biomarkers can be used in liquid biopsies and involve a combination of clinical information, including age, family history, DRE result, PSA levels, and prostate biopsy history, with genetic and epigenetic changes. Nevertheless, the technologies associated with these approaches are expensive and unavailable in many medical facilities. Other factors such as tumor heterogeneity, tumor–host interplay, complexity, multiplicity, and redundancy of tumor–cell signaling networks must be overcome to develop effective biomarkers [81].

4.2.2. Long Non-Coding RNAs

LncRNAs are RNA transcripts that are longer than 200 nucleotides and do not encode proteins. LncRNAs have been found to exhibit abnormal expression in various types of cancer, including PCa. Most lncRNAs linked to PCa are overexpressed in tumor tissues and cancer cells, contributing to tumor proliferation, invasion, and metastasis. In turn, only a small number of lncRNAs are downregulated and may function as tumor suppressors in addition to their roles as transcriptional regulators and oncogenes [106]. All these unique features make lncRNAs promising prognostic biomarkers and therapeutic targets for the diagnosis, screening, prognosis, and progression of PCa [106] (Table 2). Recent research has demonstrated that lncRNAs such as PCA3, GAS5, and HOTAIR are associated with the development and progression of PCa [106]. Given its higher specificity and sensitivity than the PSA blood test, PCA3 is one of the most well-studied lncRNAs. Additionally, its combination with PSA testing or other biomarkers will significantly improve the sensitivity, specificity, and accuracy of PCa screening and diagnosis. For instance, the use of PCA3 in conjunction with TMPRSS2-ERG tests can reduce the number of unnecessary biopsies and increase diagnostic accuracy [106]. Another putative PCa diagnostic marker is MALAT1, whose increased expression has been linked to high PSA levels and Gleason scores, as well as with tumor stage and CRPCa [106]. Single-nucleotide polymorphisms of *MALAT1* were investigated by Hu et al. [109], who found that rs619586 and rs1194338 were significantly associated with PCa's susceptibility to both advanced Gleason grade and nodal metastasis. A noninvasive post-DRE urine assay based on the combination of the lncRNAs PCA3 and MALAT1 for the early diagnosis of PCa and high-grade tumors was developed and validated by Li and collaborators [110]. However, according to some researchers, the PCA3 test is affected by intra-individual variability, being unable to differentiate between high-grade and low-grade tumors. Hence, more data are necessary to determine PCA3's application in PCa diagnosis [106]. The lncRNAs TMPO-AS1 and FALEC have shown their potential utility as biomarkers for PCa diagnosis and progression [106,112]. Zhao et al. [108] examined the biological role of FALEC in PCa cell lines as well as its expression profile, and paired histologically normal tissues. In 85 patients, clinical PCa tissues showed significantly higher FALEC expressions when compared to adjacent normal tissues. Moreover, in vitro cell proliferation, migration, and invasion could be inhibited by the downregulation of FALEC. According to these findings, FALEC may be a useful diagnostic and therapeutic target in PCa patients [108]. Li et al. [107] investigated the expression, prognostic value, and functional role of lncRNA BDNF-AS in PCa. The authors also correlated the expression of BDNF-AS with the clinicopathological factors of patients. The results of this study demonstrate the potential use of BDNF-AS as a prognostic biomarker for PCa patients with poor prognoses and shorter overall survival, as it was downregulated in these cases. Furthermore, lncRNAs can be used to predict the recurrence of biochemical events. SChLAP1 was highly expressed in PCa tissue, which was substantially correlated with biochemical recurrence, clinical progression, and PCa-specific mortality [111]. Additionally, SChLAP1 can be easily detected in urine, an important feature for the development of an SChLAP1 assay for guided therapy (as reviewed by Xu et al. [106]). Given the roles of lncRNAs in PCa, it will be important to create specific drugs that interfere with malignant signaling networks in which lncRNAs are engaged, particularly in PCa cells. However, it is still unclear how exactly lncRNAs work at the molecular level, it being essential to further investigate the role of lncRNAs in prostate carcinogenesis [106].

4.2.3. Liquid Biopsy Biomarkers

Liquid biopsy has emerged as a complement to invasive tissue biopsy to guide cancer diagnosis and treatment [76]. Liquid biopsies rely on the detection of specific biomarkers in readily accessible body fluids, such as blood, serum, or urine [89]. The common liquid biopsy biomarkers are EVs, CTCs, ctDNA, and cfDNA, which provide specific information based on their intrinsic characteristics. CTCs are cancer cells from primary and metastatic tumors that are released into the vasculature and circulate through the body to form metastatic niches in other tissues, being detectable in cancer patients only [125]. Similarly, ctDNA is a tumor-derived short, fragmented DNA found in the bloodstream, which reflects cancer-related genetic changes. cfDNA or RNA (cfRNA) are cell-free circulating small nucleic acid fragments that are released after the lysis of apoptotic or necrotic cells. cfDNA is detectable in blood and urine samples from patients with cancer, and their analyses improve the evaluation of mutations, polymorphism, methylation, and loss of DNA integrity [76,89,129]. Numerous studies have shown the relevance of liquid biopsies in PCa screening. cfDNA and EVs seem to have a better application in the diagnosis and prognosis of PCa than CTCs [76,87,89,101] (Table 2). This occurs because early-stage or localized PCa patients have very few CTCs and their use is more effective in the later stages of this cancer [89]. The only FDA-approved liquid biopsy test for PCa, CellSearch, is based on the detection of CTCs, and there is no evidence of the wide clinical implementation of this technology in medical practice. EVs are nano-sized, double-lipid membrane vesicles, such as exosomes and microvesicles, that are secreted from cells and shed into biofluids, including blood and urine [104]. EVs are involved in intercellular communication and immune function, through proteins, lipids, mRNA, microRNAs (miRNAs), and DNA, and have been correlated to the presence of cancer for diagnostic purposes (Table 2) [76,101,130,131]. Cells exchange proteins, nucleic acids, sugars, and lipids through EVs to induce changes in the recipient cells, which makes EVs potential carriers of cancer biomarkers from tumor cells to other tumor or non-tumor cells [89]. EVs can also be used as a vehicle for drugs or nucleic acids with antineoplastic effects [87,102]. The EVs approach may improve the sensitivity of PCa biomarkers, given the protective role of the EVs' lipid layer over biomolecules, meaning that the concentration of PCa biomarkers will be higher in EVs [89]. Urine is the most used body fluid for the detection of biomarkers in EVs from liquid biopsies of PCa. Moreover, exosomal miRNAs are emerging as promising prognostic biomarkers for metastatic CRPCa patients [89]. The concentration of RNA-based biomarkers, particularly miRNA, is higher in EVs than in CTCs from urine samples. Nevertheless, the application of miRNA as a diagnostic marker has been limited due to a lack of specificity, and in turn, many studies have emerged to investigate EV-mRNA as a diagnostic and prognostic biomarker for PCa management [76]. McKiernan et al. [104] developed an exosome-derived gene expression signature from normalized PCA3 and ERG RNA from urine predictive of initial biopsy results. Exosomes in post-DRE urine of PCa patients contain both PCA3 and TMPRSS2: ERG mRNA. In their study, the authors were able to develop a molecular signature predictive of PCa combined with serum PSA in a diagnostic test, which was able to discriminate between benign disease and high- and low-grade tumors, reducing the total number of unnecessary biopsies [104]. Ji et al. [105] developed a strategy for exosomal mRNA detection based on features of mRNA of circulating exosomes and identified a PCa exosomal mRNA signature for PCa screening and diagnosis. With this strategy, the authors were able to distinguish PCa patients from healthy controls [105]. Despite the beneficial properties of EVs for the diagnosis of PCa, their clinical application still presents a few challenging issues [76]. EVs are released from all cells in the body, which makes it difficult to determine which EVs are tumor-derived, meaning that new technologies for the specific detection and isolation of tumor-derived EVs need to be developed [76]. Recent EVs isolation technologies have been developed to improve isolation performance, yield, purity, usability, hands-on procedures, and processing time [76]. However, EVs isolation is still difficult, especially in EVs from blood plasma, due to the purity and efficiency achieved by laboratory procedures. Moreover, there is no wide clinical application of liquid biopsies of PCa with EVs [89], and automated analysis platforms are yet to be developed for large-scale clinical studies [76]. Overall, the use of CTCs and EVs as biomarkers of PCa in liquid biopsies is being hindered by some issues, such as the inexistence of specific guidelines for the biomarker's isolation and detection. Additionally, the validation and standardization of the microfluidic devices used in liquid biopsies has not been achieved yet [129].

4.3. Active Surveillance and Risk-Stratification Algorithms

PCa is very heterogeneous in terms of grade, phenotypes, and genetics, displaying complex features [2]. This tumor often has indolent growth, which does not compromise the patient's quality of life, but its diagnosis and subsequent treatments have a high impact on the physical and mental status of patients, significantly affecting their quality of life [81]. The main goal of early detection is to identify PCa in a phase whereat it needs less aggressive treatments with fewer side effects and has a higher chance of cure, even in the cases of locally advanced and metastatic PCa. Many early diagnoses can be safely managed by active surveillance, preventing overtreatment, thereby improving or maintaining the patient's quality of life and avoiding adverse outcomes [132].

Active surveillance consists of the serial monitoring of disease progression, through PSA tests, DRE, and biopsies, to track cancer growth. This has become the preferred approach for men with low-grade PCa [2,133], as men can avoid immediate treatment and prospective side effects [2]. When discussing therapy choices and in the selection criteria for active surveillance programs [134], external factors, such as obesity, BMI, and the hormonal profile (e.g., testosterone levels), should be considered by the clinical practice, since all these factors influence the PSA levels [135,136]. Recent studies suggest that the conjugation of PSA screening with other methodologies, such as risk RCs, biomarkers, and imaging techniques such as MRI, can attenuate overdiagnosis and underdetection issues [137]. Van Poppel et al. [137] proposed a risk-stratified algorithm, combining MRI, RC, and PSA tests, that improves the efficiency of "PSA-only" screening and reduces unnecessary biopsies and overdiagnosis. The combination of these tools improves the individual balance between the harms and benefits of early detection in well-informed men who are at risk of having PCa [137]. Based on the initial PSA test result and age, different time intervals for repeated PSA testing are proposed, reflecting the likelihood of a future diagnosis of clinically significant cancer. This strategy helps to avoid false-positive biopsies, as low-risk men can go through individualized PSA tests and, if necessary, repeated MRIs to track cancer growth. Then, RCs seem to be the most appropriate approach to assessing the risk of developing PCa after PSA testing. RCs are accessible to every clinician, easy to use, inexpensive, and non-invasive. Moreover, MRI results can be integrated into an RC that includes PSA density as a continuous variable, to determine the need for a prostate biopsy in men with intermediate- and high-risk [137,138]. PSA density has been described to improve the specificity of the PSA test [138,139]. It is defined as the level of serum PSA divided by the prostate volume and presents a cut-off of 0.15 ng/mL^2 [139]. PSA density can be used as a prognostic biomarker to determine which patients need to undergo definitive therapy from those who may be managed by active surveillance, as well as patients with a previously negative MRI who should proceed to a prostate biopsy [139]. This allows the more accurate evaluation of individual risk, which is essential for properly interpreting the MRI results. Consequently, only men who present a high risk of clinically significant PCa, according to an RC, will be proposed for a systemic biopsy after MRI [137].

Evidence shows that performing an MRI before a biopsy allows one-third of men to avoid an immediate biopsy and reduces overdiagnosis, with 40% fewer clinically unimportant cancers and approximately 15% more clinically significant cancers detected [137,140]. However, the implementation of MRI in the risk assessment of PCa is not yet fully realized in the whole of Europe [137], which in turn reflects the geographical differences in the incidence rates between European countries. To further reduce unnecessary biopsy procedures, the decision process of a biopsy in men with a PI-RADS of 3 should be carefully examined. The PI-RADS classification is based on a scale of values from 1 to 5, and determines the likelihood of clinically significant PCa. While PI-RADS values of 4 and 5 indicate that a biopsy is required, it is challenging to establish whether a biopsy should be performed or not in patients with a score of 3 [141]. Additionally, the PI-RADS score does not measure PCa aggressiveness, meaning that a biopsy is still needed. Research has found that excluding men with PI-RADS 1–2 or PI-RADS 3 lesions based on a low PSA density only increases the likelihood that clinically significant tumors will be undiagnosed due to nonvisual PCa or misinterpretation of the reader [137]. The European Association of Urology (EAU) guidelines strongly recommend performing an mpMRI before a biopsy to modify the management approach accordingly. This imaging approach presents preferable detection rates and reduces the number of biopsy procedures, particularly when MRI-negative men are excluded from prostate biopsy, due to its capacity to differentiate between significant and insignificant tumors [132]. Furthermore, the PI-RADS guidelines have recommended systematized mpMRI acquisition and the global standardization of reporting. Nevertheless, there is a lack of consensus on detailed aspects of mpMRI acquisition protocols [141].

Artificial intelligence (AI) methods have been proposed for a wide range of applications in the PCa diagnostic pathway [137,141–143]. AI can be used to improve the initial evaluation of prostate mpMRI cases and the image quality, as well as the detection and differentiation of clinically significant from insignificant cancers on a voxel level, and the classification of entire lesions into PI-RADS categories (reviewed by Belue and Turkbey [142] and Sunoqrot et al. [143]). Studies on MRI AI have revealed the role of AI in improving the clinical management of localized PCa, the interpretation of MRI and the data processing for biopsies, by reducing inter-reader variation and supporting the radiological workflow [142]. Nevertheless, AI requires caution in its use, as the proficiency of this method is still below that of an expert [141]. Moreover, more prospective studies with multicenter designs are required to understand the impact of AI on improving radiologists' performance and the clinical management of PCa [137,142].

4.4. Volatilomics

Emerging studies demonstrate that combining PSA screening with other methodologies, such as RCs, biomarkers, and imaging tests, e.g., MRI or fusion biopsies, might attenuate overdiagnosis and underdetection, eventually reducing the number of unnecessary biopsies [137]. Volatilomics, a subset of metabolomics, has recently emerged as a simple, effective, and non-invasive method with great potential for cancer screening. Volatilomics focuses on volatile organic metabolites (VOMs), which are low-molecular weight metabolites (<500 Da) with high volatility and a carbon-based chemical group [144]. VOMs are present in readily accessible biofluids, including saliva, urine, and exhaled breath, as they are produced by the metabolism of cells, reflecting their biological activity [145]. The progressive accumulation of genetic, epigenetic, and post-translational changes that support cancer growth can lead to changes in VOMs levels and, as a result, affect an individual's volatilomic profile (Figure 5). Hence, VOMs are a rich source of data on health, since they can reflect the metabolic and biochemical alterations triggered by cancer progression. From this perspective, a volatilomic biosignature for diagnostic purposes can be defined using these changes [77,86].

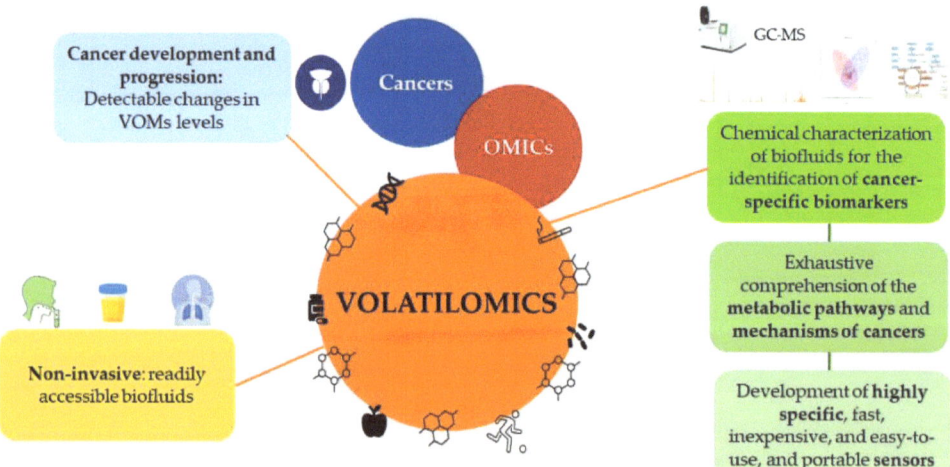

Figure 5. Cancer development and progression can lead to changes in the levels of volatile organic metabolites, which can be used to define a volatilomic biosignature for diagnostic purposes.

Even though the volatilomics approach is relatively recent in PCa compared to other cancers [77,88,146,147], empirical data have confirmed its potential use in cancer screening, the monitoring of disease progression and effectiveness of treatment, as well as for the discrimination between different cancer types [86,148–150]. Different approaches involving volatilomic studies have been proposed to establish connections between cancer and the body's VOMs signature using highly sensitive analytical techniques. In these studies, biofluids are chemically characterized to identify cancer-specific biomarkers using mass spectrometry-based techniques combined with multivariate statistical analysis. Another approach includes the identification of cancer-characteristic odor fingerprints through electronic noses (e-noses) [151]. However, since several VOMs have been suggested as PCa biomarkers and contradictory results on the same metabolites have emerged from different reports, it is difficult to establish reliable biomarkers, and no exhaustive studies have yet been published [151,152]. Additionally, a few restrictions hinder the implementation of these approaches in real-time diagnostic applications, and consequently, in clinical practice (reviewed by Berenguer et al. [144]). For instance, the ability to compare the outcomes of various studies between different laboratories is hampered by variations in sample preparation, analytical procedures, and statistical platforms [88]. Hence, methods must be standardized from sample collection to data processing, as well as assess the impact of confounding factors, such as epigenetics, diet, medication, genetics, and environmental exposure. Epigenetic factors play an important role in determining the clinical phenotypes of PCa. Therefore, due to genetic, environmental, and toxicological factors, as well as the different dietary habits around the world and their influence on the development of cancer, the volatilomic biosignatures and potential biomarkers will differ according to the region of the world [77,88,144,146,147].

Despite these limitations, volatilomics offers a wealth of informational potential that will allow a thorough understanding of the metabolic pathways, and a clarification of the mechanisms of cancers and how they impact the generation of VOMs [153]. Further analysis of the VOMs' origin and a more accurate assessment of the impact of confounding factors on the volatilomic profile will be possible as a result of these findings [147]. Additionally, the definition of cancer biomarkers will be made possible through the detection and quantification of specific metabolites due to the standardization of procedures and the creation of highly focused sensors. These findings will foster the development of highly specific, fast, inexpensive, easy-to-use, and portable sensors that can be implemented in clinical practice [145,154], demonstrating the importance of the volatilomics approach [151,155]. Hopefully, the progress in volatilomics studies will unveil biomarkers suitable for the diagnosis of PCa, to be used as a supplement to the current approaches for the classification and screening of cancer [129], with possible applications in the active surveillance of patients and individualized care [81,144].

5. Conclusions

PCa is the second leading cause of oncological death worldwide. Changes in the metabolic profile caused by metabolic disorders such as obesity are often associated with PCa, and some conditions can lead to more aggressive tumors. Lifestyle factors are modifiable and may provide an effective method for reducing PCa risk. Nevertheless, the research into nutrient intake and PCa needs to be further elucidated to understand how men can change their dietary habits to prevent cancer growth. The current screening methods are invasive and have a low sensitivity to detect PCa, leading to overdiagnosis and overtreatment. Several studies have focused on the development of new methods to overcome these limitations and provide more accurate tools for PCa detection and management. Moreover, the development of testing strategies to maintain most of the benefits of screening, while reducing the harms, has become an important need. These strategies focus on the diagnosis of potentially fatal cancers at a point where treatment is still effective, while not involving the treatment of indolent cancers, saving patients and healthcare systems from the burden of unnecessary, invasive, and costly medical procedures [83]. Furthermore, the combination of the PSA test with different techniques for the diagnosis of PCa, such as MRI, RCs, and biomarkers, has been proposed to obtain a more effective stratification of the patients and provide more personalized treatment.

Author Contributions: Conceptualization, C.V.B., F.P. and J.S.C.; investigation, C.V.B.; writing—original draft preparation C.V.B.; review and editing, J.A.M.P., F.P. and J.S.C.; visualization, J.A.M.P. and J.S.C.; supervision, J.S.C. and J.A.M.P.; funding acquisition J.S.C. All authors have read and agreed to the published version of the manuscript.

Funding: This work was supported by FCT-Fundação para a Ciência e a Tecnologia through the CQM Base Fund UIDB/00674/2020 and Programmatic Fund UIDP/00674/2020, and by ARDITI-Agência

Regional para o Desenvolvimento da Investigação Tecnologia e Inovação through the project M1420-01-0145-FEDER-000005-Centro de Química da Madeira-CQM+ (Madeira 14-20 Program). Jorge A. M. Pereira was supported by a post-doctoral fellowship given by ARDITI (Project M1420-09-5369-FSE-000001), and Cristina V. Berenguer acknowledges Núcleo Regional da Madeira da Liga Portuguesa contra o Cancro (LPCC-NRM) and Bolsa Rubina Barros for the support of this project. The authors also acknowledge the financial support from Fundação para a Ciência e Tecnologia and Madeira 14-2020 program given to the Portuguese Mass Spectrometry Network through the PROEQUIPRAM program, M14-20 M1420-01-0145-FEDER-000008.

Institutional Review Board Statement: Not applicable.

Informed Consent Statement: Not applicable.

Data Availability Statement: Not applicable.

Conflicts of Interest: The authors declare no conflict of interest.

References

1. Sung, H.; Ferlay, J.; Siegel, R.L.; Laversanne, M.; Soerjomataram, I.; Jemal, A.; Bray, F. Global Cancer Statistics 2020: GLOBOCAN Estimates of Incidence and Mortality Worldwide for 36 Cancers in 185 Countries. *CA A Cancer J. Clin.* **2021**, *71*, 209–249. [CrossRef] [PubMed]
2. Rawla, P. Epidemiology of Prostate Cancer. *World J. Oncol.* **2019**, *10*, 63–89. [CrossRef]
3. Pernar, C.H.; Ebot, E.M.; Wilson, K.M.; Mucci, L.A. The Epidemiology of Prostate Cancer. *Cold Spring Harb. Perspect. Med.* **2018**, *8*, a030361. [CrossRef] [PubMed]
4. Bhanji, Y.; Isaacs, W.B.; Xu, J.; Cooney, K.A. Prostate Cancer Predisposition. *Urol. Clin. N. Am.* **2021**, *48*, 283–296. [CrossRef] [PubMed]
5. Culp, M.B.; Soerjomataram, I.; Efstathiou, J.A.; Bray, F.; Jemal, A. Recent Global Patterns in Prostate Cancer Incidence and Mortality Rates. *Eur. Urol.* **2020**, *77*, 38–52. [CrossRef]
6. Tikkinen, K.A.O.; Dahm, P.; Lytvyn, L.; Heen, A.F.; Vernooij, R.W.M.; Siemieniuk, R.A.C.; Wheeler, R.; Vaughan, B.; Fobuzi, A.C.; Blanker, M.H.; et al. Prostate cancer screening with prostate-specific antigen (PSA) test: A clinical practice guideline. *BMJ* **2018**, *362*, k3581. [CrossRef]
7. Braga, R.; Costa, A.R.; Pina, F.; Moura-Ferreira, P.; Lunet, N. Prostate cancer screening in Portugal: Prevalence and perception of potential benefits and adverse effects. *Eur. J. Cancer Prev.* **2020**, *29*, 248–251. [CrossRef]
8. Center, M.M.; Jemal, A.; Lortet-Tieulent, J.; Ward, E.; Ferlay, J.; Brawley, O.; Bray, F. International variation in prostate cancer incidence and mortality rates. *Liver Int.* **2012**, *61*, 1079–1092. [CrossRef]
9. Marhold, M.; Kramer, G.; Krainer, M.; Le Magnen, C. The prostate cancer landscape in Europe: Current challenges, future opportunities. *Cancer Lett.* **2022**, *526*, 304–310. [CrossRef]
10. Gandaglia, G.; Leni, R.; Bray, F.; Fleshner, N.; Freedland, S.J.; Kibel, A.; Stattin, P.; Van Poppel, H.; La Vecchia, C. Epidemiology and Prevention of Prostate Cancer. *Eur. Urol. Oncol.* **2021**, *4*, 877–892. [CrossRef]
11. Coughlin, S.S. A review of social determinants of prostate cancer risk, stage, and survival. *Prostate Int.* **2020**, *8*, 49–54. [CrossRef]
12. Loeb, S.; Katz, M.S.; Langford, A.; Byrne, N.; Ciprut, S. Prostate cancer and social media. *Nat. Rev. Urol.* **2018**, *15*, 422–429. [CrossRef]
13. Nossiter, J.; Morris, M.; Parry, M.G.; Sujenthiran, A.; Cathcart, P.; van der Meulen, J.; Aggarwal, A.; Payne, H.; Clarke, N.W. Impact of the COVID-19 pandemic on the diagnosis and treatment of men with prostate cancer. *BJU Int.* **2022**, *130*, 262–270. [CrossRef] [PubMed]
14. Markozannes, G.; Tzoulaki, I.; Karli, D.; Evangelou, E.; Ntzani, E.; Gunter, M.J.; Norat, T.; Ioannidis, J.P.; Tsilidis, K.K. Diet, body size, physical activity and risk of prostate cancer: An umbrella review of the evidence. *Eur. J. Cancer* **2016**, *69*, 61–69. [CrossRef]
15. Tonon, L.; Fromont, G.; Boyault, S.; Thomas, E.; Ferrari, A.; Sertier, A.S.; Kielbassa, J.; Le Texier, V.; Kamoun, A.; Elarouci, N.; et al. Mutational Profile of Aggressive, Localised Prostate Cancer from African Caribbean Men Versus European Ancestry Men. *Eur. Urol.* **2019**, *75*, 11–15. [CrossRef] [PubMed]
16. Rebbeck, T.R. Prostate Cancer Disparities by Race and Ethnicity: From Nucleotide to Neighborhood. *Cold Spring Harb. Perspect. Med.* **2018**, *8*, a030387. [CrossRef] [PubMed]
17. Taitt, H.E. Global Trends and Prostate Cancer: A Review of Incidence, Detection, and Mortality as Influenced by Race, Ethnicity, and Geographic Location. *Am. J. Men's Health* **2018**, *12*, 1807–1823. [CrossRef] [PubMed]
18. McAllister, B.J. The association between ethnic background and prostate cancer. *Br. J. Nurs.* **2019**, *28*, S4–S10. [CrossRef]
19. Brown, C.R.; Hambleton, I.; Hercules, S.M.; Unwin, N.; Murphy, M.M.; Nigel Harris, E.; Wilks, R.; MacLeish, M.; Sullivan, L.; Sobers-Grannum, N. Social determinants of prostate cancer in the Caribbean: A systematic review and meta-analysis. *BMC Public Health* **2018**, *18*, 900. [CrossRef]
20. Grossman, D.C.; Curry, S.J.; Owens, D.K.; Bibbins-Domingo, K.; Caughey, A.B.; Davidson, K.W.; Doubeni, C.A.; Ebell, M.; Epling, J.W.; Kemper, A.R.; et al. Screening for prostate cancer USPreventive servicestaskforcerecommendation statement. *JAMA J. Am. Med. Assoc.* **2018**, *319*, 1901–1913. [CrossRef]

21. Vietri, M.T.; D'Elia, G.; Caliendo, G.; Resse, M.; Casamassimi, A.; Passariello, L.; Albanese, L.; Cioffi, M.; Molinari, A.M. Hereditary Prostate Cancer: Genes Related, Target Therapy and Prevention. *Int. J. Mol. Sci.* **2021**, *22*, 3753. [CrossRef] [PubMed]
22. Brandão, A.; Paulo, P.; Teixeira, M.R. Hereditary Predisposition to Prostate Cancer: From Genetics to Clinical Implications. *Int. J. Mol. Sci.* **2020**, *21*, 5036. [CrossRef] [PubMed]
23. Bree, K.K.; Hensley, P.J.; Pettaway, C.A. Germline Predisposition to Prostate Cancer in Diverse Populations. *Urol. Clin. N. Am.* **2021**, *48*, 411–423. [CrossRef] [PubMed]
24. Coughlin, S.S.; Vernon, M.; Klaassen, Z.; Tingen, M.S.; Cortes, J.E. Knowledge of prostate cancer among African American men: A systematic review. *Prostate* **2021**, *81*, 202–213. [CrossRef] [PubMed]
25. Ventimiglia, E.; Salonia, A.; Briganti, A.; Montorsi, F. Re: Family History and Probability of Prostate Cancer, Differentiated by Risk Category—A Nationwide Population-based Study. *Eur. Urol.* **2017**, *71*, 143–144. [CrossRef]
26. Takata, R.; Takahashi, A.; Fujita, M.; Momozawa, Y.; Saunders, E.J.; Yamada, H.; Maejima, K.; Nakano, K.; Nishida, Y.; Hishida, A.; et al. 12 new susceptibility loci for prostate cancer identified by genome-wide association study in Japanese population. *Nat. Commun.* **2019**, *10*, 4422. [CrossRef]
27. Vidal, A.C.; Freedland, S.J. Obesity and Prostate Cancer: A Focused Update on Active Surveillance, Race, and Molecular Subtyping. *Eur. Urol.* **2017**, *72*, 78–83. [CrossRef]
28. Wilson, R.L.; Taaffe, D.R.; Newton, R.U.; Hart, N.H.; Lyons-Wall, P.; Galvao, D.A. Obesity and prostate cancer: A narrative review. *Crit. Rev. Oncol. Hematol.* **2022**, *169*, 103543. [CrossRef]
29. Adesunloye, B.A. Mechanistic Insights into the Link between Obesity and Prostate Cancer. *Int. J. Mol. Sci.* **2021**, *22*, 3935. [CrossRef]
30. Bandini, M.; Gandaglia, G.; Briganti, A. Obesity and prostate cancer. *Curr. Opin. Urol.* **2017**, *27*, 415–421. [CrossRef]
31. Fujita, K.; Hayashi, T.; Matsushita, M.; Uemura, M.; Nonomura, N. Obesity, Inflammation, and Prostate Cancer. *J. Clin. Med.* **2019**, *8*, 201. [CrossRef]
32. Wilson, K.M.; Mucci, L.A. Diet and Lifestyle in Prostate Cancer. *Prostate Cancer Cell. Genet. Mech. Dis. Dev. Progress.* **2019**, *1210*, 1–27. [CrossRef]
33. Kaiser, A.; Haskins, C.; Siddiqui, M.M.; Hussain, A.; D'Adamo, C. The evolving role of diet in prostate cancer risk and progression. *Curr. Opin. Oncol.* **2019**, *31*, 222–229. [CrossRef] [PubMed]
34. Darcey, E.; Boyle, T. Tobacco smoking and survival after a prostate cancer diagnosis: A systematic review and meta-analysis. *Cancer Treat. Rev.* **2018**, *70*, 30–40. [CrossRef] [PubMed]
35. Sato, N.; Shiota, M.; Shiga, K.I.; Kashiwagi, E.; Takeuchi, A.; Inokuchi, J.; Yokomizo, A.; Naito, S.; Eto, M. Effect of Smoking on Oncological Outcome among Prostate Cancer Patients after Radical Prostatectomy with Neoadjuvant Hormonal Therapy. *Cancer Investig.* **2020**, *38*, 559–564. [CrossRef]
36. Khan, S.; Thakkar, S.; Drake, B. Smoking history, intensity, and duration and risk of prostate cancer recurrence among men with prostate cancer who received definitive treatment. *Ann. Epidemiol.* **2019**, *38*, 4–10. [CrossRef]
37. Jochems, S.H.J.; Fritz, J.; Häggström, C.; Järvholm, B.; Stattin, P.; Stocks, T. Smoking and Risk of Prostate Cancer and Prostate Cancer Death: A Pooled Study. *Eur. Urol.* **2022**, *82*, 571–579. [CrossRef]
38. Foerster, B.; Pozo, C.; Abufaraj, M.; Mari, A.; Kimura, S.; D'Andrea, D.; John, H.; Shariat, S.F. Association of Smoking Status With Recurrence, Metastasis, and Mortality Among Patients With Localized Prostate Cancer Undergoing Prostatectomy or Radiotherapy: A Systematic Review and Meta-analysis. *JAMA Oncol.* **2018**, *4*, 953–961. [CrossRef]
39. Fraser, G.E.; Jacobsen, B.K.; Knutsen, S.F.; Mashchak, A.; Lloren, J.I. Tomato consumption and intake of lycopene as predictors of the incidence of prostate cancer: The Adventist Health Study-2. *Cancer Causes Control* **2020**, *31*, 341–351. [CrossRef]
40. Li, N.; Wu, X.; Zhuang, W.; Xia, L.; Chen, Y.; Wu, C.; Rao, Z.; Du, L.; Zhao, R.; Yi, M.; et al. Tomato and lycopene and multiple health outcomes: Umbrella review. *Food Chem.* **2021**, *343*, 128396. [CrossRef]
41. Soares, N.; Elias, M.B.; Lima Machado, C.; Trindade, B.B.; Borojevic, R.; Teodoro, A.J. Comparative Analysis of Lycopene Content from Different Tomato-Based Food Products on the Cellular Activity of Prostate Cancer Cell Lines. *Foods* **2019**, *8*, 201. [CrossRef] [PubMed]
42. Puah, B.P.; Jalil, J.; Attiq, A.; Kamisah, Y. New Insights into Molecular Mechanism behind Anti-Cancer Activities of Lycopene. *Molecules* **2021**, *26*, 3888. [CrossRef]
43. Oczkowski, M.; Dziendzikowska, K.; Pasternak-Winiarska, A.; Włodarek, D.; Gromadzka-Ostrowska, J. Dietary Factors and Prostate Cancer Development, Progression, and Reduction. *Nutrients* **2021**, *13*, 496. [CrossRef] [PubMed]
44. Beynon, R.A.; Richmond, R.C.; Santos Ferreira, D.L.; Ness, A.R.; May, M.; Smith, G.D.; Vincent, E.E.; Adams, C.; Ala-Korpela, M.; Würtz, P.; et al. Investigating the effects of lycopene and green tea on the metabolome of men at risk of prostate cancer: The ProDiet randomised controlled trial. *Int. J. Cancer* **2019**, *144*, 1918–1928. [CrossRef] [PubMed]
45. Maksymchuk, O.V.; Kashuba, V.I. Altered expression of cytochrome P450 enzymes involved in metabolism of androgens and vitamin D in the prostate as a risk factor for prostate cancer. *Pharmacol. Rep.* **2020**, *72*, 1161–1172. [CrossRef] [PubMed]
46. Capiod, T.; Barry Delongchamps, N.; Pigat, N.; Souberbielle, J.C.; Goffin, V. Do dietary calcium and vitamin D matter in men with prostate cancer? *Nat. Rev. Urol.* **2018**, *15*, 453–461. [CrossRef]
47. Grant, W.B. Review of Recent Advances in Understanding the Role of Vitamin D in Reducing Cancer Risk: Breast, Colorectal, Prostate, and Overall Cancer. *Anticancer. Res.* **2020**, *40*, 491–499. [CrossRef]

48. Ardura, J.A.; Álvarez-Carrión, L.; Gutiérrez-Rojas, I.; Alonso, V. Role of Calcium Signaling in Prostate Cancer Progression: Effects on Cancer Hallmarks and Bone Metastatic Mechanisms. *Cancers (Basel)* **2020**, *12*, 1071. [CrossRef]
49. Applegate, C.C.; Rowles, J.L.; Ranard, K.M.; Jeon, S.; Erdman, J.W. Soy Consumption and the Risk of Prostate Cancer: An Updated Systematic Review and Meta-Analysis. *Nutrients* **2018**, *10*, 40. [CrossRef]
50. Tsugane, S. Why has Japan become the world's most long-lived country: Insights from a food and nutrition perspective. *Eur. J. Clin. Nutr.* **2021**, *75*, 921–928. [CrossRef]
51. Rogovskii, V.S.; Popov, S.V.; Sturov, N.V.; Shimanovskii, N.L. The Possibility of Preventive and Therapeutic Use of Green Tea Catechins in Prostate Cancer. *Anticancer. Agents Med. Chem.* **2019**, *19*, 1223–1231. [CrossRef] [PubMed]
52. Musial, C.; Kuban-Jankowska, A.; Gorska-Ponikowska, M. Beneficial Properties of Green Tea Catechins. *Int. J. Mol. Sci.* **2020**, *21*, 1744. [CrossRef] [PubMed]
53. Miyata, Y.; Shida, Y.; Hakariya, T.; Sakai, H. Anti-Cancer Effects of Green Tea Polyphenols Against Prostate Cancer. *Molecules* **2019**, *24*, 193. [CrossRef] [PubMed]
54. Ferreira, P.M.P.; Rodrigues, L.; de Alencar Carnib, L.P.; de Lima Sousa, P.V.; Nolasco Lugo, L.M.; Nunes, N.M.F.; do Nascimento Silva, J.; da Silva Araûjo, L.; de Macêdo Gonçalves Frota, K. Cruciferous Vegetables as Antioxidative, Chemopreventive and Antineoplasic Functional Foods: Preclinical and Clinical Evidences of Sulforaphane Against Prostate Cancers. *Curr. Pharm. Des.* **2018**, *24*, 4779–4793. [CrossRef]
55. Gunderson, K.; Wang, C.Y.; Wang, R. Global prostate cancer incidence and the migration, settlement, and admixture history of the Northern Europeans. *Cancer Epidemiol.* **2011**, *35*, 320–327. [CrossRef] [PubMed]
56. Kheirandish, P.; Chinegwundoh, F. Ethnic differences in prostate cancer. *Br. J. Cancer* **2011**, *105*, 481–485. [CrossRef]
57. Haiman, C.A.; Chen, G.K.; Blot, W.J.; Strom, S.S.; Berndt, S.I.; Kittles, R.A.; Rybicki, B.A.; Isaacs, W.B.; Ingles, S.A.; Stanford, J.L.; et al. Characterizing genetic risk at known prostate cancer susceptibility loci in African Americans. *PLoS Genet.* **2011**, *7*, e1001387. [CrossRef]
58. Rebbeck, T.R.; Devesa, S.S.; Chang, B.-L.; Bunker, C.H.; Cheng, I.; Cooney, K.; Eeles, R.; Fernandez, P.; Giri, V.N.; Gueye, S.M.; et al. Global Patterns of Prostate Cancer Incidence, Aggressiveness, and Mortality in Men of African Descent. *Prostate Cancer* **2013**, *2013*, 560857. [CrossRef]
59. Suuriniemi, M.; Agalliu, I.; Schaid, D.J.; Johanneson, B.; McDonnell, S.K.; Iwasaki, L.; Stanford, J.L.; Ostrander, E.A. Confirmation of a Positive Association between Prostate Cancer Risk and a Locus at Chromosome 8q24. *Cancer Epidemiol. Biomark. Prev.* **2007**, *16*, 809–814. [CrossRef]
60. Okobia, M.N.; Zmuda, J.M.; Ferrell, R.E.; Patrick, A.L.; Bunker, C.H. Chromosome 8q24 variants are associated with prostate cancer risk in a high risk population of African ancestry. *Prostate* **2011**, *71*, 1054–1063. [CrossRef]
61. Freedman, M.L.; Haiman, C.A.; Patterson, N.; McDonald, G.J.; Tandon, A.; Waliszewska, A.; Penney, K.; Steen, R.G.; Ardlie, K.; John, E.M.; et al. Admixture mapping identifies 8q24 as a prostate cancer risk locus in African-American men. *Proc. Natl. Acad. Sci. USA* **2006**, *103*, 14068–14073. [CrossRef] [PubMed]
62. Grammatikopoulou, M.G.; Gkiouras, K.; Papageorgiou, S.; Myrogiannis, I.; Mykoniatis, I.; Papamitsou, T.; Bogdanos, D.P.; Goulis, D.G. Dietary Factors and Supplements Influencing Prostate Specific-Antigen (PSA) Concentrations in Men with Prostate Cancer and Increased Cancer Risk: An Evidence Analysis Review Based on Randomized Controlled Trials. *Nutrients* **2020**, *12*, 2985. [CrossRef] [PubMed]
63. Matsushita, M.; Fujita, K.; Nonomura, N. Influence of Diet and Nutrition on Prostate Cancer. *Int. J. Mol. Sci.* **2020**, *21*, 1447. [CrossRef]
64. Ahmad, F.; Cherukuri, M.K.; Choyke, P.L. Metabolic reprogramming in prostate cancer. *Br. J. Cancer* **2021**, *125*, 1185–1196. [CrossRef] [PubMed]
65. Gathirua-Mwangi, W.G.; Zhang, J. Dietary factors and risk for advanced prostate cancer. *Eur. J. Cancer Prev.* **2014**, *23*, 96–109. [CrossRef] [PubMed]
66. Liu, X.; Allen, J.D.; Arnold, J.T.; Blackman, M.R. Lycopene inhibits IGF-I signal transduction and growth in normal prostate epithelial cells by decreasing DHT-modulated IGF-I production in co-cultured reactive stromal cells. *Carcinogenesis* **2008**, *29*, 816–823. [CrossRef] [PubMed]
67. Daniyal, M.; Siddiqui, Z.A.; Akram, M.; Asif, H.M.; Sultana, S.; Khan, A. Epidemiology, etiology, diagnosis and treatment of prostate cancer. *Asian Pac. J. Cancer Prev.* **2014**, *15*, 9575–9578. [CrossRef]
68. Rodriguez, C.; McCullough, M.L.; Mondul, A.M.; Jacobs, E.J.; Fakhrabadi-Shokoohi, D.; Giovannucci, E.L.; Thun, M.J.; Calle, E.E. Calcium, dairy products, and risk of prostate cancer in a prospective cohort of United States men. *Cancer Epidemiol. Biomark. Prev.* **2003**, *12*, 597–603.
69. Sinha, R.; Park, Y.; Graubard, B.I.; Leitzmann, M.F.; Hollenbeck, A.; Schatzkin, A.; Cross, A.J. Meat and meat-related compounds and risk of prostate cancer in a large prospective cohort study in the United States. *Am. J. Epidemiol.* **2009**, *170*, 1165–1177. [CrossRef]
70. Berquin, I.M.; Min, Y.; Wu, R.; Wu, J.; Perry, D.; Cline, J.M.; Thomas, M.J.; Thornburg, T.; Kulik, G.; Smith, A.; et al. Modulation of prostate cancer genetic risk by omega-3 and omega-6 fatty acids. *J. Clin. Investig.* **2007**, *117*, 1866–1875. [CrossRef]
71. Banez, L.L.; Hamilton, R.J.; Partin, A.W.; Vollmer, R.T.; Sun, L.; Rodriguez, C.; Wang, Y.; Terris, M.K.; Aronson, W.J.; Presti, J.C., Jr.; et al. Obesity-related plasma hemodilution and PSA concentration among men with prostate cancer. *JAMA* **2007**, *298*, 2275–2280. [CrossRef]

72. Kaaks, R.; Stattin, P. Obesity, Endogenous Hormone Metabolism, and Prostate Cancer Risk: A Conundrum of "Highs" and "Lows". *Cancer Prev. Res.* **2010**, *3*, 259. [CrossRef] [PubMed]
73. Huncharek, M.; Sue Haddock, K.; Reid, R.; Kupelnick, B. Smoking as a risk factor for prostate cancer: A meta-analysis of 24 prospective cohort studies. *Am. J. Public Health* **2010**, *100*, 693–701. [CrossRef]
74. Rohrmann, S.; Genkinger, J.M.; Burke, A.; Helzlsouer, K.J.; Comstock, G.W.; Alberg, A.J.; Platz, E.A. Smoking and Risk of Fatal Prostate Cancer in a Prospective U.S. Study. *Urology* **2007**, *69*, 721–725. [CrossRef] [PubMed]
75. Parker, C.; Castro, E.; Fizazi, K.; Heidenreich, A.; Ost, P.; Procopio, G.; Tombal, B.; Gillessen, S. Prostate cancer: ESMO Clinical Practice Guidelines for diagnosis, treatment and follow-up. *Ann. Oncol.* **2020**, *31*, 1119–1134. [CrossRef] [PubMed]
76. Kim, C.-J.; Dong, L.; Amend, S.R.; Cho, Y.-K.; Pienta, K.J. The role of liquid biopsies in prostate cancer management. *Lab A Chip* **2021**, *21*, 3263–3288. [CrossRef] [PubMed]
77. Lima, A.R.; Pinto, J.; Amaro, F.; Bastos, M.d.L.; Carvalho, M.; de Pinho, P.G. Advances and Perspectives in Prostate Cancer Biomarker Discovery in the Last 5 Years through Tissue and Urine Metabolomics. *Metabolites* **2021**, *11*, 181. [CrossRef] [PubMed]
78. Louie, K.S.; Seigneurin, A.; Cathcart, P.; Sasieni, P. Do prostate cancer risk models improve the predictive accuracy of PSA screening? A meta-analysis. *Ann. Oncol.* **2015**, *26*, 848–864. [CrossRef]
79. Das, C.J.; Razik, A.; Sharma, S.; Verma, S. Prostate biopsy: When and how to perform. *Clin. Radiol.* **2019**, *74*, 853–864. [CrossRef]
80. McDunn, J.E.; Li, Z.; Adam, K.P.; Neri, B.P.; Wolfert, R.L.; Milburn, M.V.; Lotan, Y.; Wheeler, T.M. Metabolomic signatures of aggressive prostate cancer. *Prostate* **2013**, *73*, 1547–1560. [CrossRef]
81. Salciccia, S.; Capriotti, A.L.; Lagana, A.; Fais, S.; Logozzi, M.; De Berardinis, E.; Busetto, G.M.; Di Pierro, G.B.; Ricciuti, G.P.; Del Giudice, F.; et al. Biomarkers in Prostate Cancer Diagnosis: From Current Knowledge to the Role of Metabolomics and Exosomes. *Int. J. Mol. Sci.* **2021**, *22*, 4367. [CrossRef]
82. Dimakakos, A.; Armakolas, A.; Koutsilieris, M. Novel Tools for Prostate Cancer Prognosis, Diagnosis, and Follow-Up. *BioMed. Res. Int.* **2014**, *2014*, 890697. [CrossRef]
83. Barry, M.J. Prevention of Prostate Cancer Morbidity and Mortality Primary Prevention and Early Detection. *Med. Clin. NA* **2017**, *101*, 787–806. [CrossRef]
84. Pal, R.P.; Maitra, N.U.; Mellon, J.K.; Khan, M.A. Defining prostate cancer risk before prostate biopsy. *Urol. Oncol.* **2013**, *31*, 1408–1418. [CrossRef]
85. Rigau, M.; Olivan, M.; Garcia, M.; Sequeiros, T.; Montes, M.; Colás, E.; Llauradó, M.; Planas, J.; Torres, I.D.; Morote, J.; et al. The present and future of prostate cancer urine biomarkers. *Int. J. Mol. Sci.* **2013**, *14*, 12620–12649. [CrossRef] [PubMed]
86. Lima, A.R.; Pinto, J.; Azevedo, A.I.; Barros-Silva, D.; Jerónimo, C.; Henrique, R.; de Lourdes Bastos, M.; de Pinho, P.G.; Carvalho, M. Identification of a biomarker panel for improvement of prostate cancer diagnosis by volatile metabolic profiling of urine. *Br. J. Cancer* **2019**, *121*, 857–868. [CrossRef] [PubMed]
87. Gaglani, S.; Gonzalez-Kozlova, E.; Lundon, D.J.; Tewari, A.K.; Dogra, N.; Kyprianou, N. Exosomes as A Next-Generation Diagnostic and Therapeutic Tool in Prostate Cancer. *Int. J. Mol. Sci.* **2021**, *22*, 10131. [CrossRef]
88. Lima, A.R.; Bastos, M.d.L.; Carvalho, M.; Guedes de Pinho, P. Biomarker Discovery in Human Prostate Cancer: An Update in Metabolomics Studies. *Transl. Oncol.* **2016**, *9*, 357–370. [CrossRef]
89. Campos-Fernández, E.; Barcelos, L.S.; de Souza, A.G.; Goulart, L.R.; Alonso-Goulart, V. Research landscape of liquid biopsies in prostate cancer. *Am. J. Cancer Res.* **2019**, *9*, 1309–1328.
90. Andriole, G.L.; Crawford, E.D.; Grubb, R.L., III; Buys, S.S.; Chia, D.; Church, T.R.; Fouad, M.N.; Isaacs, C.; Kvale, P.A.; Reding, D.J.; et al. Prostate cancer screening in the randomized Prostate, Lung, Colorectal, and Ovarian Cancer Screening Trial: Mortality results after 13 years of follow-up. *J. Natl. Cancer Inst.* **2012**, *104*, 125–132. [CrossRef] [PubMed]
91. Spur, E.M.; Decelle, E.A.; Cheng, L.L. Metabolomic imaging of prostate cancer with magnetic resonance spectroscopy and mass spectrometry. *Eur. J. Nucl. Med. Mol. Imaging* **2013**, *40* (Suppl. S1), S60–S71. [CrossRef] [PubMed]
92. Parsi, M.; Desai, M.H.; Desai, D.; Singhal, S.; Khandwala, P.M.; Potdar, R.R. PSMA: A game changer in the diagnosis and treatment of advanced prostate cancer. *Med. Oncol.* **2021**, *38*, 89. [CrossRef]
93. Uijen, M.J.M.; Derks, Y.H.W.; Merkx, R.I.J.; Schilham, M.G.M.; Roosen, J.; Privé, B.M.; van Lith, S.A.M.; van Herpen, C.M.L.; Gotthardt, M.; Heskamp, S.; et al. PSMA radioligand therapy for solid tumors other than prostate cancer: Background, opportunities, challenges, and first clinical reports. *Eur. J. Nucl. Med. Mol. Imaging* **2021**, *48*, 4350–4368. [CrossRef]
94. Seifert, R.; Alberts, I.L.; Afshar-Oromieh, A.; Rahbar, K. Prostate Cancer Theranostics: PSMA Targeted Therapy. *PET Clin.* **2021**, *16*, 391–396. [CrossRef]
95. Hofman, M.S.; Violet, J.; Hicks, R.J.; Ferdinandus, J.; Thang, S.P.; Akhurst, T.; Iravani, A.; Kong, G.; Ravi Kumar, A.; Murphy, D.G.; et al. [(177)Lu]-PSMA-617 radionuclide treatment in patients with metastatic castration-resistant prostate cancer (LuPSMA trial): A single-centre, single-arm, phase 2 study. *Lancet Oncol.* **2018**, *19*, 825–833. [CrossRef]
96. Hofman, M.; Violet, J.A.; Hicks, R.J.; Ferdinandus, J.; Thang, S.P.; Iravani, A.; Kong, G.; Ravi Kumar, A.; Akhurst, T.J.; Mooi, J.; et al. Results of a 50 patient single-center phase II prospective trial of Lutetium-177 PSMA-617 theranostics in metastatic castrate-resistant prostate cancer. *J. Clin. Oncol.* **2019**, *37*, 228. [CrossRef]
97. Calais, J.; Fendler, W.P.; Eiber, M.; Lassmann, M.; Dahlbom, M.; Esfandiari, R.; Gartmann, J.; Nguyen, K.; Thin, P.; Lok, V.; et al. RESIST-PC phase 2 trial: 177Lu-PSMA-617 radionuclide therapy for metastatic castrate-resistant prostate cancer. *J. Clin. Oncol.* **2019**, *37*, 5028. [CrossRef]

98. Moradi, F.; Farolfi, A.; Fanti, S.; Iagaru, A. Prostate cancer: Molecular imaging and MRI. *Eur. J. Radiol.* **2021**, *143*, 109893. [CrossRef] [PubMed]
99. Mena, E.; Black, P.C.; Rais-Bahrami, S.; Gorin, M.; Allaf, M.; Choyke, P. Novel PET imaging methods for prostate cancer. *World J. Urol.* **2021**, *39*, 687–699. [CrossRef]
100. Thomas, L.; Balmus, C.; Ahmadzadehfar, H.; Essler, M.; Strunk, H.; Bundschuh, R.A. Assessment of Bone Metastases in Patients with Prostate Cancer-A Comparison between (99m)Tc-Bone-Scintigraphy and [(68)Ga]Ga-PSMA PET/CT. *Pharmaceuticals (Basel)* **2017**, *10*, 68. [CrossRef]
101. Oey, O.; Ghaffari, M.; Li, J.J.; Hosseini-Beheshti, E. Application of extracellular vesicles in the diagnosis and treatment of prostate cancer: Implications for clinical practice. *Crit. Rev. Oncol. Hematol.* **2021**, *167*, 103495. [CrossRef] [PubMed]
102. Ludwig, M.; Rajvansh, R.; Drake, J.M. Emerging Role of Extracellular Vesicles in Prostate Cancer. *Endocrinology* **2021**, *162*, bqab139. [CrossRef]
103. Lorenc, T.; Klimczyk, K.; Michalczewska, I.; Słomka, M.; Kubiak-Tomaszewska, G.; Olejarz, W. Exosomes in Prostate Cancer Diagnosis, Prognosis and Therapy. *Int. J. Mol. Sci.* **2020**, *21*, 2118. [CrossRef]
104. McKiernan, J.; Donovan, M.J.; O'Neill, V.; Bentink, S.; Noerholm, M.; Belzer, S.; Skog, J.; Kattan, M.W.; Partin, A.; Andriole, G.; et al. A Novel Urine Exosome Gene Expression Assay to Predict High-grade Prostate Cancer at Initial Biopsy. *JAMA Oncol.* **2016**, *2*, 882–889. [CrossRef] [PubMed]
105. Ji, J.; Chen, R.; Zhao, L.; Xu, Y.; Cao, Z.; Xu, H.; Chen, X.; Shi, X.; Zhu, Y.; Lyu, J.; et al. Circulating exosomal mRNA profiling identifies novel signatures for the detection of prostate cancer. *Mol. Cancer* **2021**, *20*, 58. [CrossRef] [PubMed]
106. Xu, Y.H.; Deng, J.L.; Wang, G.; Zhu, Y.S. Long non-coding RNAs in prostate cancer: Functional roles and clinical implications. *Cancer Lett.* **2019**, *464*, 37–55. [CrossRef]
107. Li, W.; Dou, Z.; We, S.; Zhu, Z.; Pan, D.; Jia, Z.; Liu, H.; Wang, X.; Yu, G. Long noncoding RNA BDNF-AS is associated with clinical outcomes and has functional role in human prostate cancer. *Biomed. Pharmacother.* **2018**, *102*, 1105–1110. [CrossRef]
108. Zhao, R.; Sun, F.; Bei, X.; Wang, X.; Zhu, Y.; Jiang, C.; Zhao, F.; Han, B.; Xia, S. Upregulation of the long non-coding RNA FALEC promotes proliferation and migration of prostate cancer cell lines and predicts prognosis of PCa patients. *Prostate* **2017**, *77*, 1107–1117. [CrossRef]
109. Hu, J.C.; Wang, S.S.; Chou, Y.E.; Chiu, K.Y.; Li, J.R.; Chen, C.S.; Hung, S.C.; Yang, C.K.; Ou, Y.C.; Cheng, C.L.; et al. Associations between LncRNA MALAT1 Polymorphisms and Lymph Node Metastasis in Prostate Cancer. *Diagnostics (Basel)* **2021**, *11*, 1692. [CrossRef]
110. Li, Y.; Ji, J.; Lyu, J.; Jin, X.; He, X.; Mo, S.; Xu, H.; He, J.; Cao, Z.; Chen, X.; et al. A Novel Urine Exosomal lncRNA Assay to Improve the Detection of Prostate Cancer at Initial Biopsy: A Retrospective Multicenter Diagnostic Feasibility Study. *Cancers (Basel)* **2021**, *13*, 4075. [CrossRef]
111. Kidd, S.G.; Carm, K.T.; Bogaard, M.; Olsen, L.G.; Bakken, A.C.; Løvf, M.; Lothe, R.A.; Axcrona, K.; Axcrona, U.; Skotheim, R.I. High expression of SCHLAP1 in primary prostate cancer is an independent predictor of biochemical recurrence, despite substantial heterogeneity. *Neoplasia* **2021**, *23*, 634–641. [CrossRef]
112. Huang, W.; Su, X.; Yan, W.; Kong, Z.; Wang, D.; Huang, Y.; Zhai, Q.; Zhang, X.; Wu, H.; Li, Y.; et al. Overexpression of AR-regulated lncRNA TMPO-AS1 correlates with tumor progression and poor prognosis in prostate cancer. *Prostate* **2018**, *78*, 1248–1261. [CrossRef]
113. Beltran, H.; Demichelis, F. Intrapatient heterogeneity in prostate cancer. *Nat. Rev. Urol.* **2015**, *12*, 430–431. [CrossRef] [PubMed]
114. Dudka, I.; Thysell, E.; Lundquist, K.; Antti, H.; Iglesias-Gato, D.; Flores-Morales, A.; Bergh, A.; Wikström, P.; Gröbner, G. Comprehensive metabolomics analysis of prostate cancer tissue in relation to tumor aggressiveness and TMPRSS2-ERG fusion status. *BMC Cancer* **2020**, *20*, 437. [CrossRef]
115. Coleman, R.E.; Lipton, A.; Roodman, G.D.; Guise, T.A.; Boyce, B.F.; Brufsky, A.M.; Clézardin, P.; Croucher, P.I.; Gralow, J.R.; Hadji, P.; et al. Metastasis and bone loss: Advancing treatment and prevention. *Cancer Treat. Rev.* **2010**, *36*, 615–620. [CrossRef]
116. Parker, C.; Nilsson, S.; Heinrich, D.; Helle, S.I.; O'Sullivan, J.M.; Fosså, S.D.; Chodacki, A.; Wiechno, P.; Logue, J.; Seke, M.; et al. Alpha Emitter Radium-223 and Survival in Metastatic Prostate Cancer. *N. Engl. J. Med.* **2013**, *369*, 213–223. [CrossRef] [PubMed]
117. Maffioli, L.; Florimonte, L.; Costa, D.; Castanheira Correira, J.; Grana, C.; Luster, M.; Bodei, L.; Chinol, M. New radiopharmaceutical agents for the treatment of castration-resistant prostate cancer. *Q. J. Nucl. Med. Mol. Imaging* **2015**, *59*, 420–438. [PubMed]
118. Du, Y.; Dizdarevic, S. Molecular radiotheragnostics in prostate cancer. *Clin. Med. J. R. Coll. Physicians Lond.* **2017**, *17*, 458–461. [CrossRef]
119. Retter, A.; Gong, F.; Syer, T.; Singh, S.; Adeleke, S.; Punwani, S. Emerging methods for prostate cancer imaging: Evaluating cancer structure and metabolic alterations more clearly. *Mol. Oncol.* **2021**, *15*, 2565–2579. [CrossRef]
120. Maurer, T.; Gschwend, J.E.; Rauscher, I.; Souvatzoglou, M.; Haller, B.; Weirich, G.; Wester, H.J.; Heck, M.; Kübler, H.; Beer, A.J.; et al. Diagnostic Efficacy of (68)Gallium-PSMA Positron Emission Tomography Compared to Conventional Imaging for Lymph Node Staging of 130 Consecutive Patients with Intermediate to High Risk Prostate Cancer. *J. Urol.* **2016**, *195*, 1436–1443. [CrossRef]
121. Cursano, M.C.; Iuliani, M.; Casadei, C.; Stellato, M.; Tonini, G.; Paganelli, G.; Santini, D.; De Giorgi, U. Combination radium-223 therapies in patients with bone metastases from castration-resistant prostate cancer: A review. *Crit. Rev. Oncol. Hematol.* **2020**, *146*, 102864. [CrossRef]

122. Afshar-Oromieh, A.; Babich, J.W.; Kratochwil, C.; Giesel, F.L.; Eisenhut, M.; Kopka, K.; Haberkorn, U. The Rise of PSMA Ligands for Diagnosis and Therapy of Prostate Cancer. *J. Nucl. Med.* **2016**, *57*, 79S–89S. [CrossRef]
123. Rahbar, K.; Ahmadzadehfar, H.; Kratochwil, C.; Haberkorn, U.; Schäfers, M.; Essler, M.; Baum, R.P.; Kulkarni, H.R.; Schmidt, M.; Drzezga, A.; et al. German Multicenter Study Investigating 177Lu-PSMA-617 Radioligand Therapy in Advanced Prostate Cancer Patients. *J. Nucl. Med.* **2017**, *58*, 85–90. [CrossRef] [PubMed]
124. Scarpa, L.; Buxbaum, S.; Kendler, D.; Fink, K.; Bektic, J.; Gruber, L.; Decristoforo, C.; Uprimny, C.; Lukas, P.; Horninger, W.; et al. The (68)Ga/(177)Lu theragnostic concept in PSMA targeting of castration-resistant prostate cancer: Correlation of SUV(max) values and absorbed dose estimates. *Eur. J. Nucl. Med. Mol. Imaging* **2017**, *44*, 788–800. [CrossRef]
125. Morrison, G.J.; Goldkorn, A. Development and Application of Liquid Biopsies in Metastatic Prostate Cancer. *Curr. Oncol. Rep.* **2018**, *20*, 35. [CrossRef] [PubMed]
126. Matuszczak, M.; Schalken, J.A.; Salagierski, M. Prostate Cancer Liquid Biopsy Biomarkers' Clinical Utility in Diagnosis and Prognosis. *Cancers* **2021**, *13*, 3373. [CrossRef] [PubMed]
127. Bae, J.; Yang, S.H.; Kim, A.; Kim, H.G. RNA-based biomarkers for the diagnosis, prognosis, and therapeutic response monitoring of prostate cancer. *Urol. Oncol.* **2022**, *40*, 105.e1–105.e10. [CrossRef]
128. Kan, Y.; Li, B.; Yang, D.; Liu, Y.; Liu, J.; Yang, C.; Mao, L. Emerging Roles of Long Non-coding RNAs as Novel Biomarkers in the Diagnosis and Prognosis of Prostate Cancer. *Discov. Med.* **2021**, *32*, 29–37.
129. Kretschmer, A.; Tilki, D. Biomarkers in prostate cancer—Current clinical utility and future perspectives. *Crit. Rev. Oncol. Hematol.* **2017**, *120*, 180–193. [CrossRef]
130. Hanjani, N.A.; Esmaelizad, N.; Zanganeh, S.; Gharavi, A.T.; Heidarizadeh, P.; Radfar, M.; Omidi, F.; MacLoughlin, R.; Doroudian, M. Emerging role of exosomes as biomarkers in cancer treatment and diagnosis. *Crit. Rev. Oncol. Hematol.* **2022**, *169*, 103565. [CrossRef]
131. Wang, J.; Ni, J.; Beretov, J.; Thompson, J.; Graham, P.; Li, Y. Exosomal microRNAs as liquid biopsy biomarkers in prostate cancer. *Crit. Rev. Oncol. Hematol.* **2020**, *145*, 102860. [CrossRef]
132. Van Poppel, H.; Roobol, M.J.; Chapple, C.R.; Catto, J.W.F.; N'Dow, J.; Sønksen, J.; Stenzl, A.; Wirth, M. Prostate-specific Antigen Testing as Part of a Risk-Adapted Early Detection Strategy for Prostate Cancer: European Association of Urology Position and Recommendations for 2021. *Eur. Urol.* **2021**, *80*, 703–711. [CrossRef]
133. Litwin, M.S.; Tan, H.J. The diagnosis and treatment of prostate cancer: A review. *JAMA J. Am. Med. Assoc.* **2017**, *317*, 2532–2542. [CrossRef]
134. Ossoliński, K.; Nizioł, J.; Arendowski, A.; Ossolińska, A.; Ossoliński, T.; Kucharz, J.; Wiechno, P.; Ruman, T. Mass spectrometry-based metabolomic profiling of prostate cancer—A pilot study. *J. Cancer Metastasis Treat.* **2019**, *5*, 1. [CrossRef]
135. de Cobelli, O.; Terracciano, D.; Tagliabue, E.; Raimondi, S.; Galasso, G.; Cioffi, A.; Cordima, G.; Musi, G.; Damiano, R.; Cantiello, F.; et al. Body mass index was associated with upstaging and upgrading in patients with low-risk prostate cancer who met the inclusion criteria for active surveillance. *Urol. Oncol.* **2015**, *33*, 201.e1–208.e8. [CrossRef]
136. Ferro, M.; Lucarelli, G.; Bruzzese, D.; Di Lorenzo, G.; Perdonà, S.; Autorino, R.; Cantiello, F.; La Rocca, R.; Busetto, G.M.; Cimmino, A.; et al. Low serum total testosterone level as a predictor of upstaging and upgrading in low-risk prostate cancer patients meeting the inclusion criteria for active surveillance. *Oncotarget* **2017**, *8*, 18424–18434. [CrossRef] [PubMed]
137. Van Poppel, H.; Hogenhout, R.; Albers, P.; van den Bergh, R.C.N.; Barentsz, J.O.; Roobol, M.J. A European Model for an Organised Risk-stratified Early Detection Programme for Prostate Cancer. *Eur. Urol. Oncol.* **2021**, *4*, 731–739. [CrossRef] [PubMed]
138. Yusim, I.; Krenawi, M.; Mazor, E.; Novack, V.; Mabjeesh, N.J. The use of prostate specific antigen density to predict clinically significant prostate cancer. *Sci. Rep.* **2020**, *10*, 20015. [CrossRef]
139. Omri, N.; Kamil, M.; Alexander, K.; Alexander, T.; Edmond, S.; Ariel, Z.; David, K.; Gilad, A.E.; Azik, H. Association between PSA density and pathologically significant prostate cancer: The impact of prostate volume. *Prostate* **2020**, *80*, 1444–1449. [CrossRef] [PubMed]
140. Drost, F.J.H.; Osses, D.F.; Nieboer, D.; Steyerberg, E.W.; Bangma, C.H.; Roobol, M.J.; Schoots, I.G. Prostate MRI, with or without MRI-targeted biopsy, and systematic biopsy for detecting prostate cancer. *Cochrane Database Syst. Rev.* **2019**, *6*, CD012663. [CrossRef]
141. Gravina, M.; Spirito, L.; Celentano, G.; Capece, M.; Creta, M.; Califano, G.; Collà Ruvolo, C.; Morra, S.; Imbriaco, M.; Di Bello, F.; et al. Machine Learning and Clinical-Radiological Characteristics for the Classification of Prostate Cancer in PI-RADS 3 Lesions. *Diagnostics (Basel)* **2022**, *12*, 1565. [CrossRef] [PubMed]
142. Belue, M.J.; Turkbey, B. Tasks for artificial intelligence in prostate MRI. *Eur. Radiol. Exp.* **2022**, *6*, 33. [CrossRef] [PubMed]
143. Sunoqrot, M.R.S.; Saha, A.; Hosseinzadeh, M.; Elschot, M.; Huisman, H. Artificial intelligence for prostate MRI: Open datasets, available applications, and grand challenges. *Eur. Radiol. Exp.* **2022**, *6*, 35. [CrossRef] [PubMed]
144. Berenguer, C.V.; Pereira, F.; Pereira, J.A.M.; Câmara, J.S. Volatilomics: An Emerging and Promising Avenue for the Detection of Potential Prostate Cancer Biomarkers. *Cancers* **2022**, *14*, 3982. [CrossRef] [PubMed]
145. Janfaza, S.; Khorsand, B.; Nikkhah, M.; Zahiri, J. Digging deeper into volatile organic compounds associated with cancer. *Biol. Methods Protoc.* **2019**, *4*, bpz014. [CrossRef] [PubMed]
146. Silva, C.; Perestrelo, R.; Silva, P.; Tomás, H.; Câmara, J.S. Breast Cancer Metabolomics: From Analytical Platforms to Multivariate Data Analysis. A Review. *Metabolites* **2019**, *9*, 102. [CrossRef] [PubMed]

147. Gao, Q.; Lee, W.Y. Urinary metabolites for urological cancer detection: A review on the application of volatile organic compounds for cancers. *Am. J. Clin. Exp. Urol.* **2019**, *7*, 232–248. [PubMed]
148. Khalid, T.; Aggio, R.; White, P.; De Lacy Costello, B.; Persad, R.; Al-Kateb, H.; Jones, P.; Probert, C.S.; Ratcliffe, N. Urinary Volatile Organic Compounds for the Detection of Prostate Cancer. *PLoS ONE* **2015**, *10*, e0143283. [CrossRef]
149. Struck-Lewicka, W.; Kordalewska, M.; Bujak, R.; Yumba Mpanga, A.; Markuszewski, M.; Jacyna, J.; Matuszewski, M.; Kaliszan, R.; Markuszewski, M.J. Urine metabolic fingerprinting using LC-MS and GC-MS reveals metabolite changes in prostate cancer: A pilot study. *J. Pharm. Biomed. Anal.* **2015**, *111*, 351–361. [CrossRef]
150. Gao, Q.; Su, X.; Annabi, M.H.; Schreiter, B.R.; Prince, T.; Ackerman, A.; Morgas, S.; Mata, V.; Williams, H.; Lee, W.-Y. Application of Urinary Volatile Organic Compounds (VOCs) for the Diagnosis of Prostate Cancer. *Clin. Genitourin. Cancer* **2019**, *17*, 183–190. [CrossRef]
151. Bax, C.; Taverna, G.; Eusebio, L.; Sironi, S.; Grizzi, F.; Guazzoni, G.; Capelli, L. Innovative Diagnostic Methods for Early Prostate Cancer Detection through Urine Analysis: A Review. *Cancers (Basel)* **2018**, *10*, 123. [CrossRef]
152. da Costa, B.R.B.; De Martinis, B.S. Analysis of urinary VOCs using mass spectrometric methods to diagnose cancer: A review. *Clin. Mass Spectrom.* **2020**, *18*, 27–37. [CrossRef] [PubMed]
153. Tyagi, H.; Daulton, E.; Bannaga, A.S.; Arasaradnam, R.P.; Covington, J.A. Urinary Volatiles and Chemical Characterisation for the Non-Invasive Detection of Prostate and Bladder Cancers. *Biosensors (Basel)* **2021**, *11*, 437. [CrossRef] [PubMed]
154. Lima, A.R.; Pinto, J.; Carvalho-Maia, C.; Jerónimo, C.; Henrique, R.; Bastos, M.d.L.; Carvalho, M.; Guedes de Pinho, P. A Panel of Urinary Volatile Biomarkers for Differential Diagnosis of Prostate Cancer from Other Urological Cancers. *Cancers* **2020**, *12*, 2017. [CrossRef] [PubMed]
155. Capelli, L.; Taverna, G.; Bellini, A.; Eusebio, L.; Buffi, N.; Lazzeri, M.; Guazzoni, G.; Bozzini, G.; Seveso, M.; Mandressi, A.; et al. Application and Uses of Electronic Noses for Clinical Diagnosis on Urine Samples: A Review. *Sensors (Basel)* **2016**, *16*, 1708. [CrossRef] [PubMed]

Disclaimer/Publisher's Note: The statements, opinions and data contained in all publications are solely those of the individual author(s) and contributor(s) and not of MDPI and/or the editor(s). MDPI and/or the editor(s) disclaim responsibility for any injury to people or property resulting from any ideas, methods, instructions or products referred to in the content.

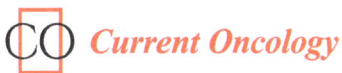

Article

Prior Negative Biopsy, PSA Density, and Anatomic Location Impact Cancer Detection Rate of MRI-Targeted PI-RADS Index Lesions

Ahmad N. Alzubaidi [1], Amy Zheng [2], Mohammad Said [3], Xuanjia Fan [2], Michael Maidaa [4], R. Grant Owens [3], Max Yudovich [1], Suraj Pursnani [1], R. Scott Owens [5], Thomas Stringer [4], Chad R. Tracy [3] and Jay D. Raman [1,*]

[1] Department of Urology, Penn State Milton S. Hershey Medical Center, Hershey, PA 17033, USA; analzubaidi@gmail.com (A.N.A.)
[2] Pennsylvania State College of Medicine, Hershey, PA 17033, USA
[3] Department of Urology, University of Iowa Hospitals and Clinics, Iowa City, IA 52242, USA; rowens@uiowa.edu (R.G.O.); chad-tracy@uiowa.edu (C.R.T.)
[4] Department of Urology, University of Florida College of Medicine, Gainesville, FL 32611, USA
[5] UPMC Central PA Hospital, Camphill, PA 17011, USA; owensrs@upmc.edu
* Correspondence: jraman@pennstatehealth.psu.edu

Abstract: Background: MRI fusion prostate biopsy has improved the detection of clinically significant prostate cancer (CSC). Continued refinements in predicting the pre-biopsy probability of CSC are essential for optimal patient counseling. We investigated potential factors related to improved cancer detection rates (CDR) of CSC in patients with PI-RADS $\geq$ 3 lesions. Methods: The pathology of 980 index lesions in 980 patients sampled by transrectal mpMRI-targeted prostate biopsy across four medical centers between 2017–2020 was reviewed. PI-RADS lesion distribution included 291 PI-RADS-5, 374 PI-RADS-4, and 315 PI-RADS-3. We compared CDR of index PI-RADS $\geq$ 3 lesions based on location (TZ) vs. (PZ), PSA density (PSAD), and history of prior negative conventional transrectal ultrasound-guided biopsy (TRUS). Results: Mean age, PSA, prostate volume, and level of prior negative TRUS biopsy were 66 years (43–90), 7.82 ng/dL (5.6–11.2), 54 cm^3 (12–173), and 456/980 (46.5%), respectively. Higher PSAD, no prior history of negative TRUS biopsy, and PZ lesions were associated with higher CDR. Stratified CDR highlighted significant variance across subgroups. CDR for a PI-RADS-5 score, PZ lesion with PSAD $\geq$ 0.15, and prior negative biopsy was 77%. Conversely, the CDR rate for a PI-RADS-4 score, TZ lesion with PSAD < 0.15, and prior negative biopsy was significantly lower at 14%. Conclusions: For index PI-RADS $\geq$ 3 lesions, CDR varied significantly based on location, prior history of negative TRUS biopsy, and PSAD. Such considerations are critical when counseling on the merits and potential yield of prostate needle biopsy.

Keywords: fusion prostate biopsy; PI-RADS; magnetic resonance imaging; PSA density

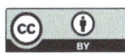

1. Introduction

Prostate cancer (PCa) is the most commonly diagnosed male malignancy worldwide. In the United States, PCa incidence increased by 3% annually from 2014 through 2019 after almost 20 years of decline. Over the last year, the United States reported approximately 290,000 cases of PCa with an estimated 35,000 cancer-related deaths [1]. Additionally, although it often has an indolent course, the proportion of prostate cancer diagnosed at an advanced stage has increased from 3.9% to 8.2% over the past decade [2].

Men with clinical suspicion of prostate cancer (with elevated PSA and/or abnormal DRE) typically undergo a transrectal (TRUS) or transperineal ultrasound-guided biopsy of the prostate during which 10 to 12 systematic cores are obtained. The transrectal ultrasound-guided approach was previously the gold standard for cancer detection when clinical suspicion is present, but it has been shown to be susceptible to underdiagnosis, grade misclassification, and complications [3,4].

Over the last decade, multiparametric magnetic resonance imaging (mpMRI) has been increasingly incorporated into prostate imaging and diagnostic evaluation. mpMRI combines anatomic (T2W phase) and functional assessment (diffusion-weighted imaging and apparent diffusion coefficient maps and dynamic contrast-enhanced) imaging to provide an objective assessment for risk of prostate cancer. This technology has been used with fusion prostate biopsy and has increasingly become the standard of care with improved detection of clinically significant prostate cancer (CSC; Grade Group $\geq$ 2) [5,6].

In 2012, after the introduction of mpMRI, the American College of Radiology (ACR) introduced a new standard reporting system named the Prostate Imaging Reporting and Data System (PI-RADS) [7], specifically pertaining to the characterization of prostate lesions. A second edition (v2.0) was released in 2016, which was further updated in 2019 and titled version (v2.1) [8,9]. It has since gained popularity among radiologists as a standardized reporting system for interpreting and dictating prostate MRI and gained widespread acceptance as a standard method of diagnosis for suspicion of clinically significant prostate cancer. The PI-RADS scoring system risk-stratifies lesions into five categories based on the size and appearance of the lesion. The categories range from PI-RADS-1 (CSC is highly unlikely) to PI-RADS-3 (CSC is equivocal) and PI-RADS-5 (CSC is highly likely). It does not factor in lesion location and any other patient-related characteristics [10]. The PRECISION trial, a multicenter international randomized controlled trial conducted in 2018 and published in the New England Journal of Medicine, randomized 500 biopsy-naïve patients with clinical suspicion for PCa to undergo mpMRI, with or without targeted biopsy, or standard TRUS biopsy. Men in the MRI group only underwent targeted biopsy if mpMRI showed a lesion with PI-RADS 3 or higher. The study concluded that in biopsy-naïve patients, PI-RADS evaluation with mpMRI could assist 28% to avoid unnecessary biopsy, as well as increase the detection of Gleason Grade (GG) $\geq$ 2 cancer when MRI-targeted biopsy was used for PI-RADS 3–5 lesions (38% vs. 26% with standard biopsy, p = 0.005) [11]. This was similar to previous findings from the PROMIS trial, which were published prior to the PIRADS system, where mpMRI allowed 27% of patients to avoid biopsy with 5% fewer clinically insignificant cancer detected [12].

Although notable improvements are observed when compared to conventional prostate biopsy, the existing literature reports variability in diagnostic yield overall and CSC [13,14]. Continued refinements in predicting the pre-biopsy probability of CSC are, therefore, essential for optimal patient counseling. Here, we aim to investigate clinical and radiographic factors that may impact the yield of cancer detection of CSC for PI-RADS $\geq$ 3 lesions. We hypothesize that lesion location, PSA density, and prior negative TRUS biopsy history may significantly impact cancer detection. Such information may be readily translated into urological practice to ensure informed decision-making for patients considering prostate biopsy.

2. Materials and Methods

Consecutive men undergoing MRI-guided prostate biopsy between 2017 and 2020 across 4 different medical centers (3 academic, 1 community) for suspected prostate cancer (elevated PSA and/or abnormal digital rectal examination) with PI-RADS $\geq$ 3 lesions were included.

2.1. MRI Protocol and Biopsies

In general, MRI images were acquired using a 3-Tesla magnet with annotation of lesions performed using the PI-RADS v2 guideline T2 weighted, diffusion-weighted (DWI), and dynamic contrast-enhanced (DCE) images. The volume (cm^3) of each region of interest was calculated using a rectangle polygon model after manually measuring the height, width, and length of each lesion. Scans were reviewed and interpreted by fellowship-trained, board-certified radiologists in conjunction with urologists.

Fusion biopsies were performed by a sub-specialized urologist at each of the 4 respective institutions using a transrectal approach. All biopsies utilized commercially available software for image registration with ultrasound segmentation via the bidimensional ultrasound probe and rendering of a three-dimensional ultrasound volume. Data acquired by ultrasound and MRI are fused together with alignment and a minimum of two biopsies were obtained from index lesions.

2.2. Cohort of Analysis

The cohort included 1054 patients with an index lesion (PI-RADS score of ≥3) on multiparametric MRI. Patients with anterior index lesions (n = 74) were excluded due to low numbers across subgroups. With such criteria, a final evaluable cohort of 980 index lesions in 980 patients was established. Index PI-RADS ≥ 3 lesions were further stratified based on location (transitional zone (TZ) vs. peripheral zone (PZ)), PSA density (cutoff of 0.15 ng/mL/cm^3), and history of prior negative conventional TRUS biopsy.

2.3. Statistical Analysis

Calculations of CDR were performed using R with subset and mean functions using no additional packages. We used the Wilcoxon rank-sum, Kruskal–Wallis tests, Chi-square, and Student *t*-test where applicable. Significance was set at a *p*-value of 0.05.

3. Results

Table 1 summarizes the clinical, radiographic, and pathologic characteristics of our cohort. Median patient age and PSA were 66 years (43–90) and 7.8 mg/dL (5.6–11.2), respectively. Approximately 50% of men in our study (456 of 980) had a prior negative biopsy. On MRI, PI-RADS index lesion distribution included 291 PI-RADS 5, 374 PI-RADS 4, and 315 PI-RADS 3. with calculated median prostate volume of 54 cm^3 (12–173). PZ index lesions were found in 58.7% (575/980) of patients, while TZ index lesions were found in 41.3% (405/980).

Table 1. Patient and tumor baseline characteristics (n = 980 index lesions).

Patient Characteristics	Median and IQR or Frequency (%)
Age at biopsy (years)	66 (61–71)
PSA (ng/dL)	7.82 (5.6–11.2)
Prostate Volume (cm^3)	54 (40–79)
PSA Density (ng/dL^3)	0.13 (0.09–0.21)
Prior Negative TRUS Biopsy	
Yes	456 (47%)
No	524 (53%)
Lesion Characteristics	
PI-RADS Score	
3	315 (32.1%)
4	374 (38.1%)
5	291 (29.7%)
Lesion Location	
Peripheral Zone	575 (58.7%)
Transition Zone	405 (41.3%)

Overall, CSC was detected in 346 lesions (35%). More specifically, CSC was detected in 164 lesions (56%), 133 lesions (36%), and 49 lesions (16%) of PI-RADS 5, PI-RADS 4, and PI-RADS 3 lesions, respectively. In aggregate, PZ lesions were more likely to harbor CSC compared to TZ lesions (42.9% vs. 24.4%, $p > 0.001$). Higher CSC was seen in those with higher PSAD above vs. below cutoff 0.15 (51.7% vs. 24.5%, $p < 0.001$). Additionally, those without a history of prior negative TRUS biopsy had higher rates of CSC (36% vs. 32%, $p < 0.001$).

Within the PZ subgroup, lesions were more likely to be classified as a PI-RADS 5 (64% (185/291) vs. PI-RADS 3 48% (151/315), $p < 0.001$). Conversely, PI-RADS 3 lesions were more likely to be found in a TZ location compared to PI-RADS 5 lesions (52% (164/315) vs. 36% (106/291), respectively, $p < 0.001$).

With respect to PSAD, PI-RADS 5 lesions had a greater percentage of occurring in the high PSAD density group (>0.15) compared to those in the PI-RADS 3 group (58% (170/291) vs. 35% (110/315), respectively, $p < 0.001$). Finally, patients with PI-RADS 5 and PI-RADS 3 were similarly likely to have had a history of prior negative TRUS biopsy (44% (128/291) vs. 45% (141/315) respectively, $p > 0.05$).

Table 2 summarizes the CDR as stratified by PSA density, lesion location, and biopsy history. Notably, significant variance in CDR was observed across subgroups. In particular, the highest CDR was seen in the cohort for a PI-RADS 5 score, PZ lesion in patients with PSAD $\geq$ 0.15, and prior negative biopsy was 77%. Conversely, the CDR rate for a PI-RADS 4 score, TZ lesion, with PSAD < 0.15, and prior negative biopsy was significantly lower at 14% ($p < 0.001$).

Table 2. Percentage of clinically significant cancer detection rates stratified by PI-RADS lesion score, tumor location, PSAD, and history of prior negative transrectal ultrasound-guided biopsy.

PI-RADS 5	CDR % 56% (164/291)	PI-RADS 4	CDR % 36% (133/374)	PI-RADS 3	CDR % 16% (49/315)
PZ	63 (117/185)	PZ	41 (97/239)	PZ	22 (33/151)
PSAD ≥ 0.15	70 (77/110)	PSAD ≥ 0.15	53 (48/91)	PSAD ≥ 0.15	30 (18/61)
Prior Negative Bx	77 (49/64)	Prior Negative Bx	57 (32/56)	Prior Negative Bx	39 (12/31)
No Prior Bx	61 (28/46)	No Prior Bx	46 (16/35)	No Prior Bx	20 (6/30)
PSAD < 0.15	53 (40/75)	PSAD < 0.15	33 (49/148)	PSAD < 0.15	16 (15/90)
Prior Negative Bx	29 (9/31)	Prior Negative Bx	26 (16/62)	Prior Negative Bx	10 (3/30)
No Prior Bx	70 (31/44)	No Prior Bx	38 (33/86)	No Prior Bx	20 (12/60)
TZ	44 (47/106)	TZ	26 (36/136)	TZ	10 (16/164)
PSAD ≥ 0.15	55 (33/60)	PSAD ≥ 0.15	43 (24/56)	PSAD ≥ 0.15	20 (10/49)
Prior Negative Bx	67 (10/15)	Prior Negative Bx	48 (12/25)	Prior Negative Bx	25 (2/8)
No Prior Bx	51 (23/45)	No Prior Bx	39 (12/31)	No Prior Bx	20 (8/41)
PSAD < 0.15	30 (14/46)	PSAD < 0.15	15 (12/80)	PSAD < 0.15	5 (6/115)
Prior Negative Bx	22 (4/18)	Prior Negative Bx	14 (6/44)	Prior Negative Bx	3 (2/72)
No Prior Bx	36 (10/28)	No Prior Bx	17 (6/36)	No Prior Bx	9 (4/43)

4. Discussion

In this study, we evaluated potential factors related to improved cancer detection rates of clinically significant cancer in patients with index PI-RADS $\geq$ 3 lesions. MRI-targeted prostate biopsy has been shown to improve the detection rate of clinically significant prostate cancer compared to conventional transrectal ultrasound-guided biopsy [6,8,15]. However, surgeon experience, number of targeted biopsy cores, radiologic interpretation, and software systems have collectively contributed to variability in cancer detection rates [14,16].

Overall, our cancer detection rates were lower for higher PI-RADS lesions compared to those of the PRECISION trial. CDRs from the PRECISION trial versus our study were 83% vs. 56% for PI-RADS 5, 60% vs. 36% for PI-RADS 4, and 12% vs. 16% for PI-RADS 3 lesions [12]. We believe these observations are critical for iterative feedback at a site-specific level to understand and improve on factors contributing to lower CDR. Nonetheless, we observed that our cohort followed similar patterns in which the percentage of CSC was highest among patients with PI-RADS 5, with a subsequent decline across different PI-RADS classifications.

Our experience across four medical institutions revealed significant discrepancies in cancer detection rates with respect to location, PSAD, and history of prior negative TRUS biopsy. Lesion location had the highest impact on CDR across PI-RADS subgroups. In aggregate, PZ lesions were more likely to harbor CSC compared to TZ lesions (42.9% vs. 24.4%, $p > 0.001$), the highest detection rate occurring in patients with PZ lesions, PSAD > 0.15, and prior negative TRUS biopsy at 77%. The next highest observed CDR was

70% within patients with PZ lesions, PSAD < 0.15, and no prior biopsy. Our results differ from those of a recent study of 263 U.S. veteran patients, which noted that the location of the lesion was not statistically associated with CSC in PI-RADS 3 lesions [17]. In contrast, lesion location was noted to be associated with PI-RADS scoring by a German population study that retrospectively reviewed MRIs of 293 patients. Mahjoub et al. suggested different PI-RADS size cut-offs based on location, with smaller and more defined separation of CSC found in the PZ compared to TZ [18]. Future optimization of PI-RADS could address location variations by accounting for gland heterogeneity, benign prostate hyperplasia, and size criterion [19,20]. Until then, given that most prostate cancers occur in the PZ, clinicians should consider the importance of location, and thus clinical suspicion of CSC in PZ lesions, in assessing the need for biopsy.

Conversely, the lowest CDRs occurred with PI-RADS 3 and 4 patients with a history of prior negative TRUS and PSAD < 0.15 at 3% and 14%, respectively. This observation adds to the debate on whether biopsy is indicated for PI-RADS scoring with a minority of CSC in the context of wide variation and low positive predictive value of PI-RADS scoring across medical centers [21]. It is generally accepted that PI-RADS 1 and 2 scores are considered likely benign and do not require additional testing. Likewise, PI-RADS 4 and 5 scores are likely associated with CSC and biopsy should be recommended. For equivocal scoring, decision-making is more ambiguous. Biopsy is reasonably indicated if there is continued clinical suspicion for CSC. Yet, close active surveillance is also a reasonable decision for patients who would prefer to avoid biopsy and are able to adhere to monitoring protocols [22]. In a prospective study of 723 men with MRI-visible prostate lesions, a combination of MRI-targeted biopsy and standard systematic biopsy was suggested to be beneficial in eliminating the risk of missing any CSC in PI-RADS 3 or 4 lesions [3]. Minimal changes in CDR occurred for the PI-RADS 5 group, suggesting that MRI-targeted biopsy alone may be sufficient for high-grade lesions [22]. However, the value of systematic biopsy allowed for significant additional detection of 7.5% and 8.0% for the PI-RADS 3 and 4 groups, respectively, compared to MRI-targeted biopsy alone, which yielded 17.2% and 35.8% of CSC, respectively. In contrast, in a study of 92 biopsied PI-RADS 3 lesions by Liddell et al., a low risk of prostate cancer (6.5%) was reported and, therefore, the authors supported ongoing surveillance [23]. Such variability in CDR has made determining the significance and management of seemingly low-risk lesions difficult.

PSAD, which is obtained by the total PSA (ng/mL) divided by the prostate volume, may serve as an adjunct in cancer detection of ambiguous PI-RADS lesions and has been associated with more aggressive prostate cancer long before the advent of MRI fusion biopsy [24]. Similar to our results, Natale et al. found that PSAD was a significant predictor of CSC in multivariate analyses, with patients with PSAD > 0.15 being five times more likely to have clinically significant disease compared to PSAD < 0.15 [17]. Other studies demonstrated that incorporation of PSAD resulted in higher CDR than PI-RADS alone (50.0–66.7% vs. 48%) for PI-RADS $\geq$ 3 and a 20% reduction in unnecessary biopsies for indeterminate PI-RAD lesions [25,26]. Contrary to most recent findings, some studies revealed the combination of methods held no significant improvement in diagnostic performance, though this may be dependent on lesion location [27,28]. Despite inconsistent conclusions in the literature, our study supports the use of MRI as a powerful tool in the detection of clinically significant prostate cancer and the impact of PSAD on CDR, where PSAD > 0.15 has significantly higher CDR for all lesions regardless of PI-RADS score. Upcoming predictive models with the integration of PSAD, among other biomarkers and patient features, with PI-RADS have shown promising results by significantly and efficiently reducing unnecessary prostate biopsies within risk thresholds of >10–20% [29,30].

Several limitations exist within our study. There may have been patient-related and prostate-specific covariates that we did not stratify for or identify, e.g., family history of prostate cancer, due to the study's retrospective nature. Results were collected from four different medical centers, including a community hospital, across the country to account for variability and broaden generalizability. Additionally, there may be variation in PI-RADS lesion classification among interpreting radiologists across institutions, though interrater agreement has been suggested to be sufficient [31]. The number of cores per lesion was also taken at the discretion of the provider, which may have led to the under-detection of CSC in this sample [16]. Nonetheless, the impact of this study shows how real-world results can significantly differ compared to data emerging from trial settings, and thus, using practical data may improve patient counseling on prostate biopsy yield. Further investigation on CDR across more institutions may provide additional insights on applicability for future risk calculation.

5. Conclusions

In patients with PI-RADS $\geq$ 3 lesions, CDR varied significantly based on location, prior history of negative TRUS biopsy, and PSA density. Higher PSA density, no prior history of negative TRUS biopsy, and PZ lesions were associated with higher CDR. Utilization of these factors can improve risk stratification for CSC and therefore develop appropriate guidelines for counseling patients on their candidacy for prostate needle biopsy and prostate cancer management.

Author Contributions: Conceptualization, A.N.A. and J.D.R.; Methodology, A.N.A., X.F., S.P., M.S., M.Y. and C.R.T.; Software, X.F.; Investigation, A.N.A.; Resources, A.Z., S.P., M.Y., R.G.O., M.M., T.S., R.S.O., C.R.T. and J.D.R.; Data curation, X.F., S.P., M.S., M.Y., R.G.O., M.M., T.S., R.S.O. and C.R.T.; Writing—original draft, A.N.A. and A.Z.; Writing—review and editing, A.N.A. and J.D.R.; Supervision, J.D.R.; Funding acquisition, J.D.R. All authors have read and agreed to the published version of the manuscript.

Funding: Penn State Health No Shave November Education and Research Fund.

Institutional Review Board Statement: The study was conducted in accordance with the Declaration of Helsinki, and approved by the Institutional Review Board of Penn State Health (STUDY14940, Approval February 2020).

Informed Consent Statement: N/A retrospective review.

Data Availability Statement: Reviewed and available via standard protocol.

Conflicts of Interest: The authors declare no conflicts of interest.

References

1. Siegel, R.L.; Miller, K.D.; Wagle, N.S.; Jemal, A. Cancer statistics, 2023. *CA Cancer J. Clin.* **2023**, *73*, 17–48. [CrossRef] [PubMed]
2. Siegel, R.L.; Miller, K.D.; Fuchs, H.E.; Jemal, A. Cancer statistics, 2022. *CA Cancer J. Clin.* **2022**, *72*, 7–33. [CrossRef] [PubMed]
3. Ahdoot, M.; Lebastchi, A.H.; Long, L.; Wilbur, A.R.; Gomella, P.T.; Mehralivand, S.; Daneshvar, M.A.; Yerram, N.K.; O'Connor, L.P.; Wang, A.Z.; et al. Using Prostate Imaging-Reporting and Data System (PI-RADS) Scores to Select an Optimal Prostate Biopsy Method: A Secondary Analysis of the Trio Study. *Eur. Urol. Oncol.* **2022**, *5*, 176–186. [CrossRef] [PubMed] [PubMed Central]
4. Borghesi, M.; Ahmed, H.; Nam, R.; Schaeffer, E.; Schiavina, R.; Taneja, S.; Weidner, W.; Loeb, S. Complications After Systematic, Random, and Image-guided Prostate Biopsy. *Eur. Urol.* **2017**, *71*, 353–365. [CrossRef] [PubMed]
5. Filson, C.P.; Natarajan, S.; Margolis, D.J.; Huang, J.; Lieu, P.; Dorey, F.J.; Reiter, R.E.; Marks, L.S. Prostate cancer detection with magnetic resonance-ultrasound fusion biopsy: The role of systematic and targeted biopsies. *Cancer* **2016**, *122*, 884–892. [CrossRef] [PubMed] [PubMed Central]
6. Siddiqui, M.M.; George, A.K.; Rubin, R.; Rais-Bahrami, S.; Parnes, H.L.; Merino, M.J.; Simon, R.M.; Turkbey, B.; Choyke, P.L.; Wood, B.J.; et al. Efficiency of Prostate Cancer Diagnosis by MR/Ultrasound Fusion-Guided Biopsy vs Standard Extended-Sextant Biopsy for MR-Visible Lesions. *J. Natl. Cancer Inst.* **2016**, *108*, djw039. [CrossRef] [PubMed]
7. Maggi, M.; Panebianco, V.; Mosca, A.; Salciccia, S.; Gentilucci, A.; Di Pierro, G.; Busetto, G.M.; Barchetti, G.; Campa, R.; Sperduti, I.; et al. Prostate Imaging Reporting and Data System 3 Category Cases at Multiparametric Magnetic Resonance for Prostate Cancer: A Systematic Review and Meta-analysis. *Eur. Urol. Focus* **2020**, *6*, 463–478. [CrossRef] [PubMed]
8. Barentsz, J.O.; Richenberg, J.; Clements, R.; Choyke, P.; Verma, S.; Villeirs, G.; Rouviere, O.; Logager, V.; Fütterer, J.J.; European Society of Urogenital Radiology. ESUR prostate MR guidelines 2012. *Eur. Radiol.* **2012**, *22*, 746–757. [CrossRef] [PubMed]

9. Vargas, H.A.; Hötker, A.M.; Goldman, D.A.; Moskowitz, C.S.; Gondo, T.; Matsumoto, K.; Ehdaie, B.; Woo, S.; Fine, S.W.; Reuter, V.E.; et al. Updated prostate imaging reporting and data system (PIRADS v2) recommendations for the detection of clinically significant prostate cancer using multiparametric MRI: Critical evaluation using whole-mount pathology as standard of reference. *Eur. Radiol.* **2016**, *26*, 1606–1612. [CrossRef] [PubMed] [PubMed Central]
10. Turkbey, B.; Rosenkrantz, A.B.; Haider, M.A.; Padhani, A.R.; Villeirs, G.; Macura, K.J.; Tempany, C.M.; Choyke, P.L.; Cornud, F.; Margolis, D.J.; et al. Prostate Imaging Reporting and Data System Version 2.1: 2019 Update of Prostate Imaging Reporting and Data System Version 2. *Eur. Urol.* **2019**, *76*, 340–351. [CrossRef]
11. Available online: https://www.acr.org/-/media/ACR/Files/RADS/PI-RADS/PIRADS-V2-1 (accessed on 16 October 2023).
12. Kasivisvanathan, V.; Rannikko, A.S.; Borghi, M.; Panebianco, V.; Mynderse, L.A.; Vaarala, M.H.; Briganti, A.; Budäus, L.; Hellawell, G.; Hindley, R.G.; et al. MRI-Targeted or Standard Biopsy for Prostate-Cancer Diagnosis. *N. Engl. J. Med.* **2018**, *378*, 1767–1777. [CrossRef] [PubMed]
13. El-Shater Bosaily, A.; Parker, C.; Brown, L.C.; Gabe, R.; Hindley, R.G.; Kaplan, R.; Emberton, M.; Ahmed, H.U.; PROMIS Group. PROMIS—Prostate MR imaging study: A paired validating cohort study evaluating the role of multi-parametric MRI in men with clinical suspicion of prostate cancer. *Contemp. Clin. Trials* **2015**, *42*, 26–40. [CrossRef] [PubMed] [PubMed Central]
14. Stabile, A.; Giganti, F.; Kasivisvanathan, V.; Giannarini, G.; Moore, C.M.; Padhani, A.R.; Panebianco, V.; Rosenkrantz, A.B.; Salomon, G.; Turkbey, B.; et al. Factors Influencing Variability in the Performance of Multiparametric Magnetic Resonance Imaging in Detecting Clinically Significant Prostate Cancer: A Systematic Literature Review. *Eur. Urol. Oncol.* **2020**, *3*, 145–167. [CrossRef]
15. Siddiqui, M.M.; Rais-Bahrami, S.; Turkbey, B.; George, A.K.; Rothwax, J.; Shakir, N.; Okoro, C.; Raskolnikov, D.; Parnes, H.L.; Linehan, W.M.; et al. Comparison of MR/ultrasound fusion-guided biopsy with ultrasound-guided biopsy for the diagnosis of prostate cancer. *JAMA* **2015**, *313*, 390–397. [CrossRef]
16. Tracy, C.R.; Flynn, K.J.; Sjoberg, D.D.; Gellhaus, P.T.; Metz, C.M.; Ehdaie, B. Optimizing MRI-targeted prostate biopsy: The diagnostic benefit of additional targeted biopsy cores. *Urol. Oncol.* **2021**, *39*, 193.e1–193.e6. [CrossRef]
17. Natale, C.; Koller, C.R.; Greenberg, J.W.; Pincus, J.; Krane, L.S. Considering Predictive Factors in the Diagnosis of Clinically Significant Prostate Cancer in Patients with PI-RADS 3 Lesions. *Life* **2021**, *11*, 1432. [CrossRef]
18. Mahjoub, S.; Baur, A.D.J.; Lenk, J.; Lee, C.H.; Hartenstein, A.; Rudolph, M.M.; Cash, H.; Hamm, B.; Asbach, P.; Haas, M.; et al. Optimizing size thresholds for detection of clinically significant prostate cancer on MRI: Peripheral zone cancers are smaller and more predictable than transition zone tumors. *Eur. J. Radiol.* **2020**, *129*, 109071. [CrossRef]
19. Rudolph, M.M.; Baur, A.D.J.; Haas, M.; Cash, H.; Miller, K.; Mahjoub, S.; Hartenstein, A.; Kaufmann, D.; Rotzinger, R.; Lee, C.H.; et al. Validation of the PI-RADS language: Predictive values of PI-RADS lexicon descriptors for detection of prostate cancer. *Eur. Radiol.* **2020**, *30*, 4262–4271. [CrossRef]
20. Westphalen, A.C.; McCulloch, C.E.; Anaokar, J.M.; Arora, S.; Barashi, N.S.; Barentsz, J.O.; Bathala, T.K.; Bittencourt, L.K.; Booker, M.T.; Braxton, V.G.; et al. Variability of the Positive Predictive Value of PI-RADS for Prostate MRI across 26 Centers: Experience of the Society of Abdominal Radiology Prostate Cancer Disease-focused Panel. *Radiology* **2020**, *296*, 76–84. [CrossRef] [PubMed]
21. Gómez Rivas, J.; Giganti, F.; Álvarez-Maestro, M.; Freire, M.J.; Kasivisvanathan, V.; Martinez-Piñeiro, L.; Emberton, M. Prostate Indeterminate Lesions on Magnetic Resonance Imaging-Biopsy Versus Surveillance: A Literature Review. *Eur. Urol. Focus* **2019**, *5*, 799–806. [CrossRef]
22. Drobish, J.N.; Bevill, M.D.; Tracy, C.R.; Sexton, S.M.; Rajput, M.; Metz, C.M.; Gellhaus, P.T. Do patients with a PI-RADS 5 lesion identified on magnetic resonance imaging require systematic biopsy in addition to targeted biopsy? *Urol. Oncol.* **2021**, *39*, 235.e1–235.e4. [CrossRef] [PubMed]
23. Liddell, H.; Jyoti, R.; Haxhimolla, H.Z. mp-MRI Prostate Characterised PIRADS 3 Lesions are Associated with a Low Risk of Clinically Significant Prostate Cancer—A Retrospective Review of 92 Biopsied PIRADS 3 Lesions. *Curr. Urol.* **2015**, *8*, 96–100. [CrossRef] [PubMed]
24. Kundu, S.D.; Roehl, K.A.; Yu, X.; Antenor, J.A.; Suarez, B.K.; Catalona, W.J. Prostate specific antigen density correlates with features of prostate cancer aggressiveness. *J. Urol.* **2007**, *177*, 505–509. [CrossRef] [PubMed]
25. Distler, F.A.; Radtke, J.P.; Bonekamp, D.; Kesch, C.; Schlemmer, H.-P.; Wieczorek, K.; Kirchner, M.; Pahernik, S.; Hohenfellner, M.; Hadaschik, B.A. The Value of PSA Density in Combination with PI-RADS™ for the Accuracy of Prostate Cancer Prediction. *J. Urol.* **2017**, *198*, 575–582. [CrossRef] [PubMed]
26. Wang, Z.B.; Wei, C.G.; Zhang, Y.Y.; Pan, P.; Dai, G.-C.; Tu, J.; Shen, J.-K. The Role of PSA Density among PI-RADS v2.1 Categories to Avoid an Unnecessary Transition Zone Biopsy in Patients with PSA 4-20 ng/mL. *Biomed. Res. Int.* **2021**, *2021*, 3995789. [CrossRef] [PubMed]
27. Cuocolo, R.; Stanzione, A.; Rusconi, G.; Petretta, M.; Ponsiglione, A.; Fusco, F.; Longo, N.; Persico, F.; Cocozza, S.; Brunetti, A.; et al. PSA-density does not improve bi-parametric prostate MR detection of prostate cancer in a biopsy naïve patient population. *Eur. J. Radiol.* **2018**, *104*, 64–70. [CrossRef] [PubMed]
28. Wen, J.; Tang, T.; Ji, Y.; Zhang, Y. PI-RADS v2.1 Combined with Prostate-Specific Antigen Density for Detection of Prostate Cancer in Peripheral Zone. *Front. Oncol.* **2022**, *12*, 861928. [CrossRef] [PubMed]
29. Ma, Z.; Wang, X.; Zhang, W.; Gao, K.; Wang, L.; Qian, L.; Mu, J.; Zheng, Z.; Cao, X. Developing a predictive model for clinically significant prostate cancer by combining age, PSA density, and mpMRI. *World J. Surg. Oncol.* **2023**, *21*, 83. [CrossRef]

30. Siddiqui, M.R.; Li, E.V.; Kumar, S.K.S.R.; Busza, A.; Lin, J.S.; Mahenthiran, A.K.; Aguiar, J.A.; Shah, P.V.; Ansbro, B.; Rich, J.M.; et al. Optimizing detection of clinically significant prostate cancer through nomograms incorporating mri, clinical features, and advanced serum biomarkers in biopsy naïve men. *Prostate Cancer Prostatic Dis.* **2023**, *26*, 588–595. [CrossRef]
31. Muller, B.G.; Shih, J.H.; Sankineni, S.; Marko, J.; Rais-Bahrami, S.; George, A.K.; de la Rosette, J.J.M.C.H.; Merino, M.J.; Wood, B.J.; Pinto, P.; et al. Prostate Cancer: Interobserver Agreement and Accuracy with the Revised Prostate Imaging Reporting and Data System at Multiparametric MR Imaging. *Radiology* **2015**, *277*, 741–750. [CrossRef]

Disclaimer/Publisher's Note: The statements, opinions and data contained in all publications are solely those of the individual author(s) and contributor(s) and not of MDPI and/or the editor(s). MDPI and/or the editor(s) disclaim responsibility for any injury to people or property resulting from any ideas, methods, instructions or products referred to in the content.

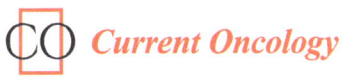

Article

Appropriateness of Imaging for Low-Risk Prostate Cancer—Real World Data from the Pennsylvania Urologic Regional Collaboration (PURC)

Raidizon Mercedes [1], Dennis Head [1], Elizabeth Zook [1], Eric Eidelman [1], Jeffrey Tomaszewski [2], Serge Ginzburg [3], Robert Uzzo [4], Marc Smaldone [4], John Danella [5], Thomas J. Guzzo [6], Daniel Lee [6], Laurence Belkoff [7], Jeffrey Walker [7], Adam Reese [8], Mihir S. Shah [9], Bruce Jacobs [10] and Jay D. Raman [1,*]

1. Department of Urology, Penn State College of Medicine, Hershey, PA 17033, USA
2. Department of Urology, Cooper University Health Care, Camden, NJ 08103, USA
3. Department of Urology, Einstein Healthcare Network, Philadelphia, PA 19141, USA
4. Department of Urology, Fox Chase Cancer Center, Philadelphia, PA 19111, USA
5. Department of Urology, Geisinger Health, Danville, PA 17822, USA
6. Department of Urology, University of Pennsylvania Health System, Philadelphia, PA 19104, USA
7. MidLantic Urology, Bala Cynwyd, PA 19008, USA
8. Department of Urology, Temple University Hospital, Philadelphia, PA 19140, USA
9. Department of Urology, Thomas Jefferson University Hospital, Philadelphia, PA 19107, USA; mihir.shah@jefferson.edu
10. Department of Urology, University of Pittsburgh Medical Center, Pittsburgh, PA 15219, USA
* Correspondence: jraman@pennstatehealth.psu.edu

Abstract: Imaging for prostate cancer defines the extent of disease. Guidelines recommend against imaging low-risk prostate cancer patients with a computed tomography (CT) scan or bone scan due to the low probability of metastasis. We reviewed imaging performed for men diagnosed with low-risk prostate cancer across the Pennsylvania Urologic Regional Collaborative (PURC), a physician-led data sharing and quality improvement collaborative. The data of 10 practices were queried regarding the imaging performed in men diagnosed with prostate cancer from 2015 to 2022. The cohort included 13,122 patients with 3502 (27%) low-risk, 2364 (18%) favorable intermediate-risk, 3585 (27%) unfavorable intermediate-risk, and 3671 (28%) high-risk prostate cancer, based on the AUA guidelines. Amongst the low-risk patients, imaging utilization included pelvic MRI (59.7%), bone scan (17.8%), CT (16.0%), and PET-based imaging (0.5%). Redundant imaging occurred in 1022 patients (29.2%). There was variability among the PURC sites for imaging used in the low-risk patients, and iterative education reduced the need for CT and bone scans. Approximately 15% of low-risk patients had staging imaging performed using either a CT or bone scan, and redundant imaging occurred in almost one-third of men. Such data underscore the need for continued guideline-based education to optimize the stewardship of resources and reduce unnecessary costs to the healthcare system.

Keywords: over-imaging; redundant; risk stratification; CT; MRI; PET

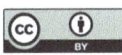

1. Introduction

Imaging studies aim to assess the extent of disease locally and identify any nodal or distant metastases, which helps guide treatment decisions. Newly diagnosed prostate cancer patients are stratified into risk groups that consider the likelihood of metastatic disease to help dictate imaging and patient management. For asymptomatic patients with low-risk prostate cancer, defined by the American Urological Association (AUA) guidelines, the probability of distant metastasis is low (<1.5%) [1–4]. The current AUA guidelines recommend that clinicians should not routinely perform abdomino-pelvic computed tomography (CT) or bone scans in asymptomatic patients with low- or intermediate-risk prostate cancer, and those imaging types should be reserved for patients with high-risk disease [4]. Additionally, the current AUA guidelines recommend that patients with prostate cancer who have a high risk of metastatic disease and negative conventional imaging may obtain prostate-specific membrane antigen positron emission tomography (PSMA PET) to evaluate for metastatic disease [5]. This guideline statement is based on expert opinion due to the lack of prospective evidence, so molecular imaging may also be obtained at the discretion of the treating physician without obtaining a negative conventional imaging first [5]. In the context of low-risk prostate cancer, magnetic resonance imaging (MRI) has been recognized as a valuable tool as it can help in determining the appropriate treatment approach for low-risk prostate cancer patients and aid in both radiotherapy and surgical planning [6].

The AUA guidelines align with the Choosing Wisely Campaign, launched in 2012, that aimed to facilitate the decision between healthcare providers and patients on unnecessary medical tests, treatments, and procedures. This campaign sought to decrease inappropriate staging imaging for men with low-risk prostate cancer and encourage the stewardship of resources [7]. Routine imaging tests like CTs, MRIs, or bone scans for early-stage low-risk prostate cancer do not offer clinical benefits but come with significant costs [8]. Both the American Society of Clinical Oncology and the AUA have stressed the importance of reducing inappropriate imaging for low-risk prostate cancer within the Choosing Wisely Campaign in order to cut down on unnecessary imaging, decrease healthcare resource overuse, and enhance quality of care [9].

In this study, we reviewed imaging performed for men diagnosed with low-risk prostate cancer across a large regional quality collaborative. Our primary objective was to evaluate real-world data concerning the use of imaging modalities, specifically MRIs, CTs, bone scans, and PSMA PET scans, in this patient population. By examining trends over time, we aimed to understand how imaging practices have evolved and whether education can aid in compliance with current guidelines.

2. Materials and Methods

The Pennsylvania Urologic Regional Collaborative (PURC) is a prospective quality improvement collaborative of diverse urology practices across Pennsylvania and New Jersey, with the goal of improving the quality of care provided during the diagnosis, management, and treatment of patient with prostate cancer or undergoing prostate biopsy. This study was performed with a dataset that was obtained through a shared data use agreement with PURC. At the time of writing this manuscript, PURC consisted of 13 practices and 170 physicians with data on over 22,000 men with prostate cancer.

The PURC data registry was queried for patients over the age of 18 who were diagnosed with low-risk prostate cancer, according to the AUA guidelines, between the years 2015 and 2022. For this study, ten practices had data available for query regarding the imaging performed. We excluded men who were diagnosed with prostate cancer but had no imaging data.

The dataset obtained from the PURC registry contained detailed information for each patient entered into the system by data abstractors. AUA risk stratification for each patient was calculated in PURC. The exported data were cleaned in Stata 18 statistical software to optimize fidelity and accuracy. Summary statistics and summary tables for low-risk prostate cancer patients were analyzed in Stata, then exported into Microsoft Excel for graphics generation.

Our primary outcome measure was the type of imaging modality (MRI, CT scan, bone scan, PSMA PET scan) obtained by the patient with low-risk prostate cancer. Additionally, we assessed the occurrence of redundant imaging, defined as patients receiving multiple imaging studies. We analyzed the distribution of imaging modalities within our cohort of interest. Secondary analyses investigated the variability of imaging practices across the 10 participating sites. Furthermore, we examined temporal trends in the utilization of CT and bone scans to assess changes in imaging practices over time.

3. Results

The study cohort comprised 13,122 patients, categorized into the following four risk groups: 3502 (27%) classified as low risk, 2364 (18%) as favorable intermediate risk, 3585 (27%) as unfavorable intermediate risk, and 3671 (28%) as high risk. Figure 1 summarizes the distribution of imaging studies obtained. Among the low-risk cohort, the predominant imaging modality utilized was pelvic MRI, which was performed in 2091 patients (59.7%). Additionally, conventional bone scans were conducted in 622 patients (17.8%), CT scans in 562 patients (16.0%), and PET-based imaging in 17 patients (0.5%).

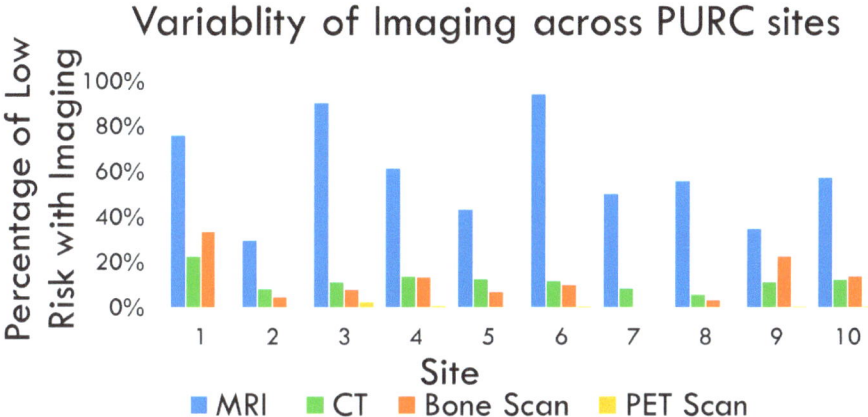

Figure 1. Distribution of imaging modalities among low-risk prostate cancer patients across the 10 participating sites. MRI (blue) was the most common imaging across all sites, while the PSMA PET scan (yellow) was the least common. CT (green) and bone scans (orange) varied depending on sites.

A total of 718 patients underwent an MRI along with an additional imaging test. Specifically, 415 patients received both an MRI and a bone scan, 290 patients had an MRI and a CT scan, and 13 patients underwent an MRI and a PSMA PET scan. Among the patients who received a CT scan, 290 also had a bone scan, and 6 were additionally imaged with a PSMA PET scan. Furthermore, eight patients who had bone scans also underwent PSMA PET imaging.

Figure 1 highlights the variability across the 10 participating sites. MRI emerged as the most frequently used imaging modality for low-risk prostate cancer patients. However, there was considerable variability in its usage among the sites from 29.5% to 94.2%. The use of CT scans varied between 5.7% and 22.3%, while bone scan utilization ranged from 0% at one site to as high as 33.3% at others. Despite its limited utility in low-risk prostate cancer cases, PSMA PET scan usage also showed variability, ranging from 0% to 2.2%.

Figure 2 depicts the trend in the use of CT scans and bone scans throughout the study period. The percentage of patients receiving CT scans decreased from 17.4% in 2015 to 1.0% in 2022. Similarly, the use of bone scans declined from 20.6% to 1.5% over the same period.

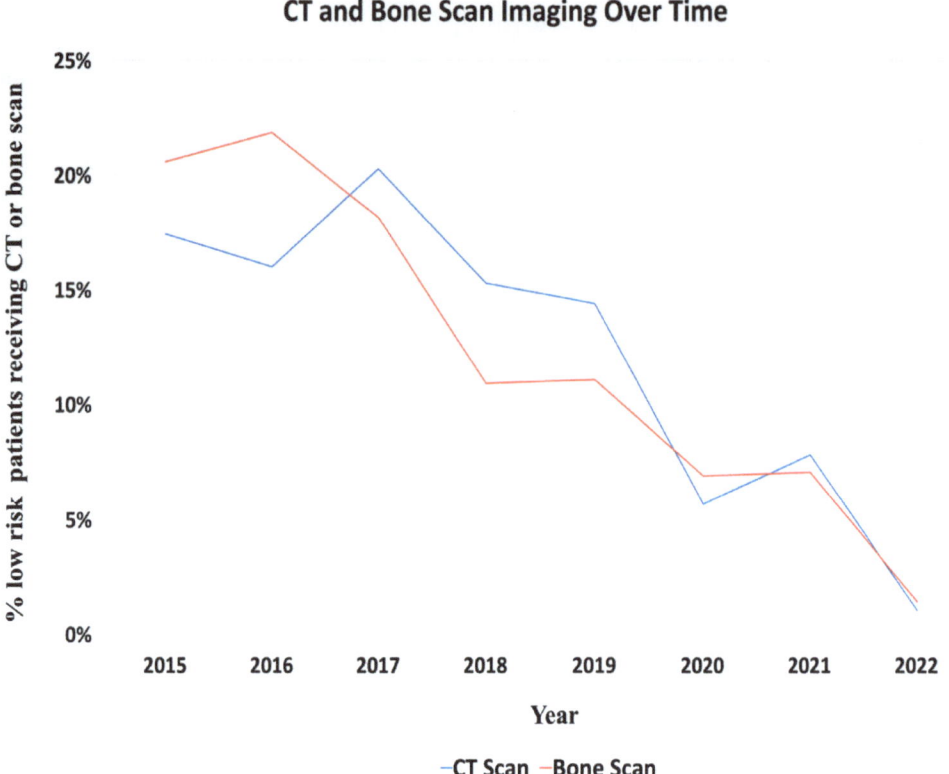

Figure 2. Distribution of total CT (Blue) and bone scans (Red) throughout the study period. The majority of CT and bone scans were obtained early in the study, with a reduction to 1.0% for CT scans and 1.5% for bone scans by 2022.

4. Discussion

Our study found that MRI is the most commonly used imaging modality for men with low-risk prostate cancer. It is important to note that these MRI are primarily utilized for biopsy guidance and lesion identification rather than for whole-body imaging and staging. This aligns with the need for precise surgical planning in this patient group. Interestingly, we observed that a significant number of patients with low-risk prostate cancer were being staged with CT scans (24.5% of the cohort), bone scans (18.0% of cohort), and, in rare cases, PSMA PET scans (0.5% of the cohort). These practices are contrary to the current AUA guidelines and recommendations, which advise against such extensive imaging in low-risk cases.

Redundant imaging remains prevalent, with 1022 patients (29.2%) undergoing multiple imaging modalities. This indicates a substantial deviation from the guideline-based care and highlights the need for continued efforts to optimize imaging practices in this population. As highlighted in Figure 2, the portion of patients receiving CT and bone scans have decreased over time, a trend likely attributable to iterative educational efforts. Physicians from the practices within PURC regularly meet to analyze data and trends, collaboratively developing best practices and practice patterns. These continuous educational interventions have likely contributed to the observed reduction in the use of CT and bone scans over the study period.

Our study aligns with the goals of the Choosing Wisely campaign, which aims to reduce inappropriate imaging for men with low-risk prostate cancer. Since the initiation of this campaign, there has been a notable decline in the use of bone scans and CT imaging for staging newly diagnosed low-risk prostate cancer [10]. Discouraging unnecessary imaging tests not only reduces wasteful testing but also alleviates the financial burden associated with downstream care that may not offer substantial benefits to patients [9]. This trend is reflected in our findings, where continuous educational interventions and regular analysis of data by the PURC physicians contributed to a reduction in CT and bone scan utilization over time. Despite this progress, redundant imaging remains prevalent, with 1022 patients (29.2%) undergoing multiple imaging modalities. This indicates a substantial deviation from guideline-based care and underscores the need for ongoing efforts to optimize imaging practices in this population.

Low-risk prostate cancer management has evolved to prioritize the use of MRI over CT scans or bone scans due to the superior diagnostic capabilities of MRI in this context. Studies have consistently shown that CT scans are not necessary for low-risk prostate cancer patients, as they offer limited benefits in detecting disease progression or metastases in this population [11]. MRIs provide detailed imaging of the prostate gland, enabling the accurate visualization of tumors and aiding in treatment planning decisions [12]. It is particularly effective in guiding targeted biopsies, assessing tumor aggressiveness, and determining the need for active surveillance, surgery, or radiotherapy in low-risk prostate cancer patients [12]. The MRI utilization rate of 60% in patients who were stratified to the low-risk group could be explained by patients with contraindications to MRI and urologists still in the process of shifting practice from trans-rectal ultrasound biopsy to MRI-targeted biopsy. This shift toward MRIs aligns with our study's findings and supports the Choosing Wisely campaign's goals to reduce inappropriate imaging. Our data indicated that MRIs were the most prevalent imaging across all sites.

A major strength of our study is its alignment with other findings that emphasize the prioritization of MRIs for low-risk prostate cancer management. Our data are consistent with previous studies, reinforcing that MRI remains the most commonly used imaging modality, while the use of CT and bone scans has decreased. Comprehensive data from a large regional quality collaborative enhances the generalizability of our results, providing a real-world snapshot of imaging practices and trends over a significant period.

However, our study also has several limitations. Being a retrospective analysis, it is subject to the inherent limitations of such studies. The data were extracted from a database, which may contain inaccuracies or incomplete entries that could affect the reliability of our findings. The variability in data recording practices across different sites may also introduce inconsistencies. Additionally, in certain instances, a PSMA PET scan may have been used as an alternative to a prostate MRI, for example, when a patient has an implanted device that is not MRI compatible, and this may account for some instances of PET utilization in our study [13]. Despite these limitations, the large sample size and the extended study period provide valuable insights into imaging practices for low-risk prostate cancer, highlighting areas for improvement and the impact of ongoing educational initiatives.

5. Conclusions

Low-risk prostate cancer accounted for approximately 25% of new diagnoses within this large collaborative. Despite guidelines advising against extensive imaging for low-risk patients, approximately 15% of these patients underwent staging imaging using either CT or bone scans. Additionally, redundant imaging occurred in almost one-third of the men, indicating a substantial deviation from recommended practices. These findings underscore the critical need for continued education based on established guidelines to optimize resource stewardship and reduce unnecessary costs to the healthcare system.

Expanding efforts to educate both clinicians and patients about the appropriate use of imaging modalities could further align practices with current recommendations, ultimately enhancing the quality of care. Future research should focus on identifying the barriers to adherence to the imaging guidelines and developing strategies to address these challenges. By continuing to refine and disseminate best practices, we can improve patient outcomes and achieve more cost-effective care for low-risk prostate cancer patients.

Author Contributions: Conceptualization, J.D.R., R.M., D.H., E.Z., E.E., J.T., S.G., R.U., M.S., J.D., T.J.G., D.L., L.B., J.W., A.R., M.S.S. and B.J.; methodology, J.D.R., R.M., E.Z. and E.E.; software, R.M. and E.Z.; validation, R.M. and E.Z.; formal analysis, R.M. and E.Z.; investigation, J.D.R., R.M., D.H., E.Z. and E.E.; data curation, R.M.; writing—original draft preparation, R.M. and D.H.; writing—review and editing, J.D.R., R.M. and D.H.; visualization, J.D.R., R.M., D.H., E.Z., E.E., J.T., S.G., R.U., M.S., J.D., T.J.G., D.L., L.B., J.W., A.R., M.S.S. and B.J.; supervision, J.D.R. and R.M. All authors have read and agreed to the published version of the manuscript.

Funding: This research received no external funding.

Institutional Review Board Statement: The study was conducted in accordance with the Declaration of Helsinki, and approved by the Institutional Review Board of Penn State College of Medicine STUDY 00005537 (Approved since 16 September 2016).

Informed Consent Statement: Patient consent was waived as this study evaluated aggregate de-identified data with a cohort analysis.

Data Availability Statement: Data were provided with permission from the Pennsylvania Urologic Regional Collaborative (PURC) participating urology practices. PURC is a quality improvement initiative led by the Health Care Improvement Foundation which brings urology practices together in a physician-led data sharing and improvement collaborative aimed at advancing the quality of diagnosis and care for men with prostate cancer.

Conflicts of Interest: The authors declare no conflicts of interest.

References

1. Merdan, S.; Womble, P.R.; Miller, D.C.; Barnett, C.; Ye, Z.; Linsell, S.M.; Montie, J.E.; Denton, B.T. Toward better use of bone scans among men with early-stage prostate cancer. *Urology* **2014**, *84*, 793–798. [CrossRef] [PubMed]
2. Risko, R.; Merdan, S.; Womble, P.R.; Barnett, C.; Ye, Z.; Linsell, S.M.; Montie, J.E.; Miller, D.C.; Denton, B.T. Clinical predictors and recommendations for staging computed tomography scan among men with prostate cancer. *Urology* **2014**, *84*, 1329–1334. [CrossRef] [PubMed]
3. Makarov, D.V.; Trock, B.J.; Humphreys, E.B.; Mangold, L.A.; Walsh, P.C.; Epstein, J.I.; Partin, A.W. Updated nomogram to predict pathologic stage of prostate cancer given prostate-specific antigen level, clinical stage, and biopsy Gleason score (Partin tables) based on cases from 2000 to 2005. *Urology* **2007**, *69*, 1095–1101. [CrossRef] [PubMed]
4. Courtney, P.T.; Deka, R.; Kotha, N.V.; Cherry, D.R.; Salans, M.A.; Nelson, T.J.; Kumar, A.; Luterstein, E.; Yip, A.T.; Nalawade, V.; et al. Metastasis and Mortality in Men With Low- and Intermediate-Risk Prostate Cancer on Active Surveillance. *J. Natl. Compr. Canc. Netw.* **2022**, *20*, 151–159. [CrossRef]
5. Eastham, J.A.; Auffenberg, G.B.; Barocas, D.A.; Chou, R.; Crispino, T.; Davis, J.W.; Eggener, S.; Horwitz, E.M.; Kane, C.J.; Kirkby, E.; et al. Clinically Localized Prostate Cancer: AUA/ASTRO Guideline, Part I: Introduction, Risk Assessment, Staging, and Risk-Based Management. *J. Urol.* **2022**, *208*, 10–18. [CrossRef]
6. Alshehri, S.Z.; Safar, O.; Almsaoud, N.A.; Al-Ghamdi, M.A.; Alqahtani, A.M.; Almurayyi, M.M.; Autwdi, A.S.; Al-Ghamdi, S.A.; Zogan, M.M.; Alamri, A.M. The role of multiparametric magnetic resonance imaging and magnetic resonance-guided biopsy in active surveillance for low-risk prostate cancer: A systematic review. *Ann. Med. Surg.* **2020**, *57*, 171–178. [CrossRef]
7. Lange, S.M.; Choudry, M.M.; Hunt, T.C.; Ambrose, J.P.; Haaland, B.A.; Lowrance, W.T.; Hanson, H.A.; O'Neil, B.B. Impact of choosing wisely on imaging in men with newly diagnosed prostate cancer. *Urol. Oncol.* **2023**, *41*, 48.e19–48.e26. [CrossRef] [PubMed]
8. Schnipper, L.; Smith, T.; Raghavan, D.; Blayney, D.; Ganz, P.; Mulvey, T.; Wollins, D. American society of clinical oncology identifies five key opportunities to improve care and reduce costs: The top five list for oncology. *J. Clin. Oncol.* **2012**, *30*, 1715–1724. [CrossRef] [PubMed]
9. Makarov, D.V.; Loeb, S.; Ulmert, D.; Drevin, L.; Lambe, M.; Stattin, P. Prostate cancer imaging trends after a nationwide effort to discourage inappropriate prostate cancer imaging. *JNCI J. Natl. Cancer Inst.* **2013**, *105*, 1306–1313. [CrossRef]
10. Pettit, S.; Mikhail, D.; Feuerstein, M. Systematic review of interventions that improve provider compliance to imaging guidelines for prostate cancer. *Can. Urol. Assoc. J.* **2022**, *16*, E490. [CrossRef] [PubMed]
11. Prasad, S.M.; Gu, X.; Lipsitz, S.R.; Nguyen, P.L.; Hu, J.C. Inappropriate utilization of radiographic imaging in men with newly diagnosed prostate cancer in the united states. *Cancer* **2011**, *118*, 1260–1267. [CrossRef] [PubMed]

12. Shao, W.; Bhattacharya, I.; Soerensen SJ, C.; Kunder, C.A.; Wang, J.B.; Fan, R.E.; Ghanouni, P.; Brooks, J.D.; Sonn, G.A. Weakly supervised registration of prostate mri and histopathology images. In Proceedings of the Medical Image Computing and Computer Assisted Intervention–MICCAI 2021: 24th International Conference, Strasbourg, France, 27 September–1 October 2021. [CrossRef]
13. Pepe, P.; Pepe, L.; Cosentino, S.; Ippolito, M.; Pennisi, M.; Fraggetta, F. Detection Rate of 68Ga-PSMA PET/CT vs. mpMRI Targeted Biopsy for Clinically Significant Prostate Cancer. *Anticancer. Res.* **2022**, *42*, 3011–3015. [CrossRef] [PubMed]

Disclaimer/Publisher's Note: The statements, opinions and data contained in all publications are solely those of the individual author(s) and contributor(s) and not of MDPI and/or the editor(s). MDPI and/or the editor(s) disclaim responsibility for any injury to people or property resulting from any ideas, methods, instructions or products referred to in the content.

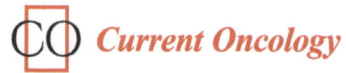 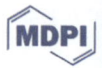

Article

Differences in the Volatilomic Urinary Biosignature of Prostate Cancer Patients as a Feasibility Study for the Detection of Potential Biomarkers

Giulia Riccio [1,2], Cristina V. Berenguer [3], Rosa Perestrelo [3], Ferdinando Pereira [4], Pedro Berenguer [5,6], Cristina P. Ornelas [7], Ana Célia Sousa [5], João Aragão Vital [4], Maria do Carmo Pinto [4], Jorge A. M. Pereira [3], Viviana Greco [1,2] and José S. Câmara [3,8,*]

[1] Department of Basic Biotechnological Sciences, Intensivological and Perioperative Clinics, Univesità Cattolica del Sacro Cuore, 00168 Rome, Italy
[2] Unity of Chemistry, Biochemistry and Clinical Molecular Biology, Department of Diagnostic and Laboratory Medicine, Fondazione Policlinico Universitario A. Gemelli IRCCS, 00168 Rome, Italy
[3] CQM—Centro de Química da Madeira, NPRG, Universidade da Madeira, Campus da Penteada, 9020-105 Funchal, Portugal; rmp@staff.uma.pt (R.P.)
[4] Serviço de Urologia, Hospital Dr. Nélio Mendonça, SESARAM, EPERAM—Serviço de Saúde da Região Autónoma da Madeira, Avenida Luís de Camões, n°57, 9004-514 Funchal, Portugal
[5] Centro de Investigação Dra Maria Isabel Mendonça, Hospital Dr. Nélio Mendonça, SESARAM, EPERAM, Avenida Luís de Camões, n°57, 9004-514 Funchal, Portugal
[6] RO-RAM—Registo Oncológico da Região Autónoma da Madeira, Hospital Dr. Nélio Mendonça, SESARAM, EPERAM, Avenida Luís de Camões, n°57, 9004-514 Funchal, Portugal
[7] Centro de Saúde do Bom Jesus, SESARAM, EPERAM, Rua das Hortas, n°67, 9050-024 Funchal, Portugal
[8] Departamento de Química, Faculdade de Ciências Exatas e Engenharia, Universidade da Madeira, Campus da Penteada, 9020-105 Funchal, Portugal
* Correspondence: jsc@staff.uma.pt

Abstract: Prostate cancer (PCa) continues to be the second most common malignant tumour and the main cause of oncological death in men. Investigating endogenous volatile organic metabolites (VOMs) produced by various metabolic pathways is emerging as a novel, effective, and non-invasive source of information to establish the volatilomic biosignature of PCa. In this study, headspace solid-phase microextraction combined with gas chromatography–mass spectrometry (HS-SPME/GC-MS) was used to establish the urine volatilomic profile of PCa and identify VOMs that can discriminate between the two investigated groups. This non-invasive approach was applied to oncological patients (PCa group, $n = 26$) and cancer-free individuals (control group, $n = 30$), retrieving a total of 147 VOMs from various chemical families. This included terpenes, norisoprenoid, sesquiterpenes, phenolic, sulphur and furanic compounds, ketones, alcohols, esters, aldehydes, carboxylic acid, benzene and naphthalene derivatives, hydrocarbons, and heterocyclic hydrocarbons. The data matrix was subjected to multivariate analysis, namely partial least-squares discriminant analysis (PLS-DA). Accordingly, this analysis showed that the group under study presented different volatomic profiles and suggested potential PCa biomarkers. Nevertheless, a larger cohort of samples is required to boost the predictability and accuracy of the statistical models developed.

Keywords: prostate cancer; volatilomics; urine; biomarkers

Citation: Riccio, G.; Berenguer, C.V.; Perestrelo, R.; Pereira, F.; Berenguer, P.; Ornelas, C.P.; Sousa, A.C.; Vital, J.A.; Pinto, M.d.C.; Pereira, J.A.M.; et al. Differences in the Volatilomic Urinary Biosignature of Prostate Cancer Patients as a Feasibility Study for the Detection of Potential Biomarkers. *Curr. Oncol.* **2023**, *30*, 4904–4921. https://doi.org/10.3390/curroncol30050370

Received: 7 March 2023
Revised: 18 April 2023
Accepted: 25 April 2023
Published: 10 May 2023

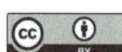

Copyright: © 2023 by the authors. Licensee MDPI, Basel, Switzerland. This article is an open access article distributed under the terms and conditions of the Creative Commons Attribution (CC BY) license (https://creativecommons.org/licenses/by/4.0/).

1. Introduction

According to the most recent data, prostate cancer (PCa) is the second most common cancer in men and the fourth most common tumour [1]. PCa occurs mostly after 60 years old, with an average age at the time of diagnosis of 66 years old [2]. The psychological and functional states of patients are greatly impacted by PCa and following treatments, considerably affecting their quality of life [3]. The current diagnostic techniques are aggressive, costly, and uncomfortable for patients. The prostate-specific antigen (PSA) biomarker test has a low level of selectivity for diagnosing PCa and tracking cancer development [4], whereas prostate biopsies can lead to both false-positive and false-negative results [2,5,6]. Consequently, these limitations lead to overdiagnosis and overtreatment of patients [7]. Hence, there is an urgent need to identify specific and noninvasive diagnostic tools for the detection of PCa.

Volatilomics studies volatile organic metabolites (VOMs), low-molecular-weight organic chemicals with a high vapour pressure at room temperature [8], corresponding to the volatile fraction of the metabolome [9]. VOMs are a useful source of information on the general state of health or disease status since they are produced by the metabolism of cells. Genetic, protein, and gut microbiota changes directly influence the profile of VOMs production [10]. Consequently, their production and release may be altered in some diseases, such as cancer [5,11]. Therefore, VOMs represent a patient's metabolic fingerprint, comprising endogenous and exogenous factors, and for these reasons, have been proposed as a promising class of disease biomarkers (Figure 1) [8,12].

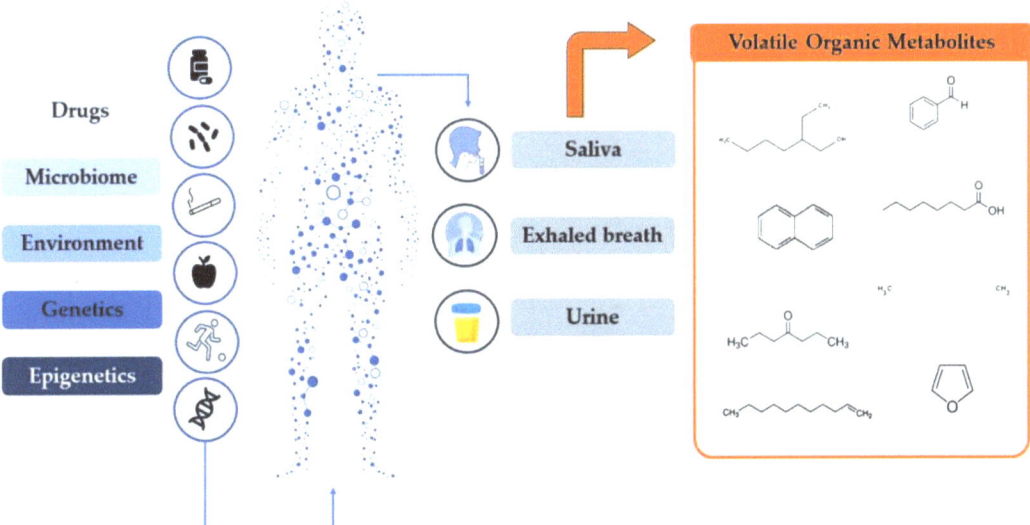

Figure 1. Genetic and epigenetic factors, as well as food, drugs, environment, and habits, influence the volatomic pattern in the biological fluids most used to establish the volatomic fingerprints.

VOMs have been highlighted in recent studies because of their ease of use and non-invasiveness, as they can be identified in easily accessible biofluids such as urine, saliva, and exhaled breath [13,14]. VOMs contain valuable information about the biochemical metabolization of cancer cells, and each cancer type is thought to have a specific VOM pattern. Moreover, previous research has shown that VOMs can be used to distinguish between oncological and healthy individuals (Table 1) [11]. Volatilomic analysis involves sensitive analytical techniques such as mass spectrometry (MS), electronic nose (e-nose), or sensor techniques combined with multivariate statistical analysis to characterise the chemical composition of biological fluids [11,15]. MS techniques identify and quantify the levels of VOMs, whereas e-nose sensor arrays are linked to pattern recognition algorithms or chemical sensor systems [10,12].

Table 1. Recent studies on volatile organic metabolites for the identification of cancer biomarkers found in urine, exhaled breath, and saliva.

Cancer Type	Analytical Approach	Biomarker's Candidates/ Findings	Prediction Model	Validation Characteristics	Reference
Urine					
Pancreatic	TD-GC-TOF-MS GC-IMS	2,6-Dimethyl-octane, nonanal, 4-ethyl-1,2-dimethyl-benzene, 2-pentanone	Repeated 10-Fold CV	NA	[16]
Bladder, prostate	GC-TOF-MS and GC-IMS	35 VOMs	ROC, Repeated 10-Fold CV	GC-IMS Sens: 87% Spec: 92% AUC: 0.95	[17]
Prostate	Urine HS conditioning, followed by e-nose analysis	The e-nose detected alterations in the urine volatilome associated with PCa	ROC	Sens: 85% Spec: 79% AUC: 0.82	[18]
Prostate	Urine HS conditioning, followed by e-nose analysis (Cyranose C320)	The e-nose discriminated the urine smell prints of patients with PCa from healthy controls	PCA, ROC	Sens: 83% Spec: 88% AUC: 0.90	[19]
Prostate	Urine HS conditioning, followed by e-nose analysis	The e-nose discriminated patients with PCa from healthy controls	PCA	Sens: 82% Spec: 87% AUC: NA	[20]
Pancreatic ductal adenocarcinoma	HiSorb probes coupled with GC-TOF-MS	2-Pentanone, hexanal, 3-hexanone, p-cymene	PLS-DA	AUC: 0.82 CER: 0.18	[21]
Breast	GC-MS analysis of the urine HS. Sample's smell print by the e-nose prototype	The e-nose software discriminated between early stage breast cancer and healthy controls	Artificial intelligence-based algorithm: CNN	Sens: 100% Spec: 50% Classification rate: 75%	[22]
Bladder	HS-SPME/GCxGC TOF-MS	Butyrolactone, 2-methoxyphenol, 3-methoxy-5-methylphenol, 1-(2,6,6-trimethylcyclohexa-1,3-dien-1-yl)-2-buten-1-one, nootkatone, 1-(2,6,6-trimethyl-1-cyclohexenyl)-2-buten-1-one	ANN	NA	[23]

Cancer Type	Analytical Approach	Biomarker's Candidates/ Findings	Prediction Model	Validation Characteristics	Reference
Lung	GC-IMS	2-Pentanone, 2-hexenal, 2-hexen-1-ol, hept-4-en-2-ol, 2-heptanone, 3-octen-2-one, 4-methylpentanol, 4-methyl-octane	SVM	GC-IMS Sens: 85% Spec: 90% AUC: 0.91	[24]

Exhaled breath

Table 1. Cont.

Cancer Type	Analytical Approach	Biomarker's Candidates/ Findings	Prediction Model	Validation Characteristics	Reference
Colorectal	Thermal desorption-GC-TOF-MS	10 VOMs distinguished advanced adenomas from negative controls. Colorectal cancer patients and advanced adenoma combined were discriminated from controls	RF	Colorectal cancer vs. controls Sens: 80% Spec: 70%	[25]
Gastric	PTR-TOF-MS	Propanal, aceticamide, isoprene, 1,3-propanediol	ROC	Sens: 61% Spec: 94% AUC: 0.842	[26]
Breast	SIFT-MS	3,7-Dimethyl-2,6-octadien-1-ol, ethanolamine, ethyl nonanoate	PCA, MLR	Sens: 86.3% Spec: 55.6%	[27]
Hepatocellular	SPME/GC-MS	Phenol 2,2 methylene bis [6-(1,1-dimethyl ethyl)-4-methyl] (MBMBP)	PCA	NA	[28]
Lung	HPPI-TOFMS	Isoprene, hexanal, pentanal, propylcyclohexane, nonanal, 2,2-dimethyldecane, heptanal, decanal	Hosmer-Lemeshow test	Sens: 86% Spec: 87.2% Acc: 86.9% AUC: 0.931	[29]
Hepatocellular carcinoma	HS-SPME/GC-MS	Acetone, 1,4-pentadiene, methylene chloride, benzene, phenol, allyl methyl sulfide	SVM	Sens: 44% Spec: 75% Acc: 55.4%	[30]

Table 1. *Cont.*

Cancer Type	Analytical Approach	Biomarker's Candidates/Findings	Prediction Model	Validation Characteristics	Reference
		Saliva			
Oral	HS-SPME/GC-MS	1-Octen-3-ol, hexanoic acid, E-2-octenal, heptanoic acid, octanoic acid, E-2-nonenal, nonanoic acid, 2,4-decadienal, 9-undecenoic acid	PCA	Sens: 100% Spec: 100% AUC: 1	[31]
Stomach and colorectal cancer	Capillary GC-FID	Acetaldehyde, acetone, 2-propanol, ethanol	CART	Sens: 95.7% Spec: 90.9%	[32]
Oral squamous cell carcinoma	Thin-film microextraction based on a ZSM-5/polydimethylsiloxane hybrid film coupled with GC-MS	12 VOMs	PCA	Sens: 95.8% Spec: 94%	[33]

Legend: Acc: accuracy; ANN: artificial neural networks; AUC: area under the receiver operating characteristic (ROC) curve; CART: classification and regression tree; CER: classification error rate; CNN: convolutional neural network; CV: cross-validation; GC-IMS: gas chromatography–ion migration spectroscopy; GC-MS: gas chromatography–mass spectrometry; GC-TOF-MS: gas chromatography coupled to time-of-flight mass spectrometry; HPPI-TOFMS: high-pressure photon ionization time-of-flight mass spectrometry; HS: headspace; HS-SPME: headspace solid-phase microextraction; MLR: multiple logistic regression; NA: not analyzed; PCa: prostate cancer; PCA: principal component analysis; PLS-DA: partial least-squares discriminant analysis; PTR-TOF-MS: proton-transfer-reaction time-of-flight mass spectrometry; RF: random forest; ROC: receiver operating characteristic; Sens: sensitivity; SIFT-MS: selected ion flow tube–mass spectrometry; Spec: specificity; SVM: support vector machine; TD-GC-MS: thermal desorption gas chromatography–mass spectrometry; TD-GC-TOF-MS: two-dimensional gas chromatography with time-of-flight mass spectrometer.

Owing to the enrichment of volatile compounds, ranging in polarity and complexity, urine is the preferred biological fluid for volatilomic research. In addition to its reproducibility and patient acceptability, urine has fewer interfering proteins or lipids [12,34,35]. Taverna et al. [18], Filianoti et al. [19], and Capelli et al. [20] proposed different e-noses for PCa diagnosis through urinary volatilomic profiling (Table 1). The e-noses developed were able to detect alterations in the urine volatilome associated with PCa and thereby discriminated oncological patients from healthy controls, with sensitivity and specificity superior to 81% and 79%, respectively. Wen and collaborators [21] developed an extraction technique using HiSorb sorptive extraction combined with gas chromatography coupled to time-of-flight mass spectrometry (GC-TOF-MS) for urine analysis of PCa patients. The authors identified four candidate urinary biomarkers, 2-pentanone, hexanal, 3-hexanone, and *p*-cymene, which were able to discriminate patients with pancreatic ductal adenocarcinoma from non-cancer individuals. Benet et al. [22] implemented an e-nose to detect breast cancer in urine samples, which was tested using an artificial intelligence-based classification algorithm after GC-MS analysis, resulting in a sensitivity of 100% and a specificity of 50%. Exhaled breath reflects the status and condition of the metabolism. It is an acceptable approach, and its sampling is easy to use via simple hand-held devices [12,34,35]. Cheng et al. [25] proposed a prospective study consisting of the analysis of the exhaled breath of colorectal cancer patients. The samples were analysed using thermal desorption-GC-MS (TD-GC-MS), and the data were examined with machine learning techniques. The results revealed ten discriminatory VOMs in which advanced adenomas could be distinguished from negative controls with a sensitivity and specificity of 79% and 70%, respectively. Combined cancer patients and advanced adenomas could be discriminated from controls with a sensitivity and specificity of 77% and 70%, respectively. Patients with colorectal cancer were also discriminated from controls with a sensitivity of 80% and a specificity of 70%. Jung and collaborators [26] aimed to identify specific VOMs related to gastric cancer by PTR-TOF-MS. Four VOMs, propanal, aceticamide, isoprene and 1,3-propanediol, showed gradual increases as the tumour advanced, from controlled to early or advanced gastric cancer. Sukaram et al. [30] investigated the VOMs profile in the exhaled breath of hepatocellular carcinoma patients through headspace solid-phase microextraction (HS-SPME) combined with GC-MS and Support Vector Machine algorithm. A panel of six VOMs consisting of acetone, 1,4-pentadiene, methylene chloride, benzene, phenol, and allyl methyl sulfide, was correlated with the hepatocellular carcinoma stages, exhibiting an increased distance from the classification boundary when the stage advanced. Saliva collection is the easiest method for sampling biofluids. [12,34,35]. Its volatile composition reflects the oral composition, allowing relevant metabolic information [12,34,35]. Bel'skaya et al. [32] determined the volatilomic composition of saliva in stomach and colorectal cancer patients. The samples were analysed using capillary GC and showed that acetaldehyde, acetone, 2-propanol, and ethanol could discriminate between cancer and control groups with a sensitivity and specificity of 95.7 and 90.9%, respectively. Shigeyama et al. [33] established the salivary profile of patients with oral squamous cell carcinoma to investigate VOMs as potential biomarkers in the diagnosis of oral cancer. The authors combined thin-film microextraction based on a ZSM-5/polydimethylsiloxane hybrid film coupled with GC-MS and identified twelve discriminatory VOMs.

The analysis of the volatilome of PCa is still relatively recent when compared to other malignancies. Most research is based on the chemical characterisation of a biofluid or its headspace for the detection and quantification of putative PCa biomarkers through comparative analysis of samples from PCa patients and healthy controls (as reviewed by Berenguer et al. [11]). HS-SPME, developed by Arthur and Pawliszyn [36,37], combined with GC-MS, has been widely used for VOMs analysis. It is a simple, solvent-free, and sensitive extraction method that does not require a concentration step before analysis, thereby reducing the risk of interference generation [38]. Therefore, this study aimed to comprehensively characterise the urine volatilome of PCa patients by using HS-SPME/GC-MS to identify and define a set of molecular biomarkers for the diagnosis of PCa. Chromatographic data were then submitted to advanced statistical tools as a powerful way to define a pool of potential PCa biomarkers which can be used after validation for PCa diagnosis.

2. Materials and Methods

2.1. Materials and Reagents

Sodium chloride (NaCl, 99.5%) was acquired from Panreac AppliChem ITW Reagents (Barcelona, Spain) to promote salting-out of the VOMs. Ultrapure water obtained from a Milli-Q water purification system (Millipore, Bedford, PA, USA) was used to prepare the solutions hydrochloric acid (HCl, 37%) 5 M and 3-octanol (internal standard (IS), 99%) 2.5 parts per million (ppm), both from Sigma-Aldrich (St. Louis, MO, USA). For the HS-SPME procedure, the glass vials, SPME holder, and a fused silica fibre coating partially cross-linked with 50/30 μm Divinylbenzene/Carboxen/Polydimethylsiloxane (DVB/CAR/PDMS) were purchased from Supelco (Merck KGaA, Darmstadt, Germany). The DVB/CAR/PDMS fibre was used to extract a wider range of VOMs and was conditioned at 270 °C for 30 min before use, according to the manufacturer's guidelines.

2.2. Subjects

A cohort of 56 men was included in this study: 30 healthy individuals without any known pathology (control group) and 26 PCa patients (PCa group) (Table 2). The control group consisted of current non-smokers with no history of prostate malignancy. These individuals also did not take any medication for age-related comorbidities or metabolic diseases such as hypertension or diabetes. Urine samples from the control group were collected during General and Family Medicine consultations at the Centro de Saúde do Bom Jesus. Urine samples from PCa patients were collected at the Urology Unit of SESARAM, EPERAM, prior to the confirmatory prostatic biopsy; therefore, before the newly diagnosed PCa patients enrolled in any kind of treatment or medication. All participants signed an informed consent form after being fully informed of the study's objectives and protocol, which was previously approved by the local ethics committee (CES18/2022). Each urine sample was aliquoted in 8 mL vials and stored at −20 °C until analysis. All data collected from the participants were processed to ensure confidentiality, privacy, and ethical principles inherent to any research study involving human subjects.

None of the patients in this study were receiving treatment for PCa. The Urology unit follows the European Association of Urology guidelines that state that the definitive diagnosis is given by the prostatic biopsy, and no treatment should be initiated before that. Even in the cases of high-volume disease, the biopsy was taken before systemic treatment was initiated.

2.3. HS-SPME Procedure

HS-SPME extraction was performed according to previously optimized conditions for the analysis of the volatilomic composition of urine samples of other malignant tumours [35,39]. Briefly, 4 mL aliquots of urine sample, adjusted to pH 1–2 with 500 μL HCl (5 M), were transferred to an 8 mL sampling glass vial with 0.8 g NaCl and 5 μL 3-octanol (2.5 ppm). For the extraction of volatiles, the vial was placed in a thermostat bath adjusted to 50.0 ± 0.1 °C under stirring at 800 rpm for 60 min. After extraction, the SPME fibre was inserted into the injector port (250 °C) of the GC-MS for 6 min to desorb the analytes. The absence of 3-octanol in the samples of all studied groups was confirmed before its use as an IS.

2.4. GC-MS Analysis

The GC-MS analysis was performed in an Agilent Technologies 6890N Network (Palo Alto, CA, USA), equipped with a 30 m × 0.25 mm ID × 0.25 μm film thickness, BP-20 (SGE, Dortmund, Germany) fused silica column. The oven temperature was fixed at 35 °C for 2 min, increased to 220 °C (rate 2.5 °C min^{-1}), and held for 5 min, for a total run time of 77 min. Helium of purity 5.0 (Air Liquide, Algés, Portugal) was used as the carrier gas at 1.1 mL min^{-1}. The injection port was heated at 250 °C and operated in splitless mode. The temperatures of the transfer line, quadrupole, and ionisation source were 270 °C, 150 °C, and 230 °C, respectively. The analysis was performed in scan mode using a mass range of 30–300 m/z, and the electron impact mass spectra was 70 eV. The electron multiplier was set to auto-tune procedure, and the ionisation current was 10 mA. The identification of the VOMs was achieved by manual interpretation of the spectra and comparison with the Agilent MS ChemStation Software (Palo Alto, CA, USA), equipped with a NIST05 mass spectral library with a similarity threshold of 480%. The results are expressed as relative peak areas.

Table 2. Demographic and clinical data of the cancer-free controls and prostate cancer patients included in this study.

Characteristics	Control	Prostate Cancer
Number of subjects	30	26
Mean age ± SD (years)	46.21 ± 11.58	66.92 ± 9.14
BMI (kg/m^2) ± SD	27.67 ± 3.78	27.34 ± 3.40
Smoking habits		
Ever smokers	6	16
Never smokers	19	10
Unknown	5	0
PSA (ng/mL), n (%)		
<4	30 (100%)	1 (3.85%)
4–10	-	13 (50.00%)
>10	-	12 (46.15%)
Gleason score, n (%)		
≤6	-	4 (15.38%)
7	-	12 (46.15%)
≥8	-	10 (38.46%)
Grade group, n (%)		
1	-	4 (15.38%)
2	-	8 (30.77%)
3	-	4 (15.38%)
4	-	9 (34.62%)
5	-	1 (3.85%)

Legend: BMI: body mass index; SD: standard deviation.

2.5. Statistical Analysis

MetaboAnalyst 5.0 [40] was used to perform the statistical analysis. The data matrix was normalised using a cubic root transformation and mean-centered scaling. Normalised data were processed using a *t*-test (*p*-values < 0.05). Considering the statistically significant VOMs, multivariate analysis was performed through partial least-squares discriminant analysis (PLS-DA). A heatmap using Euclidean correlation was used to identify potential clustering patterns among the significantly altered VOMs in the studied groups. The important variables of the PLS-DA model were verified according to the variable importance in projection (VIP) score and used to validate the PLS-DA models by 10-fold cross-validation (CV) and permutation tests (1000 random permutations of Y-observations).

3. Results and Discussion

3.1. Characterisation of Urinary Volatile Metabolites

VOMs have been described as a promising class of biomarkers for specific diseases through the definition of volatilomic biosignatures. These sets of VOMs have the potential to be used in early detection, as diagnostic tools, and to monitor therapeutic efficacy and disease follow-up [41,42]. This study aimed to establish a urinary volatilomic profile of PCa to identify putative biomarkers for PCa diagnosis. The volatile composition of urine samples from the PCa patients (*n* = 26) and healthy subjects without any known pathology (control group, n = 30) (Table 1) was established using HS-SPME/GC-MS, according to the experimental procedure described. Following the HS-SPME/GC-MS analysis of the urine samples of the 56 recruited subjects, different chromatographic profiles were obtained from the control group and the PCa patients (Figure 2).

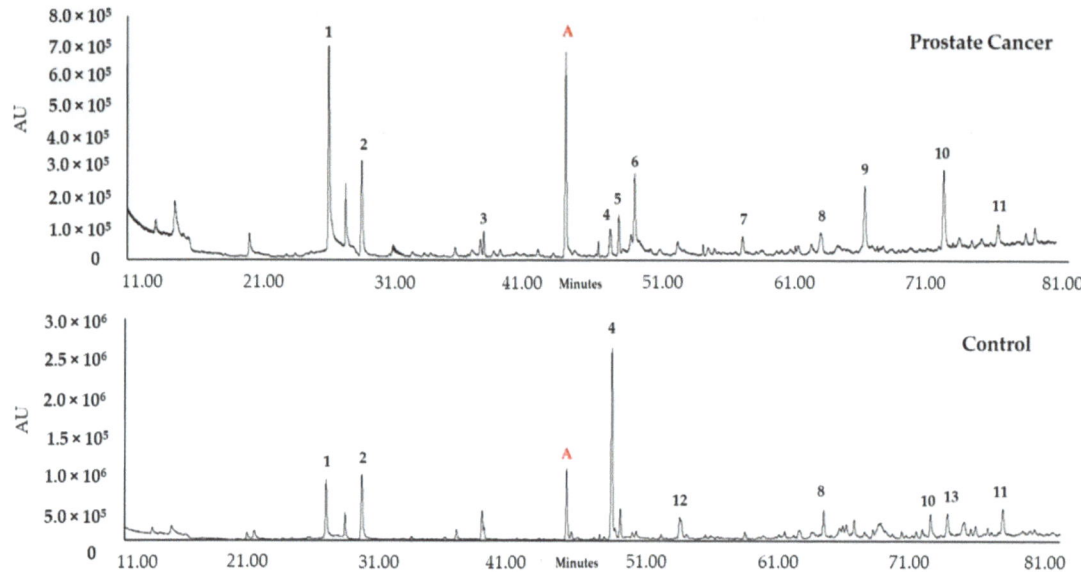

Figure 2. Example of typical GC-qMS urinary volatilomic profile of prostate cancer and control samples. Most important peaks: (1) Dimethyl disulfide; (2) 4-Heptanone; (3) o-Cymene; (4) p-Cymenene; (5) Dihydromyrcenol; (6) 2-Ethyl-1-hexanol; (7) Menthol; (8) D-Carvone; (9) β-Damascenone; (10) Phenol; (11) 4-Methyphenol; (12) β-Ionone; (13) 2-Bromophenol. (A) 3-Octanol, internal standard.

Overall, 147 VOMs were identified in the analysed samples, belonging to different chemical families, which included 13 ketones, five aldehydes, three esters, one alcohol, three carboxylic acids, seven sulfur compounds, 16 benzene derivatives, five naphthalene derivatives, 11 phenolic compounds, seven furanic compounds, 15 hydrocarbons, four heterocyclic hydrocarbons, 35 terpenes, 19 norisoprenoids, and three sesquiterpenes (Table S1, Supplementary Materials).

Detailed analysis of each sample group showed differences in terms of areas for the different chemical families (Figure 3). As a result of bacterial activity, metabolism, pH changes, or breakdown of urine constituents, the human urinary profile changes over time. It is also influenced by external factors, including health status, dietary habits, physical stress, and environmental exposure, which along with exogenous compounds, contribute to an individual's volatilomic profile [11]. Due to these factors, the human metabolism is very complex, and cancer development and progression make it even more difficult to understand all the metabolic processes that may contribute to an increase or decrease in certain metabolites [35,43,44]. Thus, it is crucial to establish a relationship between the identified VOMs and their potential endogenous origin; however, the origin of many VOMs has not been clearly defined [8].

Terpenes, phenolic compounds, and norisoprenoids were the chemical families that contributed the most to the volatilomic pattern of the studied groups (Figure 3). Norisoprenoids, phenolic, and terpenic compounds can be easily found in different exogenous sources such as food [45,46]. Nevertheless, many metabolites belonging to these chemical families originate from endogenous metabolic processes in our organism, namely p-cymenene, p-cymene, 2-bromophenol, phenol, and p-cresol [47]. Terpenes come from the mevalonic acid pathway [35,43] and can also result from the consumption of foods and beverages [47]. 3,5-Dimethylbenzaldehyde, 2-methoxy-5-methylthiophene (MMT), 1,1,6-trimethyl-1,2-dihydronapththalene (TDN), and 2-ethyl-1-hexanol were the most abundant metabolites in the PCa group. TDN is typically found in liquorice tasting, alcoholic beverages and fruits [44,47]. 2-Ethyl-1-hexanol is a fatty alcohol in lipid molecules; it can be found in foods such as different kinds of tea, cereals and cereal products, fats and oils, and alcoholic beverages [44,47]. Furthermore, 2-ethyl-1-hexanol has been detected in five types of cancer, namely lung, laryngeal, thyroid, colorectal, and breast [8]. o-Cymene has been proposed as a putative biomarker of citrus ingestion since this compound is frequently found in citrus fruits [44,47].

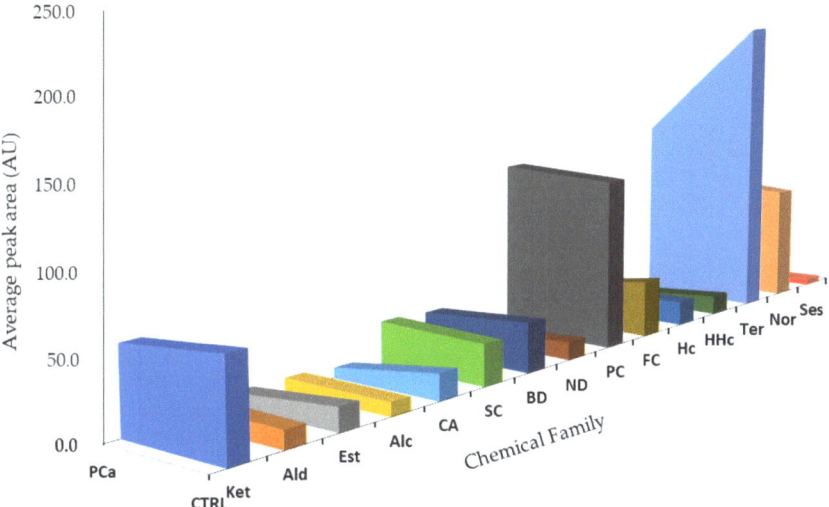

Figure 3. Chemical family distribution of the peak total area in the PCa (*n* = 26) and control (CTRL, *n* = 30) groups. Ket: Ketones; Ald: Aldehydes; Est: Esters; Alc: Alcohols; CA: Carboxylic Acid; SC: Sulfur Compounds; BD: Benzene Derivatives; ND: Naphthalene Derivatives; PC: Phenolic Compounds; FC: Furanic Compounds; Hc: Hydrocarbons; HHc: Heterocyclic Hydrocarbons; Ter: Terpenes; Nor: Norisoprenoids; Ses: Sesquiterpenes.

According to the literature, ketones are one of the most abundant chemical families in the volatile profile of urine [43,48]. They are products of different metabolic pathways, namely carbohydrate metabolism and lipid oxidation processes [49,50]. A few studies have proposed that a considerable fraction of ketones in urine arises from the action of gut bacteria, but ketones can also come from exogenous sources, such as food (beverages, foods, and flavouring ingredients) or environmental pollution [8]. 2-Pentanone, the simplest ketone identified, has been found in different foods, including fruits, cereals, milk, herbs and spice, fats, and oils. Moreover, 2-pentanone has been linked to diseases such as ulcerative colitis, non-alcoholic fatty liver disease, Crohn's disease, and also to the inborn metabolic disorder of celiac disease [47]. 4-Heptanone is one of the most common VOMs in urine; its origin is still unknown, but it may be associated with the β-oxidation of 2-ethylhexanoic acid [8]. In addition to dietary sources, 3-hexanone has been associated with several diseases, including non-alcoholic fatty liver disease, autism, and inborn metabolic disorder celiac disease [8].

Similar to ketones, sulfur compounds have been described to possess a high expression in the human urinary volatilomic profile [35,51]. Most of these metabolites are produced during the transamination pathway by the incomplete metabolism of methionine and cysteine [35,52–54]. During transamination, methionine and cysteine are transformed into methanethiol [55]. Then, methanethiol is easily oxidized to dimethyl disulfide and dimethyl trisulfide [53]. It has been described that Gram-negative bacteria may also produce considerable amounts of methanethiol and dimethyl disulfide [56]. Furthermore, these compounds can also result from dietary sources since dimethyl disulfide and dimethyl trisulfide are present in many foods and beverages. MMT is one of the most abundant sulfur compounds among the PCa group.

Alcohols can originate from different sources, such as the reduction of fatty acids in the gastrointestinal tract, pyruvate, citrate, or glycolysis pathways [57], or even the metabolism of hydrocarbons [8]. Similarly, the metabolism of microorganisms such as bacteria can also be a source of these metabolites [58]. Another source of alcohols is diet through the ingestion of food and beverages [8]. Dihydromyrcenol was previously detected in the urine samples of PCa patients [55] and was reported at lower levels than in control subjects [8].

Hydrocarbons are metabolites of great diagnostic interest because they are closely related to oxidative stress [59]. Alkanes and other methylated hydrocarbons typically result from the lipid peroxidation of polyunsaturated fatty acids found mainly in cell membranes [59]. Significant changes in the levels of alkanes and methyl alkanes in cancer patients may be related to the activity of CYP 450 enzymes [8]. In contrast, unsaturated hydrocarbons, typically alkenes, are often involved in the mevalonic acid pathway of cholesterol synthesis [59]. Polycyclic aromatic hydrocarbons (PAHs) are carcinogenic substances that humans are exposed to in the environment, at certain industrial workplaces, and from tobacco smoke [59]. Naphthalene is a PAH often associated with cancer development and is released by industrial, domestic, and natural burning processes, leading to exposure of the general population [59,60]. However, no metabolic pathway has clearly explained the origin of naphthalene derivatives in urine. Some researchers have indicated a potential relationship with steroid metabolism, while others have suggested that these compounds may come from the environment to which the individual is exposed [59,60].

Furanic compounds and benzene derivatives can be found in both exogenous and endogenous sources as metabolic products of food and different processes in the human organism [45–47]. The thermal degradation and rearrangement of carbohydrates in natural and processed food is the primary source of furanic compounds [44,46,47]. Furan was proposed as a PCa biomarker by Jiménez-Pacheco et al. [61]. 2-Methyl-5-(methylthio)furan, a furanic compound found in both the control and PCa groups, has been found in coffee, garlic, and horseradish. Benzene derivates are often related to environmental sources, such as air and environmental pollution from industrial (pesticides, dyes) or natural processes (fires). The major sources of benzene exposure are automobile service stations and tobacco smoke [48].

3.2. Chemometric Analysis of Urine Samples

MetaboAnalyst 5.0 [40] was used to perform the statistical analysis. The variables were initially normalised to obtain a homogeneous distribution and generate reliable and interpretable models. The normalised matrix was subjected to univariate analysis using a t-test ($p < 0.05$), in which the p values obtained proved that 7 of the 147 VOMs identified presented statistically significant differences between the analysed groups, the healthy subjects (control group), and oncological patients (PCa group) (Table 3). Some of these metabolites have been previously related to oncological pathologies, according to the Human Metabolome Database [8]. TDN has been detected in urine samples of colorectal, leukaemia, and lymphoma cancers, where it was found increasingly expressed in the samples of oncological patients [8]. About 3,5-dimethylbenzaldehyde, very little information has been published in the literature, but similar molecules, such as the isomer 2,5-dimethylbenzaldehyde or benzaldehyde, have already been related to prostate [41] and lung [62] cancers. For many VOMs related to the control group, such as D-carvone, 6-methylphenanthedrine, α-methylcinnamaldehyde, and 2-bromophenol, a significant decrease in concentration was observed in the PCa group. Although the origin of some of these metabolites is known, most of them still need more detailed evaluation to establish a relationship with PCa.

Table 3. Important features identified using the *t*-tests.

No.	Significant VOMs	*t*-Stat	*p*-Value	=−LOG10(p)	FDR
1	3,5-Dimethylbenzaldehyde	−7.479	6.87×10^{-10}	9.1628	3.92×10^{-8}
2	TDN	−5.7798	3.84×10^{-7}	6.4162	1.09×10^{-5}
3	D-Carvone	4.363	5.82×10^{-5}	4.235	0.001106
4	6-Methylphenanthridine	3.8847	0.000282	3.55	0.004016
5	α-Methylcinnamaldehyde	3.6128	0.000665	3.1772	0.007581
6	2-Bromophenol	3.486	0.000982	3.0079	0.009328
7	TONEA	3.3169	0.001633	2.7871	0.013294

Abbreviations: TDN: 1,1,6-Trimethyl-1,2-dihydronaphthalene; TONEA: 2,5,5,8a-tetramethyl-1,2,3,5,6,7,8,8-octahydro-1-naphthalenyl ester acetate; FDR: false discovery rate.

PLS-DA multivariate pattern recognition procedures use the information contained in the VOMs fingerprint as several variables to visualize group trends and clustering patterns, respectively, according to the separations among sample sets. The resulting PLS-DA analysis showed two well-separated groups, the PCa and the control groups (Figure 4a). Besides the significant difference between PCa patients and healthy subjects (control group) in terms of smoking habits and age, these factors did not contribute to the differences noted between both groups. When carrying out the discriminant statistical analysis by age and by smoking habits, it was verified that no cluster was formed associated with any of the target groups. Hence, it can be deduced that neither age nor the difference in the number of smokers between both groups influenced the separation obtained among the PCa cluster and control group cluster. The VIP scores plot describes the relative contribution of the metabolites to the variance between the two groups, where TDN and D-carvone showed the most significant contributions to the PCa and control groups, respectively (Figure 4b). The robustness of the generated PLS-DA model was evaluated by 10-fold CV (Figure 4c), and to assess the significance of class discrimination, a permutation test was performed (Figure 4d). The resulting PLS-DA analysis showed two well-separated groups. The VIP scores plot describes the relative contribution of the metabolites to the variance between the two groups. TDN and D-carvone showed the most significant contributions to the PCa and control groups, respectively.

Hierarchical clustering was performed, resulting in a dendrogram and heatmap (Figure 5). The heatmap created using Euclidean distance measure with the 15 statistically significant VOMs illustrated the correlations between these VOMs and the sample groups (Figure 5b). This hierarchical cluster analysis showed that each cluster of the studied groups was well-defined by a distinct panel of metabolites. For instance, D-carvone, *p*-cymenene, and 2-bromophenol *p*-tert-butylphenol were the metabolites most associated with the control group, whereas 3,5-dimethylbenzaldehyde, MMT, TDN, and 2-ethyl-1-hexanol were highly correlated with the PCa group.

To evaluate the performance of the potential biomarker models, the multivariate exploratory receiver operating characteristic (ROC) curves were generated by Monte Carlo cross-validation (MCCV), using 2/3 of the samples to evaluate feature importance, and the remaining 1/3 were used to validate the created models (Figure 6a,b). The top-ranking features in terms of importance were used to build the classification models. Figure 6a shows the ROC curves of a set of six volatiles based on the average cross-validation performance. The obtained values for the area under the curves (AUC) between 0.867 and 0.968, with a 95% confidence interval, are excellent and represent a good accuracy in discriminating both groups. Figure 6b shows the plot of the predictive accuracy of biomarker models with an increasing number of features.

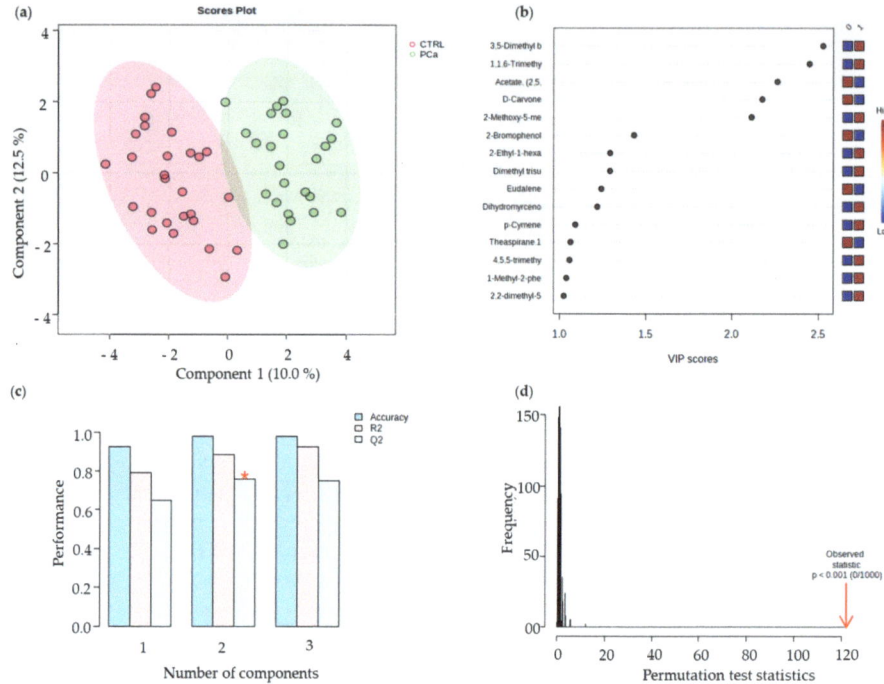

Figure 4. (**a**) Partial least-squares discriminant analysis (PLS-DA). (**b**) Variables of importance in projection (VIP) scores plot, representing the important features identified by the PLS-DA. The coloured boxes on the right indicate the relative concentrations of the corresponding metabolites in each group under study. (**c**) 10-fold CV performance of the PLS-DA classification using a different number of components (* means best Q^2 value, the best classifier). (**d**) PLS-DA model validation by permutation tests based on 1000 permutations of the VOMs obtained by GC-MS of the urine samples from the groups under study.

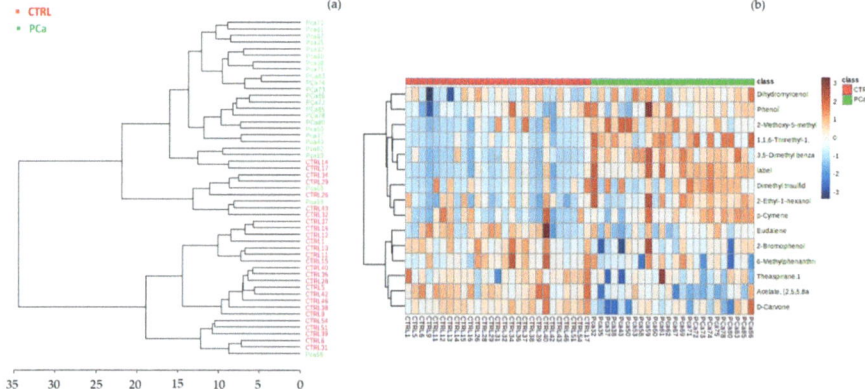

Figure 5. Hierarchical cluster analysis of CTRL (control) and Pca (prostate cancer) groups (**a**) Dendrogram analysis of the volatomic data, using Euclidean distance measure and Ward's linkage. (**b**) Clustering result shown as heatmap illustrates the concentration of the urinary volatile organic metabolites identified in each sample. Columns correspond to Pca and CTRL sample groups, respectively, whereas rows correspond to the most relevant VOMs detected. The colour of the cells corresponds to the normalised peak areas of the compounds (minimum −1, dark blue; maximum +1, dark red).

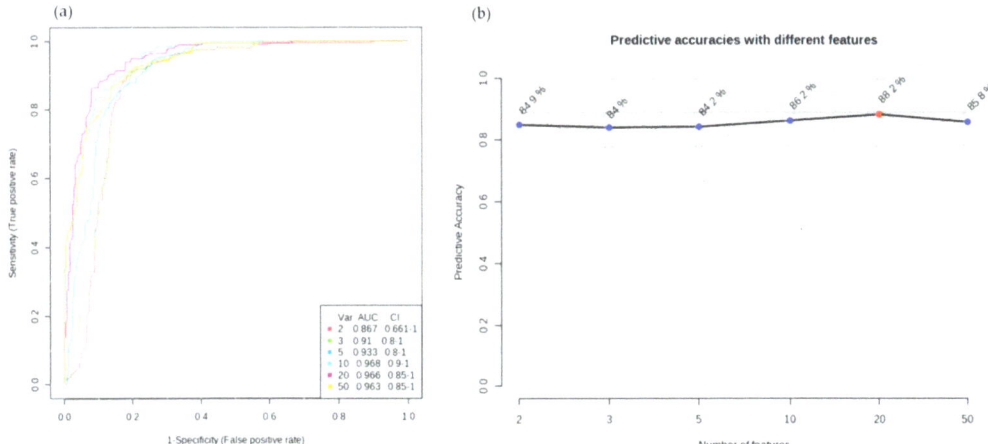

Figure 6. (a) ROC curves for the most important features with the highest ability to discriminate both groups. (b) Plot of the predictive accuracy of biomarker models with an increasing number of features. The most accurate biomarker model is highlighted with a red dot.

The performance of the classification model was assessed through a confusion matrix was performed based on the classification method: PLS-DA. The columns represent the actual classes the outcomes should have been, while the rows represent the predictions we have made. The number of correct and incorrect predictions is summarized in Figure 7.

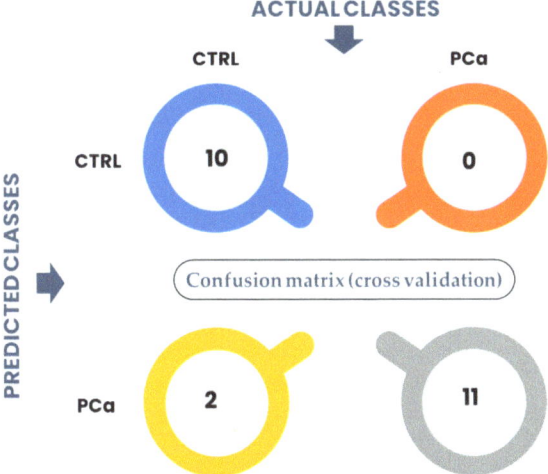

Figure 7. Structure of a 2 × 2 confusion matrix to assess the performance of a classification model.

Our model predicted that 10/12 were from control groups when there were 12/12. The accuracy corresponds to the proportion of predictions that the model classified correctly. In this case, the accuracy of the model was 91.3% as it predicted that two healthy individuals belong to the PCa group (two false positives). The precision of the model, related to the proportion of positive identifications that were correct, was 85%. The sensitivity which expresses the proportion of actual positives identified correctly was 100%, whereas the specificity associated with the proportion of actual negatives that are correctly identified was 83.3%.

4. Conclusions

A total of 147 VOMs were identified as belonging to different chemical families, and different chromatographic profiles were retrieved for the groups of subjects recruited. Terpenes, phenolic compounds, and norisoprenoids were the chemical families that contributed the most to the volatilomic profile of the three studied groups: control and PCa. The statistical analysis revealed that 7 of the 147 VOMs identified presented statistically significant differences between the recruited groups, according to the t-test ($p < 0.05$). PLS-DA was performed, and the robustness of the generated model was evaluated using 10-fold CV and permutation tests. PLS-DA showed two well-separated groups, and the VIP score showed the most relevant metabolites among the studied groups. Hierarchical cluster analysis, carried out by Euclidean distance measure and Ward's linkage, showed that each cluster of the studied groups was well defined by a distinct panel of metabolites. The metabolites D-carvone, p-cymenene, 2-bromophenol, and p-tert-butylphenol were more strongly associated with the control group, whereas 3,5-dimethylbenzaldehyde, MMT, TDN, and 2-ethyl-1-hexanol were highly correlated with the PCa group. A significant increase in the peak area of TDN and 3,5-dimethylbenzaldehyde was observed in PCa patients. On average, significantly lower abundances of D-carvone, 6-methylphenanthridine, α-methylcinnamaldehyde, 2-bromophenol, and 2,5,5,8a-tetramethyl-1,2,3,5,6,7,8,8-octahydro-1-naphthalenyl ester acetate (TONEA) were found in cancer patients. Further validation of the findings in this study is required using a much larger sample cohort to improve the predictive power and reliability of the developed statistical models. Likewise, additional research is required to determine which of the metabolites are of endogenous origin, disease-related, and which originate from exogenous sources, related to normal metabolic processes and external contaminations (environment or diet).

Supplementary Materials: The following supporting information can be downloaded at: https://www.mdpi.com/article/10.3390/curroncol30050370/s1, Table S1. Identified metabolites in urine samples of PCa patients and healthy subjects. Retention time (RT) in min, formula, CAS number and chemical family is reported for each compound. Frequency of occurrence as a percentage (%) and mean relative peak areas are reported for prostate cancer and control groups (n = 3; RSD <20%).

Author Contributions: Conceptualization, G.R., C.V.B., F.P., V.G. and J.S.C.; investigation, G.R. and R.P.; writing original draft preparation G.R., R.P. and C.V.B.; review and editing, J.A.M.P., F.P. and J.S.C.; P.B., C.P.O., A.C.S., J.A.V. and M.d.C.P. were responsible for management the sample collection, inform the patients and healthy individuals about the study and obtain the informed consent from all participants; visualization, V.G., J.A.M.P. and J.S.C.; supervision, V.G., J.S.C. and J.A.M.P.; funding acquisition J.S.C. All authors have read and agreed to the published version of the manuscript.

Funding: This work was supported by FCT-Fundação para a Ciência e a Tecnologia through the CQM Base Fund-UIDB/00674/2020 and Programmatic Fund-UIDP/00674/2020; and by ARDITI-Agência Regional para o Desenvolvimento da Investigação Tecnologia e Inovação through the project M1420-01-0145-FEDER-000005-Centro de Química da Madeira-CQM+ (Madeira 14-20 Program). Giulia Riccio was supported by a PhD scholarship given by Univesità Cattolica del Sacro Cuore, 00168 Rome, Italy. Jorge A. M. Pereira was supported by a post-doctoral fellowship given by ARDITI (Project M1420-09-5369-FSE-000001), and Cristina V. Berenguer acknowledges Núcleo Regional da Madeira da Liga Portuguesa contra o Cancro (LPCC-NRM) and Bolsa Rubina Barros for their support with this project. The authors also acknowledge the financial support from Fundação para a Ciência e Tecnologia and Madeira 14-2020 program to the Portuguese Mass Spectrometry Network through the PROEQUIPRAM program M14-20 M1420-01-0145-FEDER-000008.

Institutional Review Board Statement: Not applicable.

Informed Consent Statement: Informed consent was obtained from all subjects involved in the study.

Data Availability Statement: Not applicable.

Conflicts of Interest: The authors declare no conflict of interest.

References

1. Sung, H.; Ferlay, J.; Siegel, R.L.; Laversanne, M.; Soerjomataram, I.; Jemal, A.; Bray, F. Global Cancer Statistics 2020: GLOBOCAN Estimates of Incidence and Mortality Worldwide for 36 Cancers in 185 Countries. *CA Cancer J. Clin.* **2021**, *71*, 209–249. [CrossRef] [PubMed]
2. Rawla, P. Epidemiology of Prostate Cancer. *World J. Oncol.* **2019**, *10*, 63–89. [CrossRef] [PubMed]
3. Salciccia, S.; Capriotti, A.L.; Lagana, A.; Fais, S.; Logozzi, M.; De Berardinis, E.; Busetto, G.M.; Di Pierro, G.B.; Ricciuti, G.P.; Del Giudice, F.; et al. Biomarkers in Prostate Cancer Diagnosis: From Current Knowledge to the Role of Metabolomics and Exosomes. *Int. J. Mol. Sci.* **2021**, *22*, 4367. [CrossRef] [PubMed]
4. Kim, C.-J.; Dong, L.; Amend, S.R.; Cho, Y.-K.; Pienta, K.J. The role of liquid biopsies in prostate cancer management. *Lab. Chip* **2021**, *21*, 3263–3288. [CrossRef] [PubMed]
5. Lima, A.R.; Bastos, M.d.L.; Carvalho, M.; Guedes de Pinho, P. Biomarker Discovery in Human Prostate Cancer: An Update in Metabolomics Studies. *Transl. Oncol.* **2016**, *9*, 357–370. [CrossRef]
6. Campos-Fernández, E.; Barcelos, L.S.; de Souza, A.G.; Goulart, L.R.; Alonso-Goulart, V. Research landscape of liquid biopsies in prostate cancer. *Am. J. Cancer Res.* **2019**, *9*, 1309–1328.
7. Lee, S.; Ku, J.Y.; Kang, B.J.; Kim, K.H.; Ha, H.K.; Kim, S. A Unique Urinary Metabolic Feature for the Determination of Bladder Cancer, Prostate Cancer, and Renal Cell Carcinoma. *Metabolites* **2021**, *11*, 591. [CrossRef]
8. Janfaza, S.; Khorsand, B.; Nikkhah, M.; Zahiri, J. Digging deeper into volatile organic compounds associated with cancer. *Biol. Methods Protoc.* **2019**, *4*, bpz014. [CrossRef]
9. Mallafré-Muro, C.; Llambrich, M.; Cumeras, R.; Pardo, A.; Brezmes, J.; Marco, S.; Gumà, J. Comprehensive Volatilome and Metabolome Signatures of Colorectal Cancer in Urine: A Systematic Review and Meta-Analysis. *Cancers* **2021**, *13*, 2534. [CrossRef]
10. Berenguer, C.V.; Pereira, F.; Câmara, J.S.; Pereira, J.A.M. Underlying Features of Prostate Cancer—Statistics, Risk Factors, and Emerging Methods for Its Diagnosis. *Curr. Oncol.* **2023**, *30*, 2300–2321. [CrossRef]
11. Berenguer, C.V.; Pereira, F.; Pereira, J.A.M.; Camara, J.S. Volatilomics: An Emerging and Promising Avenue for the Detection of Potential Prostate Cancer Biomarkers. *Cancers* **2022**, *14*, 3982. [CrossRef] [PubMed]
12. Gower, H.; Danielson, K.; Dennett, A.P.E.; Deere, J. Potential role of volatile organic compound breath testing in the Australasian colorectal cancer pathway. *ANZ J. Surg.* **2023**. [CrossRef] [PubMed]
13. Silva, C.; Perestrelo, R.; Silva, P.; Tomás, H.; Câmara, J.S. Breast Cancer Metabolomics: From Analytical Platforms to Multivariate Data Analysis. A Review. *Metabolites* **2019**, *9*, 102. [CrossRef] [PubMed]
14. Gao, Q.; Lee, W.-Y. Urinary metabolites for urological cancer detection: A review on the application of volatile organic compounds for cancers. *Am. J. Clin. Exp. Urol.* **2019**, *7*, 232–248. [PubMed]
15. Bax, C.; Taverna, G.; Eusebio, L.; Sironi, S.; Grizzi, F.; Guazzoni, G.; Capelli, L. Innovative Diagnostic Methods for Early Prostate Cancer Detection through Urine Analysis: A Review. *Cancers* **2018**, *10*, 123. [CrossRef]
16. Daulton, E.; Wicaksono, A.N.; Tiele, A.; Kocher, H.M.; Debernardi, S.; Crnogorac-Jurcevic, T.; Covington, J.A. Volatile organic compounds (VOCs) for the non-invasive detection of pancreatic cancer from urine. *Talanta* **2021**, *221*, 121604. [CrossRef]
17. Tyagi, H.; Daulton, E.; Bannaga, A.S.; Arasaradnam, R.P.; Covington, J.A. Urinary Volatiles and Chemical Characterisation for the Non-Invasive Detection of Prostate and Bladder Cancers. *Biosensors* **2021**, *11*, 437. [CrossRef]
18. Taverna, G.; Grizzi, F.; Tidu, L.; Bax, C.; Zanoni, M.; Vota, P.; Lotesoriere, B.J.; Prudenza, S.; Magagnin, L.; Langfelder, G.; et al. Accuracy of a new electronic nose for prostate cancer diagnosis in urine samples. *Int. J. Urol.* **2022**, *29*, 890–896. [CrossRef]
19. Filianoti, A.; Costantini, M.; Bove, A.M.; Anceschi, U.; Brassetti, A.; Ferriero, M.; Mastroianni, R.; Misuraca, L.; Tuderti, G.; Ciliberto, G.; et al. Volatilome Analysis in Prostate Cancer by Electronic Nose: A Pilot Monocentric Study. *Cancers* **2022**, *14*, 2927. [CrossRef]
20. Capelli, L.; Bax, C.; Grizzi, F.; Taverna, G. Optimization of training and measurement protocol for eNose analysis of urine headspace aimed at prostate cancer diagnosis. *Sci. Rep.* **2021**, *11*, 20898. [CrossRef]
21. Wen, Q.; Myridakis, A.; Boshier, P.R.; Zuffa, S.; Belluomo, I.; Parker, A.G.; Chin, S.-T.; Hakim, S.; Markar, S.R.; Hanna, G.B. A Complete Pipeline for Untargeted Urinary Volatolomic Profiling with Sorptive Extraction and Dual Polar and Non-polar Column Methodologies Coupled with Gas Chromatography Time-of-Flight Mass Spectrometry. *Anal. Chem.* **2023**, *95*, 758–765. [CrossRef] [PubMed]
22. Giró Benet, J.; Seo, M.; Khine, M.; Gumà Padró, J.; Pardo Martnez, A.; Kurdahi, F. Breast cancer detection by analyzing the volatile organic compound (VOC) signature in human urine. *Sci. Rep.* **2022**, *12*, 14873. [CrossRef] [PubMed]
23. Ligor, T.; Adamczyk, P.; Kowalkowski, T.; Ratiu, I.A.; Wenda-Piesik, A.; Buszewski, B. Analysis of VOCs in Urine Samples Directed towards of Bladder Cancer Detection. *Molecules* **2022**, *27*, 5023. [CrossRef] [PubMed]
24. Gasparri, R.; Capuano, R.; Guaglio, A.; Caminiti, V.; Canini, F.; Catini, A.; Sedda, G.; Paolesse, R.; Di Natale, C.; Spaggiari, L. Volatolomic urinary profile analysis for diagnosis of the early stage of lung cancer. *J. Breath. Res.* **2022**, *16*, 046008. [CrossRef]
25. Cheng, H.R.; van Vorstenbosch, R.W.R.; Pachen, D.M.; Meulen, L.W.T.; Straathof, J.W.A.; Dallinga, J.W.; Jonkers, D.M.A.E.; Masclee, A.A.M.; Schooten, F.-J.v.; Mujagic, Z.; et al. Detecting Colorectal Adenomas and Cancer Using Volatile Organic Compounds in Exhaled Breath: A Proof-of-Principle Study to Improve Screening. *Clin. Transl. Gastroenterol.* **2022**, *13*, e00518. [CrossRef]
26. Jung, Y.J.; Seo, H.S.; Kim, J.H.; Song, K.Y.; Park, C.H.; Lee, H.H. Advanced Diagnostic Technology of Volatile Organic Compounds Real Time analysis Analysis From Exhaled Breath of Gastric Cancer Patients Using Proton-Transfer-Reaction Time-of-Flight Mass Spectrometry. *Front. Oncol.* **2021**, *11*, 560591. [CrossRef]

27. Nakayama, Y.; Hanada, M.; Koda, H.; Sugimoto, M.; Takada, M.; Toi, M. Breast cancer detection using volatile compound profiles in exhaled breath via selected ion-flow tube mass spectrometry. *J. Breath. Res.* **2023**, *17*, 016006. [CrossRef]
28. Nazir, N.U.; Abbas, S.R. Identification of phenol 2,2-methylene bis, 6 [1,1-D] as breath biomarker of hepatocellular carcinoma (HCC) patients and its electrochemical sensing: E-nose biosensor for HCC. *Anal. Chim. Acta* **2023**, *1242*, 340752. [CrossRef]
29. Wang, P.; Huang, Q.; Meng, S.; Mu, T.; Liu, Z.; He, M.; Li, Q.; Zhao, S.; Wang, S.; Qiu, M. Identification of lung cancer breath biomarkers based on perioperative breathomics testing: A prospective observational study. *eClinicalMedicine* **2022**, *47*, 101384. [CrossRef]
30. Sukaram, T.; Tansawat, R.; Apiparakoon, P.; Tiyarattanachai, T.; Marukatat, S.; Rerknimitr, R.; Chaiteerakij, R. Exhaled volatile organic compounds for diagnosis of hepatocellular carcinoma. *Sci. Rep.* **2022**, *12*, 5326. [CrossRef]
31. Monedeiro, F.; Monedeiro-Milanowski, M.; Zmysłowski, H.; De Martinis, B.S.; Buszewski, B. Evaluation of salivary VOC profile composition directed towards oral cancer and oral lesion assessment. *Clin. Oral. Investig.* **2021**, *25*, 4415–4430. [CrossRef] [PubMed]
32. Bel'skaya, L.V.; Sarf, E.A.; Shalygin, S.P.; Postnova, T.V.; Kosenok, V.K. Identification of salivary volatile organic compounds as potential markers of stomach and colorectal cancer: A pilot study. *J. Oral. Biosci.* **2020**, *62*, 212–221. [CrossRef] [PubMed]
33. Shigeyama, H.; Wang, T.; Ichinose, M.; Ansai, T.; Lee, S.-W. Identification of volatile metabolites in human saliva from patients with oral squamous cell carcinoma via zeolite-based thin-film microextraction coupled with GC–MS. *J. Chromatogr. B.* **2019**, *1104*, 49–58. [CrossRef] [PubMed]
34. Aggarwal, P.; Baker, J.; Boyd, M.T.; Coyle, S.; Probert, C.; Chapman, E.A. Optimisation of Urine Sample Preparation for Headspace-Solid Phase Microextraction Gas Chromatography-Mass Spectrometry: Altering Sample pH, Sulphuric Acid Concentration and Phase Ratio. *Metabolites* **2020**, *10*, 482. [CrossRef] [PubMed]
35. Silva, C.L.; Passos, M.; Câmara, J.S. Solid phase microextraction, mass spectrometry and metabolomic approaches for detection of potential urinary cancer biomarkers—A powerful strategy for breast cancer diagnosis. *Talanta* **2012**, *89*, 360–368. [CrossRef]
36. Arthur, C.L.; Pawliszyn, J. Solid phase microextraction with thermal desorption using fused silica optical fibers. *Anal. Chem.* **1990**, *62*, 2145–2148. [CrossRef]
37. Câmara, J.S.; Perestrelo, R.; Berenguer, C.V.; Andrade, C.F.P.; Gomes, T.M.; Olayanju, B.; Kabir, A.; Rocha, C.M.R.; Teixeira, J.A.; Pereira, J.A.M. Green Extraction Techniques as Advanced Sample Preparation Approaches in Biological, Food, and Environmental Matrices: A Review. *Molecules* **2022**, *27*, 2953. [CrossRef]
38. Živković Semren, T.; Brčić Karačonji, I.; Safner, T.; Brajenović, N.; Tariba Lovaković, B.; Pizent, A. Gas chromatographic-mass spectrometric analysis of urinary volatile organic metabolites: Optimization of the HS-SPME procedure and sample storage conditions. *Talanta* **2018**, *176*, 537–543. [CrossRef]
39. Porto-Figueira, P.; Pereira, J.; Miekisch, W.; Câmara, J.S. Exploring the potential of NTME/GC-MS, in the establishment of urinary volatomic profiles. Lung cancer patients as case study. *Sci. Rep.* **2018**, *8*, 13113. [CrossRef]
40. Pang, Z.; Chong, J.; Zhou, G.; de Lima Morais, D.A.; Chang, L.; Barrette, M.; Gauthier, C.; Jacques, P.; Li, S.; Xia, J. MetaboAnalyst 5.0: Narrowing the gap between raw spectra and functional insights. *Nucleic Acids Res.* **2021**, *49*, W388–W396. [CrossRef]
41. Lima, A.R.; Pinto, J.; Azevedo, A.I.; Barros-Silva, D.; Jerónimo, C.; Henrique, R.; de Lourdes Bastos, M.; Guedes de Pinho, P.; Carvalho, M. Identification of a biomarker panel for improvement of prostate cancer diagnosis by volatile metabolic profiling of urine. *Br. J. Cancer* **2019**, *121*, 857–868. [CrossRef] [PubMed]
42. Lima, A.R.; Pinto, J.; Amaro, F.; Bastos, M.d.L.; Carvalho, M.; Guedes de Pinho, P. Advances and Perspectives in Prostate Cancer Biomarker Discovery in the Last 5 Years through Tissue and Urine Metabolomics. *Metabolites* **2021**, *11*, 181. [CrossRef] [PubMed]
43. Silva, C.L.; Passos, M.; Camara, J.S. Investigation of urinary volatile organic metabolites as potential cancer biomarkers by solid-phase microextraction in combination with gas chromatography-mass spectrometry. *Br. J. Cancer* **2011**, *105*, 1894–1904. [CrossRef] [PubMed]
44. Taunk, K.; Porto-Figueira, P.; Pereira, J.A.M.; Taware, R.; da Costa, N.L.; Barbosa, R.; Rapole, S.; Câmara, J.S. Urinary Volatomic Expression Pattern: Paving the Way for Identification of Potential Candidate Biosignatures for Lung Cancer. *Metabolites* **2022**, *12*, 36. [CrossRef] [PubMed]
45. Hasnip, S.; Crews, C.; Castle, L. Some factors affecting the formation of furan in heated foods. *Food Addit. Contam.* **2006**, *23*, 219–227. [CrossRef]
46. Wegener, J.W.; Lopez-Sanchez, P. Furan levels in fruit and vegetables juices, nutrition drinks and bakery products. *Anal. Chim. Acta* **2010**, *672*, 55–60. [CrossRef]
47. Wishart, D.S.; Guo, A.; Oler, E.; Wang, F.; Anjum, A.; Peters, H.; Dizon, R.; Sayeeda, Z.; Tian, S.; Lee, B.L.; et al. HMDB 5.0: The Human Metabolome Database for 2022. *Nucleic Acids Res.* **2022**, *50*, D622–D631. [CrossRef]
48. De Lacy Costello, B.; Amann, A.; Al-Kateb, H.; Flynn, C.; Filipiak, W.; Khalid, T.; Osborne, D.; Ratcliffe, N.M. A review of the volatiles from the healthy human body. *J. Breath. Res.* **2014**, *8*, 014001. [CrossRef]
49. Buszewski, B.; Ulanowska, A.; Ligor, T.; Jackowski, M.; Kłodzińska, E.; Szeliga, J. Identification of volatile organic compounds secreted from cancer tissues and bacterial cultures. *J. Chromatogr. B Anal. Technol. Biomed. Life Sci.* **2008**, *868*, 88–94. [CrossRef]
50. Mills, G.A.; Walker, V. Headspace solid-phase microextraction profiling of volatile compounds in urine: Application to metabolic investigations. *J. Chromatogr. B Biomed. Sci. Appl.* **2001**, *753*, 259–268. [CrossRef]
51. Smith, S.; Burden, H.; Persad, R.; Whittington, K.; de Lacy Costello, B.; Ratcliffe, N.M.; Probert, C.S. A comparative study of the analysis of human urine headspace using gas chromatography–mass spectrometry. *J. Breath. Res.* **2008**, *2*, 037022. [CrossRef]

52. Miekisch, W.; Schubert, J.K.; Vagts, D.A.; Geiger, K. Analysis of Volatile Disease Markers in Blood. *Clin. Chem.* **2001**, *47*, 1053–1060. [CrossRef] [PubMed]
53. Tangerman, A. Measurement and biological significance of the volatile sulfur compounds hydrogen sulfide, methanethiol and dimethyl sulfide in various biological matrices. *J. Chromatogr. B Anal. Technol. Biomed. Life Sci.* **2009**, *877*, 3366–3377. [CrossRef] [PubMed]
54. Blom, H.J.; Boers, G.H.; van den Elzen, J.P.; Gahl, W.A.; Tangerman, A. Transamination of methionine in humans. *Clin. Sci.* **1989**, *76*, 43–49. [CrossRef] [PubMed]
55. Khalid, T.; Aggio, R.; White, P.; De Lacy Costello, B.; Persad, R.; Al-Kateb, H.; Jones, P.; Probert, C.S.; Ratcliffe, N. Urinary Volatile Organic Compounds for the Detection of Prostate Cancer. *PLoS ONE* **2015**, *10*, e0143283. [CrossRef]
56. Schöller, C.; Molin, S.; Wilkins, K. Volatile metabolites from some gram-negative bacteria. *Chemosphere* **1997**, *35*, 1487–1495. [CrossRef]
57. Garner, C.E.; Smith, S.; de Lacy Costello, B.; White, P.; Spencer, R.; Probert, C.S.; Ratcliffe, N.M. Volatile organic compounds from feces and their potential for diagnosis of gastrointestinal disease. *FASEB J.* **2007**, *21*, 1675–1688. [CrossRef]
58. Filipiak, W.; Sponring, A.; Baur, M.M.; Filipiak, A.; Ager, C.; Wiesenhofer, H.; Nagl, M.; Troppmair, J.; Amann, A. Molecular analysis of volatile metabolites released specifically by Staphylococcus aureus and Pseudomonas aeruginosa. *BMC Microbiol.* **2012**, *12*, 113. [CrossRef]
59. Pereira, J.; Porto-Figueira, P.; Cavaco, C.; Taunk, K.; Rapole, S.; Dhakne, R.; Nagarajaram, H.; Camara, J.S. Breath analysis as a potential and non-invasive frontier in disease diagnosis: An overview. *Metabolites* **2015**, *5*, 3–55. [CrossRef]
60. Preuss, R.; Angerer, J.; Drexler, H. Naphthalene—An environmental and occupational toxicant. *Int. Arch. Occup. Env. Health* **2003**, *76*, 556–576. [CrossRef]
61. Jiménez-Pacheco, A.; Salinero-Bachiller, M.; Iribar, M.C.; López-Luque, A.; Miján-Ortiz, J.L.; Peinado, J.M. Furan and p-xylene as candidate biomarkers for prostate cancer. *Urol. Oncol. Semin. Orig. Investig.* **2018**, *36*, 243.e221–243.e227. [CrossRef] [PubMed]
62. Bianchi, F.; Riboni, N.; Carbognani, P.; Gnetti, L.; Dalcanale, E.; Ampollini, L.; Careri, M. Solid-phase microextraction coupled to gas chromatography–mass spectrometry followed by multivariate data analysis for the identification of volatile organic compounds as possible biomarkers in lung cancer tissues. *J. Pharm. Biomed. Anal.* **2017**, *146*, 329–333. [CrossRef] [PubMed]

Disclaimer/Publisher's Note: The statements, opinions and data contained in all publications are solely those of the individual author(s) and contributor(s) and not of MDPI and/or the editor(s). MDPI and/or the editor(s) disclaim responsibility for any injury to people or property resulting from any ideas, methods, instructions or products referred to in the content.

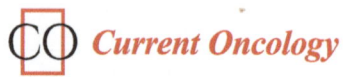

Article

Dual-Tracer PET-MRI-Derived Imaging Biomarkers for Prediction of Clinically Significant Prostate Cancer

Bernhard Grubmüller [1,2,3,4,†], Nicolai A. Huebner [1,4,†], Sazan Rasul [5], Paola Clauser [6], Nina Pötsch [6], Karl Hermann Grubmüller [2,3], Marcus Hacker [5], Sabrina Hartenbach [7], Shahrokh F. Shariat [1,8,9,10,11,12,13], Markus Hartenbach [5] and Pascal Baltzer [6,*]

1 Department of Urology, Medical University of Vienna, 1090 Vienna, Austria
2 Department of Urology and Andrology, University Hospital Krems, 3500 Krems, Austria
3 Karl Landsteiner University of Health Sciences, 3500 Krems, Austria
4 Working Group of Diagnostic Imaging in Urology, Austrian Society of Urology, 1090 Vienna, Austria
5 Department of Biomedical Imaging and Image Guided Therapy, Division of Nuclear Medicine, Medical University of Vienna, 1090 Vienna, Austria
6 Department of Biomedical Imaging and Image Guided Therapy, Division of General and Pediatric Radiology, Medical University of Vienna, 1090 Vienna, Austria
7 HistoConsultingHartenbach, 89081 Ulm, Germany
8 Comprehensive Cancer Center, Medical University of Vienna, 1090 Vienna, Austria
9 Department of Urology, Weill Medical College of Cornell University, New York, NY 10021, USA
10 Department of Urology, University of Texas Southwestern, Dallas, TX 75390, USA
11 Department of Urology, Second Faculty of Medicine, Charles University, 116 36 Prague, Czech Republic
12 Hourani Center for Applied Scientific Research, Al-Ahliyya Amman University, Amman 19328, Jordan
13 Karl Landsteiner Institute of Urology and Andrology, 1010 Vienna, Austria
* Correspondence: pascal.baltzer@meduniwien.ac.at
† These authors contributed equally to this paper.

Abstract: Purpose: To investigate if imaging biomarkers derived from 3-Tesla dual-tracer [(18)F] fluoromethylcholine (FMC) and [^{68}Ga]Ga-PSMA$^{HBED-CC}$ conjugate 11 (PSMA)-positron emission tomography can adequately predict clinically significant prostate cancer (csPC). Methods: We assessed 77 biopsy-proven PC patients who underwent 3T dual-tracer PET/mpMRI followed by radical prostatectomy (RP) between 2014 and 2017. We performed a retrospective lesion-based analysis of all cancer foci and compared it to whole-mount histopathology of the RP specimen. The primary aim was to investigate the pretherapeutic role of the imaging biomarkers FMC- and PSMA-maximum standardized uptake values (SUVmax) for the prediction of csPC and to compare it to the mpMRI-methods and PI-RADS score. Results: Overall, we identified 104 cancer foci, 69 were clinically significant (66.3%) and 35 were clinically insignificant (33.7%). We found that the combined FMC+PSMA SUVmax were the only significant parameters ($p < 0.001$ and $p = 0.049$) for the prediction of csPC. ROC analysis showed an AUC for the prediction of csPC of 0.695 for PI-RADS scoring (95% CI 0.591 to 0.786), 0.792 for FMC SUVmax (95% CI 0.696 to 0.869), 0.852 for FMC+PSMA SUVmax (95% CI 0.764 to 0.917), and 0.852 for the multivariable CHAID model (95% CI 0.763 to 0.916). Comparing the AUCs, we found that FMC+PSMA SUVmax and the multivariable model were significantly more accurate for the prediction of csPC compared to PI-RADS scoring ($p = 0.0123$, $p = 0.0253$, respectively). Conclusions: Combined FMC+PSMA SUVmax seems to be a reliable parameter for the prediction of csPC and might overcome the limitations of PI-RADS scoring. Further prospective studies are necessary to confirm these promising preliminary results.

Keywords: prostate cancer; PET/MRI; imaging biomarkers; dual tracer

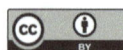

1. Introduction

Prostate cancer (PC) is among the most frequent malignancies in European men and is responsible for a significant number of cancer related deaths [1]. Nevertheless, there is evidence that a specific number of diagnosed PCs, namely "clinically insignificant" PCs (defined as ISUP grade 1), will never develop any clinical symptoms [2–4]. Indeed, many studies have consistently shown high 10-year cancer specific survival (CSS) rates of more than 90% for well-differentiated ISUP grade 1 PCs [5,6]. There is, therefore, a clinical need for accurate differentiation between "clinically significant" (defined as ISUP grade 2 or higher) (csPC) and "clinically insignificant" PCs, inducing a fundamental change in traditional diagnostic approaches [7].

Multiparametric magnetic resonance imaging (mpMRI) has, over the last years, become the most accurate local staging modality in this regard, helping in the identification of csPC. Many studies have reported a high sensitivity and specificity for both the detection and localization of csPC compared to previously used diagnostic modalities including prostate specific antigen (PSA) kinetics and standard systematic prostate biopsy [8,9].

The probability of the detection of PC with MRI-identified lesions has been standardized using the Prostate Imaging Reporting and Data System (PI-RADS) score, which has been recently updated to improve its reproducibility [10]. A published meta-analysis including 13 studies with suspected PC patients showed that the positive predictive value (PPV) for csPC with PI-RADS scores of 3, 4, and 5 were 12%, 48%, and 72%, respectively, with a high heterogeneity among the included studies [11]. This suggests that csPC can be missed with this technology due to MRI-invisible cancers, the reader's misinterpretation, and possibly technical issues during biopsy [12].

Molecular imaging and the use of specific target probes such as [(18)F]fluoromethylcholine (FMC) positron emission tomography (PET) and [^{68}Ga]Ga-PSMA$^{HBED-CC}$ conjugate 11 (PSMA)-PET promise to overcome these limitations [13,14]. In this regard, combined hybrid imaging using FMC-PET/mpMRI and PSMA-PET/mpMRI achieved very high sensitivities for detecting csPC in previously published studies, improving the diagnostic accuracy and pretherapeutic assessment of PC compared to both PET and mpMRI alone [13–15]. However, these studies were limited by their sample size, study design, and pathologic evaluation.

Therefore, our aim was to investigate if imaging biomarkers derived from the 3T dual-tracer (FMC and PSMA) PET/mpMRI can adequately predict csPC. We investigated the feasibility of pretherapeutic combined FMC- and PSMA-PET/mpMRI as the local PC staging modality and compared imaging biomarkers derived from FMC- and PSMA-PET to the mpMRI parameters and the PI-RADS score.

2. Material and Methods

2.1. Patients

This study was a retrospective analysis embedded in a prospective diagnostic trial (clinicaltrials.gov NCT02659527) including 77 consecutive patients with biopsy proven PC, who had undergone 3T dual-tracer (FMC and PSMA) PET/mpMRI followed by robotic-assisted radical prostatectomy (RP) between April 2014 and July 2017. Inclusion criteria of the aforementioned study were patients with clinical suspicion for localized prostate cancer, based on a PSA above 4.0 ng/mL and total to free PSA ratio above 22%, and/or two consecutive rising PSA values. Key exclusion criteria were previous therapy with androgen deprivation, recent prostate biopsy within 21 days, insufficient pathologic report of biopsy, or intolerance to used radiotracers. We performed a retrospective lesion-based analysis of all cancer foci within the investigated patient group and compared it to the whole-mount histopathologic RP specimen. All patients were treated with RP according to the recommendations of the guidelines. All surgical specimens were processed according to the standard pathologic procedures, staged with the AJCC TNM classification, and graded with the WHO/ISUP 2014 grading system [3] by a dedicated uro-pathologist. The primary aim of the study was to investigate the pretherapeutic role of imaging biomarkers derived from 3T dual-tracer PET/MRI (FMC- and PSMA-maximum standardized uptake values (SUVmax)) for the prediction of csPC and to compare it to the mpMRI methods (T2w, DCE, ADC) and PI-RADS score. All investigations were conducted in accordance with the Declaration of Helsinki and national regulations. The study was approved by the Ethics Committee (permit 1985/2014) and the drug authorities (EudraCT: 2014-004758-33).

2.2. Imaging Protocol and Analyses

All PET-MRI examinations were performed using a hybrid PET-MRI system (Biograph mMR, Siemens, Germany) capable of simultaneous data acquisition. The system consists of an MRI-compatible state-of-the-art PET detector integrated in a 3.0-T whole-body MRI scanner. In short, the PET detector technology relies on lutetium oxyorthosilicate scintillation crystals in combination with MRI-compatible avalanche photodiodes instead of photomultiplier tubes. The PET component uses a 3-dimensional (3D) acquisition technique and offers an axial FOV of approximately 23 cm and a transversal FOV of 45 cm. The gradient system of the MRI scanner operates with a maximum gradient strength of 45 mT/m and a slew rate of 200 T/m/s in all three axes.

Patients received dual tracer PET/MRI scans, starting with a local static 5 min emission scan with 3 MBq/kg body weight FMC and a 45 min local list mode scan immediately after the injection of 2 MBq/kg body weight PSMA intravenously. Pelvic PET acquisition in the case of FMC was started 45 min post injection of the radiotracer. While acquiring the prostate MRI sequences, PSMA was injected dynamically and acquired simultaneously in the prostate/pelvic region for 45 min using listmode acquisition.

The review of the PET/MRI images was performed separately by two experienced certified nuclear medicine physicians together with an experienced radiologist using Hermes Hybrid 3D (Hermes Medical Solutions Stockholm), while the assessment of MR images to assign PI-RADS v2.1 scores was conducted using AGFA IMPAXX EE software.

2.3. Follow-Up

Follow-up consisted of the standard follow-up after RP. In general, patients underwent physical examination and PSA testing every 3 months for the first two years, every 6 months from the second to the fifth year, then yearly.

2.4. Statistical Analyses

The primary objective of this study was the diagnostic accuracy of dual-tracer PET/MRI for csPC defined as an ISUP grade of 2 or above. Descriptive statistics of the cohort were performed. Receiver operating characteristics (ROC) analysis was used to quantify the univariable diagnostic performance using the area under the ROC curve (AUC) metric. Multivariable feature combination was modeled using the exhaustive Chi squared interaction detection (CHAID) algorithm. Minimum node size was set to 5, a minimum p-value of Bonferroni corrected 0.05 was used. Ordinally ordered terminal node categories were used to measure the multivariable model AUC in ROC analysis. The DeLong test was used to compare the AUCs, a p-value of 0.05 was considered significant. Statistical evaluation was carried out using STATA (version 14StataCorp, College Station, Texas, United States)).

3. Results

3.1. Patients

Overall, 77 patients met the inclusion criteria and were included in the study. The clinicopathologic features of patients and tumors after 3T dual-tracer PET/mpMRI followed by robotic-assisted RP are shown in Table 1. Median age was 70 at the time of RP with a median PSA of 8.1 ng/mL. Overall, 9.1%, 19.5%, 36.3%, 14.3%, and 20.8% of patients had ISUP 1, 2, 3, 4, and 5 at the time of RP, respectively. Of all the 104 cancer foci, 69 were clinically significant (66.3%) and 35 were clinically insignificant (33.7%). The median FMC SUVmax was 5 (4–6.9) and the median FMC+PSMA SUVmax was 14.3 (11.1–20.6) MBq in all of the cancer foci.

Table 1. Clinicopathologic features of 77 patients after 3T dual-tracer (FMC and PSMA) PET/mpMRI followed by robotic-assisted radical prostatectomy.

Age at RP (years), median (IQR)	70 (65–76)
PSA at RP (ng/mL), median (IQR)	8.1 (5.6–13.7)
Pathologic T staging after RP, n (%)	
2	41 (53.2)
3a	19 (24.7)
3b	17 (22.1)
Positive surgical margins, n (%)	24 (31.2)
ISUP grade on 77 RP specimen, n (%)	
1	7 (9.1)
2	15 (19.5)
3	28 (36.3)
4	11 (14.3)
5	16 (20.8)
Number of cancer foci in all 77 prostates, n (%)	104 (100)
Clinically insignificant cancer foci (ISUP 1)	35 (33.7)
Clinically significant cancer foci (≥ISUP 2),	69 (66.3)
Positive lymph nodes in histopathology, n (%)	14 (18.2)
Overall PI-RADS, n (%)	
3	2 (2.6)
4	16 (20.8)
5	59 (76.6)
FMC SUVmax of all cancer foci (MBq), median (IQR)	5 (4–6.9)
FMC + PSMA SUVmax of all cancer foci (MBq), median (IQR)	14.3 (11.1–20.6)

RP = radical prostatectomy, IQR = interquartile range, mpMRI = multiparametric magnetic resonance imaging, ISUP grade = International Society of Urological Pathology grade, FMC = fluoromethylcholine, PSMA = prostate specific membrane antigen, PI-RADS = Prostate Imaging Reporting and Data System, SUVmax = maximum standardized uptake value, MBq = megabecquerel.

3.2. Prediction of Clinically Significant Prostate Cancer

The classification and regression tree methodology including PI-RADS score, apparent diffusion coefficient (ADC), dynamic contrast enhanced imaging (DCE) curve type, FMC SUVmax, FMC+PSMA SUVmax, lesion size, and zonal location as parameters revealed that FMC SUVmax and combined FMC+PSMA SUVmax were the only significant independent contributing parameters for the prediction of csPC ($p < 0.001$ and $p = 0.049$). ROC analysis showed that the AUC for the prediction of csPC was 0.695 [standard error (SE) 0.061] for the PI-RADS score (95% CI 0.591 to 0.786), 0.755 (SE 0.055) for the ADC (95% CI 0.656 to 0.838), 0.604 (SE 0.065) for the DCE curve type (95% CI 0.498 to 0.703), 0.792 (SE 0.795) for FMC SUVmax (95% CI 0.696 to 0.869), 0.852 (SE 0.038) for FMC+PSMA SUVmax (95% CI 0.764 to 0.917), and 0.852 (SE 0.038) for the multivariable CHAID model (95% CI 0.763 to 0.916) (Figure 1). Comparing different AUCs, the FMC+PSMA SUVmax and the multivariable model were more accurate for the prediction of csPC compared to the PI-RADS score ($p = 0.0123$ and $p = 0.0253$, respectively). A rule-out csPCa criterion was exclusively present in the multivariable model, correctly identifying 10/35 (28.6%) of all non-csPCa cases while missing no csPCa.

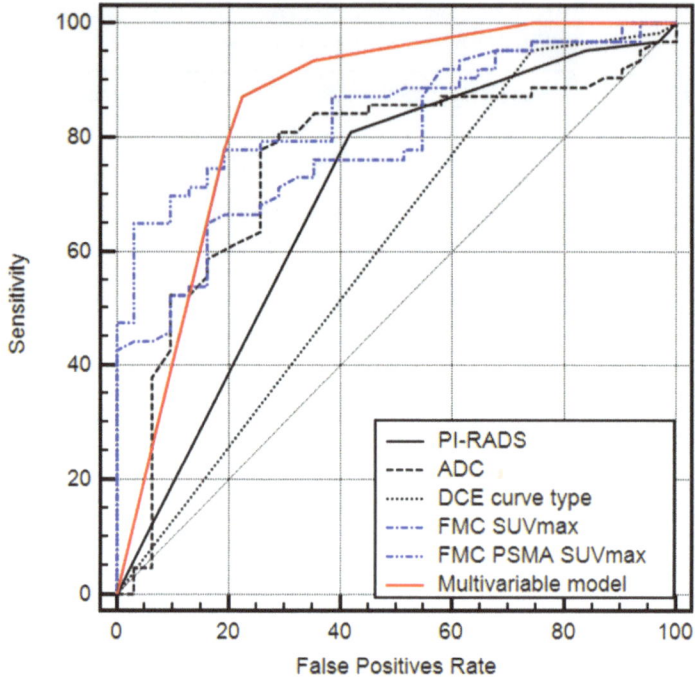

Figure 1. Receiver operating characteristic (ROC) analysis for the single parameters and the multivariable CHAID model.

4. Discussion

There were two main findings to our study. First, we found that dual-tracer molecular imaging using FMC and PSMA was better at predicting the presence of csPC than conventional mpMRI graded according to the PI-RADS classification. Second, the multivariable model showed the possibility of a rule-out criterion for csPC that correctly identified 28.6% of all insignificant cancers by imaging, without missing a single case of csPC.

The introduction of mpMRI has greatly improved the detection of prostate cancer lesions [16]. The updated PI-RADS version 2 has subsequently made the grading of lesions more uniform, which has been expanded upon by the most recent update of the PI-RADS recommendations [10]. While the implementation of mpMRI followed by ultrasound fusion biopsy as a standard of care has significantly improved cancer detection and shown the potential to reduce overdiagnosis of insignificant PC, there is still a proportion of cancers being missed on mpMRI, and there are also suspicious lesions on imaging showing insignificant PC on biopsy and whole mount pathology. Several approaches have been evaluated to improve upon the accuracy of prostate cancer diagnosis, avoid unnecessary negative biopsies, and biopsies of insignificant PC.

One of these was the evaluation of the quantitative parameters of prostate mpMRI in addition to the PI-RADS scoring system, which have previously been investigated. Polanec et al. showed that by measuring the minimum ADC-Map values in PI-RADS 4 and 5 lesions, unnecessary negative biopsy could be avoided in 33% of cases [17]. Chatterjee et al. published another study using the ADC-Map value, T2, and DCE enhancement rate as quantitative markers on a voxel by voxel basis. These quantitative risk-maps were matched to the RP specimen and could predict any cancer, csPC, defined as ISUP 2 or higher, and index lesions with an accuracy of 76.6%, 89.2%, and 100% [18]. These quantitative metrics have also been shown to be consistent over time and various scanners such as Wang et al. have published their recent results, showing good repeatability as well as reproducibility of the quantitative MRI parameters [19]. The addition of PET-based molecular imaging using different radiotracers has also shown the potential to improve upon the diagnostic accuracy of mpMRI alone. Berger et al. showed in a cohort of 50 patients undergoing RP with previous PSMA PET/MRI that with the addition of PSMA-PET, 100% of index lesions could be detected compared to 94% by MRI alone, and 93.5% vs. 51.6% of secondary cancer foci [20]. Similarly, Metser et al. also published their results, showing a significantly better diagnostic accuracy on the ROC analysis of PET/MRI vs. mpMRI (0.69 vs. 0.78; $p = 0.04$) in patients undergoing ^{18}F-DCFPyL PET/mpMR for the suspicion of csPC, using ultrasound-guided fusion biopsy as the reference [21].

Other reliable diagnostic methods of further tumor characterization are generally based on tissue analysis, thus require an invasive procedure beforehand. These tissue-based biomarkers such as the Prolaris®or Decipher®can help identify and aid in clinical decision-making in patients with insignificant PC at high risk for upgrading and clinical progression, who should consider undergoing definitive treatment, or repeat biopsy as well as favorable intermediate risk patients at low risk of progression who are good candidates for active surveillance or conservative disease management [22,23].

Some studies have also shown a correlation between genomic classifiers and imaging characteristics, in some cases even using imaging to predict genomic markers. In Hectors et al.'s analysis of 64 patients, a radiomic model of 14 features showed correlation with the genomic signatures as well as good prediction of a Decipher®score above the threshold of 0.6 with an AUC of 0.84 [24]. However, data are scarce and conflicting, oftentimes not showing any synergistic effects of combining imaging and genomic biomarkers over each individual test alone [25]. Additionally, most of the available data were gathered retrospectively, allowing in some cases, the analysis of MRI-invisible PC lesions gnomically, but this would not be the case in clinical routine, as invisible lesions would not, or only by chance, be biopsied. For this reason, the simultaneous improvement in the detection as well as ideally non-invasive tumor classification would be of great benefit for patients and clinicians treating PC.

In combining two molecular imaging tracers, knowing PSMAs but also to a degree, FMCs beneficial role in the detection of PC, we evaluated whether we could not only improve sensitivity, but further improve upon non-invasive tumor characterization. In our study, this was in fact the case, as the combined SUVmax of FMC and PSMA not only showed the best accuracy on the ROC analysis for the prediction of csPC, it also allowed for a rule-out criterion of csPC when implemented into a multivariable model, potentially allowing patients to forgo prostate biopsy, even in the case of suspicious lesions on mpMRI, and be directly entered into a program of surveillance, if proven in a larger prospective cohort. Additionally this has multiple potential uses during the follow-up of patients on active surveillance, as a confirmatory test in patients already diagnosed with low-risk PC as well as a form of longitudinal imaging follow-up in patients with elevated PSA and suspicious mpMRI. While this might seem to be very resource demanding, it is worth noting that tissue-based genomic biomarkers, which are becoming more widely available and used in patients on active surveillance, are within a very similar range of associated cost, as an instance of molecular imaging in many health care systems, while imaging retains the advantage of being a non-invasive diagnostic technique. Additionally, as multiple tracers can be applied simultaneously, the amount of time needed for such an examination is only increased marginally, depending on the tracers.

The combination of two radiotracers in molecular imaging has also shown proficiency, even in prospective studies, when guiding treatment decisions. Hofman et al. used the combination of PSMA and 2-flourine-18[18F]fluoro-2-deoxy-D-glucose (FDG) in their trial evaluating [^{177}Lu]Lutetium-PSMA-617 as a therapy in advanced metastatic castration resistant PC (mCRPC) [26]. Patients with discordant results on imaging, showing FDG positive and PSMA negative lesions, or patients with very low PSMA expression were excluded from the study. This combination imaging was chosen due to the higher sensitivity, but it also allowed for tumor characterization. As described in another study, patients with discordant lesions represent a cohort of patients with very poor prognosis as these lesions tend to harbor de-differentiated PC cells, without PSMA expression, which are in most cases not suitable for radionuclide treatment and have grown resistant to most conventional PC therapies [27]. We chose the combination of PSMA and FMC in the setting of primary cancer, again, to improve the sensitivity, and allow for the identification of possible low risk cancers.

The biggest limitation of this study is its retrospective design. While the database was maintained prospectively as part of a prospective trial, this was a retrospective analysis. Furthermore, the cohort was already scheduled for RP, so it does not represent a normally distributed cohort of primary PC patients. Additionally, only patients with proven PC were included within this analysis, thus we cannot make any assumptions about the impact of dual-tracer PET/MRI in cancer detection overall or sensitivity in a biopsy naïve cohort, and we could only calculate the prediction of csPC on the RP specimen in patients with a previous positive biopsy. We did not perform any calculations on the survival outcomes such as PC recurrence, as this would not have been feasible with a cohort of this size and relatively short follow-up. Furthermore, the single center approach precludes robust estimates of the reproducibility and repeatability of the method.

5. Conclusions

This study demonstrated that combined FMC+PSMA SUVmax in preoperative 3T dual-tracer PET/mpMRI seems to be a reliable parameter for the prediction of csPC and might overcome the limitations of MRI parameters and the interpretation according to the PI-RADS score. Further studies with bigger cohorts and a prospective randomized nature are necessary to confirm these promising but preliminary results.

Author Contributions: All authors contributed to the conception of the study. Data collection, imaging, and pathology review were performed by B.G., N.A.H., S.R., P.C., S.H., M.H. (Markus Hartenbach) and P.B.; Statistics were performed by B.G., N.A.H., and P.B. Statistics and data were reviewed by N.P., K.H.G., M.H. (Marcus Hacker) and S.F.S. The first manuscript was written by B.G., N.A.H. and P.B. All authors have made remarks and changes to the manuscript. All authors have read and agreed to the published version of the manuscript.

Funding: This research received no external funding.

Institutional Review Board Statement: This study was approved by the ethics committee of the Medical University of Vienna (permit 1985/2014). All procedures performed in this study were in accordance with the ethical standards of the institutional research committee and with the 1964 Declaration of Helsinki and its later amendments. Informed consent was obtained from all of the individual participants included in the study, and all participants also consented to the publication of the results.

Informed Consent Statement: Informed consent was obtained from all subjects involved in the study.

Data Availability Statement: The complete dataset used for this analysis is available in a pseudonymized fashion upon request, and after acquisition of IRB approval as well as data sharing agreements between institutions.

Conflicts of Interest: The authors declare no conflict of interest.

References

1. Ferlay, J.; Colombet, M.; Soerjomataram, I.; Dyba, T.; Randi, G.; Bettio, M.; Gavin, A.; Visser, O.; Bray, F. Cancer incidence and mortality patterns in Europe: Estimates for 40 countries and 25 major cancers in 2018. *Eur. J. Cancer* **2018**, *103*, 356–387. [CrossRef] [PubMed]
2. Matoso, A.; Epstein, J.I. Defining clinically significant prostate cancer on the basis of pathological findings. *Histopathology* **2019**, *74*, 135–145. [CrossRef] [PubMed]
3. Epstein, J.I.; Egevad, L.; Amin, M.B.; Delahunt, B.; Srigley, J.R.; Humphrey, P.A. The 2014 International Society of Urological Pathology (ISUP) Consensus Conference on Gleason Grading of Prostatic Carcinoma. *Am. J. Surg. Pathol.* **2016**, *40*, 244–252. [CrossRef] [PubMed]

4. Mottet, N.; van den Bergh, R.C.; Briers, E.; Van den Broeck, T.; Cumberbatch, M.G.; De Santis, M.; Fanti, S.; Fossati, N.; Gandaglia, G.; Gillessen, S.; et al. EAU-EANM-ESTRO-ESUR-SIOG Guidelines on Prostate Cancer—2020 Update. Part 1: Screening, Diagnosis, and Local Treatment with Curative Intent. *Eur. Urol.* **2020**, *79*, 243–262. [CrossRef]
5. Hayes, J.H.; Ollendorf, D.A.; Pearson, S.D.; Barry, M.J.; Kantoff, P.; Lee, P.A.; McMahon, P.M. Observation Versus Initial Treatment for Men With Localized, Low-Risk Prostate Cancer: A Cost-Effectiveness Analysis. *Ann. Intern. Med.* **2013**, *158*, 853. [CrossRef]
6. Lu-Yao, G.L.; Albertsen, P.C.; Moore, D.F.; Shih, W.; Lin, Y.; DiPaola, R.S.; Barry, M.J.; Zietman, A.; O'Leary, M.; Walker-Corkery, E.; et al. Outcomes of Localized Prostate Cancer Following Conservative Management. *JAMA* **2009**, *302*, 1202–1209. [CrossRef]
7. Ali, A.; Hoyle, A.; Baena, E.; Clarke, N.W. Identification and evaluation of clinically significant prostate cancer. *Curr. Opin. Urol.* **2017**, *27*, 217–224. [CrossRef]
8. Johnson, D.C.; Raman, S.S.; Mirak, S.A.; Kwan, L.; Bajgiran, A.M.; Hsu, W.; Maehara, C.K.; Ahuja, P.; Faiena, I.; Pooli, A.; et al. Detection of Individual Prostate Cancer Foci via Multiparametric Magnetic Resonance Imaging. *Eur. Urol.* **2019**, *75*, 712–720. [CrossRef]
9. Drost, F.H.; Osses, D.F.; Nieboer, D.; Steyerberg, E.W.; Bangma, C.H.; Roobol, M.J.; Schoots, I.G. Prostate MRI, with or without MRI-targeted biopsy, and systematic biopsy for detecting prostate cancer. *Cochrane Database Syst. Rev.* **2019**, *4*, CD012663. [CrossRef]
10. Turkbey, B.; Rosenkrantz, A.B.; Haider, M.A.; Padhani, A.R.; Villeirs, G.; Macura, K.J.; Tempany, C.M.; Choyke, P.L.; Cornud, F.; Margolis, D.J.; et al. Prostate Imaging Reporting and Data System Version 2.1: 2019 Update of Prostate Imaging Reporting and Data System Version 2. *Eur. Urol.* **2019**, *76*, 340–351. [CrossRef]
11. Barkovich, E.J.; Shankar, P.R.; Westphalen, A.C. A Systematic Review of the Existing Prostate Imaging Reporting and Data System Version 2 (PI-RADSv2) Literature and Subset Meta-Analysis of PI-RADSv2 Categories Stratified by Gleason Scores. *Am. J. Roentgenol.* **2019**, *212*, 847–854. [CrossRef] [PubMed]
12. Mehralivand, S.; Shih, J.H.; Rais-Bahrami, S.; Oto, A.; Bednarova, S.; Nix, J.W.; Thomas, J.V.; Gordetsky, J.B.; Gaur, S.; Harmon, S.A.; et al. A Magnetic Resonance Imaging–Based Prediction Model for Prostate Biopsy Risk Stratification. *JAMA Oncol.* **2018**, *4*, 678. [CrossRef] [PubMed]
13. Hartenbach, M.; Hartenbach, S.; Bechtloff, W.; Danz, B.; Kraft, K.; Klemenz, B.; Sparwasser, C.; Hacker, M. Combined PET/MRI improves diagnostic accuracy in patients with prostate cancer: A prospective diagnostic trial. *Clin. Cancer Res.* **2014**, *20*, 3244–3253. [CrossRef] [PubMed]
14. Grubmüller, B.; Baltzer, P.; Hartenbach, S.; D'Andrea, D.; Helbich, T.H.; Haug, A.R.; Goldner, G.M.; Wadsak, W.; Pfaff, S.; Mitterhauser, M.; et al. PSMA Ligand PET/MRI for Primary Prostate Cancer: Staging Performance and Clinical Impact. *Clin. Cancer Res.* **2018**, *24*, 6300–6307. [CrossRef] [PubMed]
15. EEiber, M.; Weirich, G.; Holzapfel, K.; Souvatzoglou, M.; Haller, B.; Rauscher, I.; Beer, A.J.; Wester, H.-J.; Gschwend, J.; Schwaiger, M.; et al. Simultaneous 68Ga-PSMA HBED-CC PET/MRI Improves the Localization of Primary Prostate Cancer. *Eur. Urol.* **2016**, *70*, 829–836. [CrossRef]
16. Ahmed, H.U.; El-Shater Bosaily, A.; Brown, L.C.; Gabe, R.; Kaplan, R.; Parmar, M.K.; Collaco-Moraes, Y.; Ward, K.; Hindley, R.G.; Freeman, A.; et al. Diagnostic accuracy of multi-parametric MRI and TRUS biopsy in prostate cancer (PROMIS): A paired validating confirmatory study. *Lancet* **2017**, *389*, 815–822. [CrossRef]
17. Polanec, S.H.; Helbich, T.H.; Bickel, H.; Wengert, G.J.; Pinker, K.; Spick, C.; Clauser, P.; Susani, M.; Shariat, S.; Baltzer, P.A. Quantitative Apparent Diffusion Coefficient Derived From Diffusion-Weighted Imaging Has the Potential to Avoid Unnecessary MRI-Guided Biopsies of mpMRI-Detected PI-RADS 4 and 5 Lesions. *Investig. Radiol.* **2018**, *53*, 736–741. [CrossRef]
18. Chatterjee, A.; He, D.; Fan, X.; Antic, T.; Jiang, Y.; Eggener, S.; Karczmar, G.S.; Oto, A. Diagnosis of Prostate Cancer by Use of MRI-Derived Quantitative Risk Maps: A Feasibility Study. *Am. J. Roentgenol.* **2019**, *213*, W66–W75. [CrossRef]
19. Wang, Y.; Tadimalla, S.; Rai, R.; Goodwin, J.; Foster, S.; Liney, G.; Holloway, L.; Haworth, A. Quantitative MRI: Defining repeatability, reproducibility and accuracy for prostate cancer imaging biomarker development. *Magn. Reson. Imaging* **2021**, *77*, 169–179. [CrossRef]
20. Berger, I.; Annabattula, C.; Lewis, J.; Shetty, D.V.; Kam, J.; MacLean, F.; Arianayagam, M.; Canagasingham, B.; Ferguson, R.; Khadra, M.; et al. 68Ga-PSMA PET/CT vs. mpMRI for locoregional prostate cancer staging: Correlation with final histopathology. *Prostate Cancer Prostatic Dis.* **2018**, *21*, 204–211. [CrossRef]
21. Metser, U.; Ortega, C.; Perlis, N.; Lechtman, E.; Berlin, A.; Anconina, R.; Eshet, Y.; Chan, R.; Veit-Haibach, P.; van der Kwast, T.H.; et al. Detection of clinically significant prostate cancer with 18F-DCFPyL PET/multiparametric MR. *Eur. J. Nucl. Med. Mol. Imaging* **2021**, *48*, 3702–3711. [CrossRef] [PubMed]
22. Jairath, N.K.; Pra, A.D.; Vince, R.; Dess, R.T.; Jackson, W.C.; Tosoian, J.J.; McBride, S.M.; Zhao, S.G.; Berlin, A.; Mahal, B.A.; et al. A Systematic Review of the Evidence for the Decipher Genomic Classifier in Prostate Cancer. *Eur. Urol.* **2020**, *79*, 374–383. [CrossRef] [PubMed]
23. Sommariva, S.; Tarricone, R.; Lazzeri, M.; Ricciardi, W.; Montorsi, F. Prognostic Value of the Cell Cycle Progression Score in Patients with Prostate Cancer: A Systematic Review and Meta-analysis. *Eur. Urol.* **2016**, *69*, 107–115. [CrossRef] [PubMed]
24. Hectors, S.; Cherny, M.; Yadav, K.K.; Beksaç, A.T.; Thulasidass, H.; Lewis, S.; Davicioni, E.; Wang, P.; Tewari, A.K.; Taouli, B. Radiomics Features Measured with Multiparametric Magnetic Resonance Imaging Predict Prostate Cancer Aggressiveness. *J. Urol.* **2019**, *202*, 498–505. [CrossRef] [PubMed]

25. Jambor, I.; Falagario, U.; Ratnani, P.; Msc, I.M.P.; Demir, K.; Merisaari, H.; Sobotka, S.; Haines, G.K.; Martini, A.; Beksac, A.T.; et al Prediction of biochemical recurrence in prostate cancer patients who underwent prostatectomy using routine clinical prostate multiparametric MRI and decipher genomic score. *J. Magn. Reson. Imaging* **2020**, *51*, 1075–1085. [CrossRef]
26. Hofman, M.S.; Emmett, L.; Sandhu, S.; Iravani, A.; Joshua, A.M.; Goh, J.C.; Pattison, D.A.; Tan, T.H.; Kirkwood, I.D.; Ng, S.; et al [177Lu]Lu-PSMA-617 versus cabazitaxel in patients with metastatic castration-resistant prostate cancer (TheraP): A randomised, open-label, phase 2 trial. *Lancet* **2021**, *397*, 797–804. [CrossRef]
27. Thang, S.P.; Violet, J.; Sandhu, S.; Iravani, A.; Akhurst, T.; Kong, G.; Kumar, A.R.; Murphy, D.G.; Williams, S.G.; Hicks, R.J.; et al Poor Outcomes for Patients with Metastatic Castration-resistant Prostate Cancer with Low Prostate-specific Membrane Antigen (PSMA) Expression Deemed Ineligible for 177Lu-labelled PSMA Radioligand Therapy. *Eur. Urol. Oncol.* **2019**, *2*, 670–676. [CrossRef]

Disclaimer/Publisher's Note: The statements, opinions and data contained in all publications are solely those of the individual author(s) and contributor(s) and not of MDPI and/or the editor(s). MDPI and/or the editor(s) disclaim responsibility for any injury to people or property resulting from any ideas, methods, instructions or products referred to in the content.

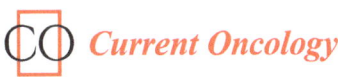

Review

An Updated Systematic and Comprehensive Review of Cytoreductive Prostatectomy for Metastatic Prostate Cancer

Takafumi Yanagisawa [1,2], Pawel Rajwa [1,3], Tatsushi Kawada [1,4], Kensuke Bekku [1,4], Ekaterina Laukhtina [1,5], Markus von Deimling [1,6], Muhammad Majdoub [1,7], Marcin Chlosta [1,8], Pierre I. Karakiewicz [9], Axel Heidenreich [1,10], Takahiro Kimura [2] and Shahrokh F. Shariat [1,5,11,12,13,14,15,*]

1. Department of Urology, Comprehensive Cancer Center, Medical University of Vienna, Wahringer Gurtel 18-20, 1090 Vienna, Austria
2. Department of Urology, The Jikei University School of Medicine, Tokyo 105-8461, Japan
3. Department of Urology, Medical University of Silesia, 41-800 Zabrze, Poland
4. Department of Urology, Okayama University Graduate School of Medicine, Dentistry and Pharmaceutical Sciences, Okayama 700-8530, Japan
5. Institute for Urology and Reproductive Health, Sechenov University, 119435 Moscow, Russia
6. Department of Urology, University Medical Center Hamburg-Eppendorf, 20251 Hamburg, Germany
7. Department of Urology, Hillel Yaffe Medical Center, 169, Hadera 38100, Israel
8. Clinic of Urology and Urological Oncology, Jagiellonian University, 30-688 Krakow, Poland
9. Cancer Prognostics and Health Outcomes Unit, Division of Urology, University of Montreal Health Center, Montreal, QC H2X 0A9, Canada
10. Department of Urology, Faculty of Medicine and University Hospital of Cologne, 50937 Cologne, Germany
11. Division of Urology, Department of Special Surgery, The University of Jordan, Amman 19328, Jordan
12. Department of Urology, University of Texas Southwestern Medical Center, Dallas, TX 75390, USA
13. Department of Urology, Second Faculty of Medicine, Charles University, 15006 Prague, Czech Republic
14. Department of Urology, Weill Cornell Medical College, New York, NY 10021, USA
15. Karl Landsteiner Institute of Urology and Andrology, 1090 Vienna, Austria
* Correspondence: shahrokh.shariat@meduniwien.ac.at; Tel.: +43-14040026150; Fax: +43-14040023320

Abstract: (1) Background: Local therapy is highly promising in a multimodal approach strategy for patients with low-volume metastatic prostate cancer (mPCa). We aimed to systematically assess and summarize the safety, oncologic, and functional outcomes of cytoreductive prostatectomy (cRP) in mPCa. (2) Methods: Three databases were queried in September 2022 for publications that analyzed mPCa patients treated with cytoreductive prostatectomy without restrictions. The outcomes of interest were progression-free survival (PFS), cancer-specific survival (CSS), overall survival (OS), perioperative complication rates, and functional outcomes following cRP. (3) Results: Overall, 26 studies were included in this systematic review. Among eight population-based studies, cRP was associated with a reduced risk of CSS and OS compared with no local therapy (NLT) after adjusting for the effects of possible confounders. Furthermore, one population-based study showed that cRP reduced the risk of CSS even when compared with radiotherapy (RT) of the prostate after adjusting for the effects of possible confounders. In addition, one randomized controlled trial (RCT) demonstrated that local therapy (comprising 85% of cRP) significantly improved the prostate-specific antigen (PSA)-PFS and OS. Overall, cRP had acceptable perioperative complication rates and functional outcomes. (4) Conclusions: Mounting evidence suggests that cRP offers promising oncological and functional outcomes and technical feasibility and that it is associated with limited complications. Well-designed RCTs that limit selection bias in patients treated with cRP are warranted.

Keywords: metastatic prostate cancer; prostatectomy; cytoreductive prostatectomy; local therapy

Citation: Yanagisawa, T.; Rajwa, P.; Kawada, T.; Bekku, K.; Laukhtina, E.; Deimling, M.v.; Majdoub, M.; Chlosta, M.; Karakiewicz, P.I.; Heidenreich, A.; et al. An Updated Systematic and Comprehensive Review of Cytoreductive Prostatectomy for Metastatic Prostate Cancer. *Curr. Oncol.* **2023**, *30*, 2194–2216. https://doi.org/10.3390/curroncol30020170

Received: 30 December 2022
Revised: 8 February 2023
Accepted: 8 February 2023
Published: 10 February 2023

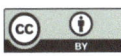

Copyright: © 2023 by the authors. Licensee MDPI, Basel, Switzerland. This article is an open access article distributed under the terms and conditions of the Creative Commons Attribution (CC BY) license (https://creativecommons.org/licenses/by/4.0/).

1. Introduction

The management of metastatic hormone-sensitive prostate cancer (mHSPC) has transformed during the past decade owing to the emergence of combination systemic therapies, such as androgen receptor signaling inhibitor and/or docetaxel plus androgen deprivation therapy (ADT) [1–6]. Further, mHSPC is a heterogeneous disease entity with varied prognoses. Tumor burden stratified as low- vs. high-volume disease (defined as the presence of visceral metastases, or four or more bone metastases, of which at least one must be located outside the vertebral column or pelvic bone) on the basis of the definition of the CHAARTED trial has been shown to stratify mHSPC into different risk categories [4,6–11]. For mHSPC patients with low-volume disease, local destructive therapy for primary prostate cancer and metastasis-directed therapy have gained widespread use [12]. For example, the STAMPEDE trial showed an OS benefit by delivering radiation therapy (RT) to the prostate in mHSPC patients treated with a standard of care for low-volume disease [13]. Since then, there has been increasing interest in local therapy (LT) as a part of the treatment strategy for mHSPC to ensure durability in efficacy and quality of life (i.e., local progression prevention). In addition to RT, cytoreductive prostatectomy (cRP) has been used in this setting. A previous meta-analysis based on population-based studies demonstrated the OS benefit of cRP even in mHSPC patients, including both low- and high-volume diseases [14]. Despite this, there are several limitations in the methodology of the published literature, primarily owing to heterogeneity in the included studies and patient selection [14–16]. One such factor is the even-increasing heterogeneity in the low-volume mHSPC group. On the basis of the increasing implementation of prostate-specific membrane antigen (PSMA)–positron emission tomography (PET) scans in clinical practice, an increasing number of oligometastatic patients with mHSPC are being identified [17]. Therefore, we conducted this systematic and comprehensive review to update and assess the safety, oncologic, and functional outcomes in mHSPC patients who underwent cRP.

2. Materials and Methods

The protocol has been registered in the International Prospective Register of Systematic Reviews database (PROSPERO: CRD42022368246).

2.1. Search Strategy

This systematic review was carried out according to the guidelines of the Preferred Reporting Items for Meta-Analyses of Observational Studies in Epidemiology Statement (Supplementary Figure S1) [18]. A literature search on the PubMed, Web of Science, and Scopus databases was performed in September 2022 to identify studies investigating the perioperative, oncologic, or functional outcomes of cRP for mPCa. The detailed search strategy was as follows: (metastatic) AND (prostate cancer) AND (prostatectomy) OR (cytoreductive). The primary outcomes of interest were overall survival (OS) and cancer-specific survival (CSS), and the secondary outcomes of interest were progression-free survival (PFS), perioperative outcomes, and urinary and erectile functional outcomes. The initial screening based on the titles and abstracts aimed to identify eligible studies and was performed by two investigators. Potentially relevant studies were subjected to a full-text review. Disagreements were resolved by consensus with the coauthors.

2.2. Inclusion and Exclusion Criteria

Studies were included if they investigated metastatic PCa (mPCa) patients (patients), who underwent cRP (interventions) compared with those treated with RT or without LT (comparisons), to assess the differential oncologic, perioperative, and functional outcomes (outcome) in randomized controlled studies (RCTs) and in nonrandomized, observational, population-based, or cohort studies (Study design). We excluded studies that compared the differential outcomes of LT vs. non-LT (NLT), not separately reporting the outcomes of cRP or RT unless more than 80% of patients treated with LT were cRP. Studies lacking original patient data, reviews, letters, editorial comments, replies from authors, case reports, and articles not written in English were excluded. References of all papers included were scanned for additional studies of interest.

2.3. Data Extraction

Two authors independently extracted the following data: the first author's name, publication year, country, inclusion criteria, number of patients, follow-up duration, age, performance status or comorbidity, clinical stage, biopsy Gleason score (GS), pretreatment of prostate-specific antigen (PSA), metastatic site, surgical approach of cRP, lymph node dissection (LND) and number of removed lymph nodes (LNs), estimated blood loss, operation time, catheterization periods, length of hospital stay, all and severe (≥Clavien-Dindo classification III) postoperative complication rates, positive surgical margin (PSM), LN involvement, pathologic stage, GS in the resected specimen, continence rates, erectile function, patient-reported quality of life (QOL), OS, CSS, PFS, time to castration-resistant prostate cancer (CRPC), and CRPC-free survival. Subsequently, the hazard ratios (HRs) and 95% confidence intervals (CIs) from Cox regression models for OS and CSS were retrieved. All discrepancies were resolved by consensus with the coauthors.

2.4. Risk-of-Bias Assessment

The study quality and risk of bias were assessed according to the Risk of Bias in Non-randomized Studies of Interventions (ROBINS-I) tool and the risk-of-bias (RoB version2), referring to the Cochrane Handbook for Systematic Reviews of Interventions [18]. Each bias domain and the overall risk of bias were judged as 'low', 'moderate', 'serious' or 'critical'. The presence of possible confounders was determined by consensus and a literature review. The ROBINS-I and risk-of-bias assessment of each study were independently conducted by two authors (Supplementary Figure S2 and Table S1).

3. Results

3.1. Study Selection and Characteristics

Our initial search identified 6980 records. After removing duplicates, 4110 records remained for screening titles and abstracts (Figure 1). After screening, a full-text review of 142 articles was performed. According to our inclusion criteria, we finally identified 27 studies eligible for systematic review [19–45]. The demographics of each included study are shown in Tables 1 and 2. Of the 27 studies, 9 were population-based designs, 11 were comparative (including case-control cohorts and RCTs), and seven included only cRP patients. This section may be divided by subheadings. It should provide a concise and precise description of the experimental results, their interpretation, and the experimental conclusions that can be drawn.

3.2. Oncologic Outcomes

3.2.1. Population-Based Studies

We identified seven studies by using the Surveillance, Epidemiology, and End Results (SEER) database and one study each by using the Munich Cancer Registry database and the National Cancer Database (NCDB). SEER and NCDB reflect the real-world survival data of patients diagnosed with mPCa in the US. However, variables unavailable from SEER, such as patient performance status, comorbidity, and metastatic burden (i.e., including both high- and low-volume disease), undoubtedly limited the granularity and generalizability of the analyses and precluded controlling for the often-existent selection bias [20]. Patient demographics of included population-based studies are summarized in Supplementary Table S2.

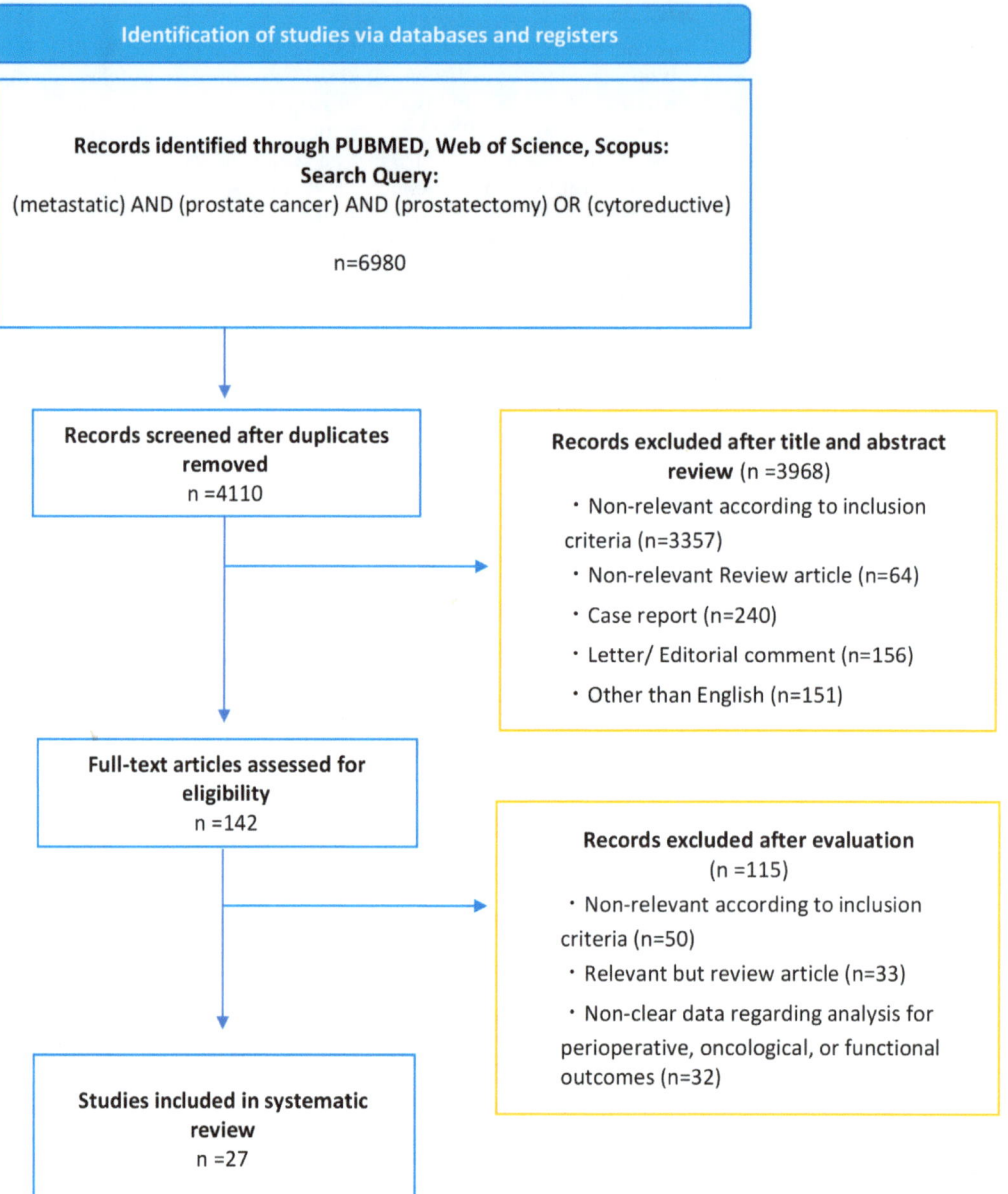

Figure 1. The Preferred Reporting Items for Systematic Reviews and Meta-analyses (PRISMA) flow chart, detailing the article-selection process.

Table 1. Demographics and oncologic outcomes of population-based study.

Author	Year	Comparisons	No. of Patients	Recruitment Year	Inclusion Criteria	Confounders for Matching	Follow-Up	Cancer-Specific Mortality	Overall Mortality
Culp et al. [20] (SEER)	2014	NLI	7811	2004–2010	Stage IV (M1a-c) PCa (adenocarcinoma) at diagnosis identified using SEER and divided on the basis of definitive treatment of the RP or BT or NLI	ND	Median: 16 mo. (IQR: 7–31)	5-yearCSS: 48.7%	5-year OS: 22.5% (95% CI: 21.1–23.9)
		cRP	245					5-yearCSS: 75.8%	5-year OS: 67.4% (95% CI: 58.7–74.7)
		BT	129					5-yearCSS: 61.3%	5-year OS: 52.6% (95% CI: 39.8–63.9)
Gratzke et al. [21] (Munich Cancer Registry)	2014	NLI	1075	1998–2010	ND	ND	ND	ND	5-year OS: 21%
		cRP	74						5-year OS: 55%
		RT	389						ND
Antwi et al. [19] (SEER)	2014	NLI	7516	2004–2010	Stage IV (M1a-c) PCa (adenocarcinoma) at diagnosis identified using SEER and divided on the basis of definitive treatment of the RP or BT or NLI	Age, race, marital status, tumor grade, PSA level, and cancer registry	ND	Reference	Reference
		cRP	222					Adjusted HR: 0.28 (95% CI: 0.20–0.39)	Adjusted HR: 0.27 (95% CI: 0.20–0.38)
		BT	120					Adjusted HR: 0.46 (95% CI: 0.33–0.64)	Adjusted HR: 0.43 (95% CI: 0.31–0.59)
Satkunasivam et al. [26] (SEER)	2015	NLI	3827	2004–2009	Stage IV (M1a-c) PCa (adenocarcinoma) at diagnosis identified using SEER and divided on the basis of definitive treatment of the RP or IMRT or CRT or NLI. Included only patients > age 65 years	Age at diagnosis, diagnosis year, race, marital status, pretreatment PSA (categorical variable), clinical tumor stage and grade, CCI, ADT, and bone radiation within 6 months of diagnosis	Median: 20 mo. (IQR: 10–36)	3-year CSS: 46%	3-year OS: 34% Reference
		cRP	47					3-year CSS: 79% Adjusted HR: 0.48 (95% CI: 0.27–0.85)	3-year OS: 73% Adjusted HR: 0.43 (95% CI: 0.26–0.70)
		IMRT	88					3-year CSS: 82% Adjusted HR: 0.38 (95% CI: 0.24–0.61)	3-year OS: 72% Adjusted HR: 0.45 (95% CI: 0.31–0.65)
		CRT	107					3-year CSS: 49% Adjusted HR: 0.85 (95% CI: 0.64–1.14)	3-year OS: 37% ND
Parikh et al. [25] (NCDB)	2017	NLI	5224	2004–2013	Stage IV (M1a-c) PCa (adenocarcinoma) at diagnosis identified using NCDB and divided on the basis of definitive treatment of the RP or IMRT or CRT or NLI	Race, age, CCI score, T-stage, N-stage, insurance stattus, income quartile, facility type, and use of ADT	Median: 22 mo.	ND	5-year OS: 17.1% Reference
		cRP	622						5-year OS: 51.4% Adjusted HR: 0.51 (95% CI: 0.45–0.59)
		CRT	153						Adjusted HR: 1.04 (95% CI: 0.86–1.27)
		IMRT	52						5-year OS: 26.8% Adjusted HR: 0.47 (95% CI: 0.31–0.72)

Table 1. Cont.

Author	Year	Comparisons	No. of Patients	Recruitment Year	Inclusion Criteria	Confounders for Matching	Follow-Up	Cancer-Specific Mortality	Overall Mortality
Jin S et al. [24] (SEER)	2020	NLT	5628	2010–2014	Stage IV (M1a-c) PCa (adenocarcinoma) at diagnosis identified using SEER and divided on the basis of definitive treatment of the RP or BT or NLT	ND	ND	Reference	Reference
		cRP	159					Adjusted HR: 0.56 (95% CI: 0.37–0.86)	Adjusted HR: 0.60 (95% CI: 0.42–0.87)
		BT	62					Adjusted HR: 0.71 (95% CI: 0.43–1.18)	Adjusted HR: 0.72 (95% CI: 0.46–1.14)
Jin K et al. [23] (SEER)	2020	NLT	18,857	2004–2015	Stage IV (M1a-c) PCa (adenocarcinoma) at diagnosis identified using SEER and divided on the basis of definitive treatment of the RP or RT or NLT. Patients who received EBRT with unknown region were excluded	marital status, race, age, clinical TNM stages, GS, and PSA level	ND	Reference	Reference
		cRP	435					Adjusted HR (Cox regression): 0.61 (95% CI: 0.42–0.91) Adjusted HR (PSM): 0.49 (95% CI: 0.32–0.73)	Adjusted HR (Cox regression): 0.60 (95% CI: 0.43–0.83) Adjusted HR (PSM): 0.45 (95% CI: 0.32–0.65)
		RT	320					Adjusted HR (Cox regression): 0.39 (95% CI: 0.34–0.45) Adjusted HR (PSM): 0.50 (95% CI: 0.41–0.60) Adjusted HR (Covariate adjustment PS): 0.57 (95% CI: 0.49–0.66)	Adjusted HR (Cox regression): 0.39 (95% CI: 0.35–0.44) Adjusted HR (PSM): 0.51 (95% CI: 0.44–0.60) Adjusted HR (Covariate adjustment PS): 0.57 (95% CI: 0.50–0.65)
Guo et al. [22] (SEER)	2021	cRP	481 (148) *	2004–2016	Stage IV (M1a-c) PCa (adenocarcinoma) at diagnosis identified using SEER and divided on the basis of definitive treatment of the RP or RT. Patients with incomplete clinicopathological data, such as T-stage, PSA value, and GS were excluded	Age, year of diagnosis, PSA level, clinical tumor stage, biopsy GS, and the M stage	Median (IQR): 37 mo. (14.0–83.5)	10-year CSS: 73.8% Adjusted HR (PSM): 0.77 (95% CI: 0.46–1.30) Adjusted HR (SMRW): 0.83 (95% CI: 0.52–1.32)	10-year OS: 60.8% Adjusted HR (PSM): 0.73 (95% CI: 0.48–1.11) Adjusted HR (SMRW): 0.75 (95% CI: 0.52–1.09)
		RT	203 (148) *				Median (IQR): 56.5 mo. (18.0–110.0)	10-year CSS: 66.7% Reference	10-year OS: 45.6% Reference

Table 1. Cont.

Author	Year	Comparisons	No. of Patients	Recruitment Year	Inclusion Criteria	Confounders for Matching	Follow-Up	Cancer-Specific Mortality		Overall Mortality
Stolzenbach et al. [27] (SEER)	2021	cRP	954	2004–2016	Stage IV (M1a-b) PCa (adenocarcinoma) at diagnosis identified using SEER and divided on the basis of definitive treatment of the RP or RT. On the basis of the composition of the STAMPEDE trial and on the basis of the definition of low-volume mPCa, M1c patients were excluded	Age at diagnosis, initial PSA, biopsy GGG, and clinical T, N and M1 stages	Median (range): 23 mo. (11–46)	PSM cohort 5-year CSM: 47% ($p = 0.003$)	Adjusted HR (PSM and CRR): 0.79 (95% CI: 0.68–0.90)	ND
		RT	3326				Median (range): 21 mo. (10–42)	PSM cohort 5-year CSM: 53% ($p = 0.003$)	Reference	ND

No.: number, Pts.: patients, NCDB: National Cancer Database, SEER; surveillance, epidemiology and end results, LT; local therapy, NLT: no local therapy, RT; radiotherapy, EBRT; external beam radiotherapy, BT; brachytherapy, IMRT; intensity-modulated radiotherapy, CRT; conformal radiation therapy, PS; propensity score, PSM; propensity-score matching, CRR; competing risks regression, SMRW; standardized mortality ratio weighting, cRP; cytoreductive radical prostatectomy, IQR; interquartile range, NA; not applicable, ND; No data, PSA; prostate-specific antigen, GS; Gleason score, GGG: Gleason grade group, CSS; cancer-specific survival, CSM; cancer-specific mortality, ACM; all-cause mortality, OS; overall survival, HR; hazard ratio, CI; confidence interval, PCa; prostate cancer, CCI; Charlson comorbidity index. * Described as number of PSM cohorts.

Table 2. Study demographics and oncologic outcomes of cohort studies.

Author	Year	Comparisons	No. of pts.	Recruitment Year	Country (Institution)	Inclusion Criteria	Treatment after cRP	Follow-Up Duration	Progression-Free	Time to CRPC/CRPC-Free Survival	Cancer-Specific Survival	Overall Survival
						Comparative studies between cRP and no cRP						
Heidenreich et al. [33]	2015	cRP	23	ND	Germany	Patients with biopsy-proven PCa, minimal bone metastases (3 or fewer hot spots on bone scan), absence of visceral or extensive LN metastases and PSA decrease to less than 1.0 ng/mL after neoadjuvant ADT	No treatment: 9 (39) ADT only: 5 (21); ABI: 5 (21) DOC: 2 (21)	Median (range): 34.5 mo. (7–75)	Median (range): 38.6 mo. (12–52)	Median (range): 40 mo. (9–65)	Median: 47 mo. (range: 9–71) 95.6%	91.3%
		No cRP	38			Patients with mPCa treated with ADT without LT served as the control group		Median (range): 37.0 mo. (28–96)	Median (range): 26.5 mo. (12–48)	Median (range): 29 mo. (16–54)	Median: 40.5 mo. (range: 19–75) 84.2%	78.9%
Poelaert et al. [40] (LoMP trial)	2017	cRP	17	2014-	Multicenter	RP was performed in asymptomatic patients with a resectable tumor and who were fit to undergo surgery (group A, n = 17)	No treatment: 4 (24) ADT: 13 (76)	Mean ± SD: 13 ± 8 mo.	ND	No patients develop CRPC	2-yr: 100%	2-yr: 100%
		No cRP	29			Only SOC was administered to patients with mPCa ineligible or unwilling to undergo cRP (group B, n = 29)		Mean ± SD: 16 ± 10 mo.		Median (range): 14 mo. (2–26)	2-yr: 61%	2-yr: 55%
Moschini et al. [39]	2017	cRP	31	2007–2014	USA (Mayo)	31 (66%) underwent cRP with or without adjuvant therapies and 16 (34%) underwent ADT only	M1a: minimum 6 mo. ADT M1b: minimum 6 mo. ADT + MDT	Median: 38.8 mo.	ND	ND	1-yr: 100% 3-yr: 91.3% 5-yr: 61.9%	ND
		No cRP	16				NA				1-yr: 93.8% 3-yr: 76.9% 5-yr: 46.2%	
Steuber et al. [42]	2017	cRP	43	2000–2011	Germany (Martini-Klinik Prostate Cancer Center)	Patients with low-volume bone metastases (1–3 lesions) undergoing cRP	All patients received ADT or CAB	Median: 32.7 mo.	ND	No significant differences in CRPC-free survival: p = 0.92	ND	No significant differences in overall survival: p = 0.92
		No cRP	40			Patients receiving best systemic therapy		Median: 82.2 mo.				

Table 2. Cont.

Author	Year	Comparisons	No. of pts.	Recruitment Year	Country (Institution)	Inclusion Criteria	Treatment after cRP	Follow-Up Duration	Progression-Free	Time to CRPC/CRPC-Free Survival	Cancer-Specific Survival	Overall Survival
Buelens et al. [29] (LoMP trial)	2022	cRP	40	2014–2018	Multicenter	Asymptomatic patients: cRP was offered to all fit patients with resectable tumors, resulting in 40 patients; standard of care was administered to 40 patients who were ineligible or unwilling to undergo surgery	All patients received ADT ± DOC/ABI	Median (IQR): 38 (32–50) mo.	ND	Median CRPC-free survival: 53 mo. (95% CI: 14–92) 3-yr: 59% (95% CI: 43–74)	ND	ND
		No cRP	40					Median (IQR): 31 (15–46) mo.		Median CRPC-free survival: 21 mo. (95% CI: 15–27) 3-yr: 40% (95% CI: 25–55)		
Mistretta et al. [38]	2022	cRP	40	2010–2018	Italy	Patients affected by cM1a-b oligometastatic PCa (defined as <5 metastatic lesions at diagnosis involving M1a and/or bone (M1b), with locally resectable cT1-T3 tumors)	Adjuvant ADT at least 12 mo.	Median: 55 mo.	radiological progression: 83.1%	mCRPC rate: 24.0%	CSM: 5.9%	ND
		No cRP	34				NA	Median: 50 mo.	radiological progression: 62.5%	mCRPC rate: 62.5%	CSM: 37.1%	
Sooriakumaran et al. [41] (TRoMbone)	2022	cRP	25	ND	UK (multicenter)	RCT (Phase1/2) for cRP vs. No cRP Patients diagnosed with oligometastatic PCa (defined as one to three skeletal lesions on bone imaging, no visceral metastases); locally resectable tumor (clinical/radiological stage T1–T3; ECOG-PS 01); and suitable for RP within 3 months of starting SOC	All patients received ADT ± DOC	ND	ND	ND	ND	ND
		No cRP	25			All patients received SOC systemic therapy of ADT + DOC						

Table 2. Cont.

Author	Year	Comparisons	No. of pts.	Recruitment Year	Country (Institution)	Inclusion Criteria	Treatment after cRP	Follow-Up Duration	Progression-Free	Time to CRPC/CRPC-Free Survival	Cancer-Specific Survival	Overall Survival
						Comparative studies between cRP and RT						
Knipper et al. [35]	2020	cRP	78	2008–2018	Germany (Martini-Klinik Prostate Cancer Center)	Patients with newly diagnosed mPCa with low-volume (<4 bone metastases and no visceral metastases according to STAMPEDE definition), confirmed on bone scan and CT/MRI, who underwent RP with PLND	All patients received ADT	Median (IQR): 36 (15–48) mo.	3-yr metastatic PFS: 63%	ND	3-yr CSS: 92%	3-yr OS: 91%
		STAMPEDE arm H (low volume with RT)	410			NA	NA	ND	3-yr metastatic PFS: 67%		3-yr CSS: 86%	3-yr OS: 81%
						RCT (Phase2) assessing LT (including 85% of cRP) vs. NLI						
Dai et al. [31]	2022	LT	100 (85) *	2015–2019	China	Patients with newly diagnosed oligometastasis PCa defined as five or fewer bone or extrapelvic LN metastases and no visceral metastases	All patients received ADT (94% received CAB)	Median (IQR): 48 (43–50) mo.	Median rPFS: not reached 3-yr rPFS: 79% HR: 0.43, 95% CI: 0.27–0.70	ND	ND	3-yr OS: 88% HR: 0.44, 95% CI: 0.24–0.81
		NLI	100						Median rPFS: 40 mo. 3-yr rPFS: 56%			3-yr OS: 70%
						Comparative studies between cRP, RT, and NLI						
Lumen et al. [36] (LoMP trial)	2021	cRP	48	2014–	Multicenter	RP was performed in asymptomatic patients with a resectable tumor and who were fit to undergo surgery; only SOC was administered to patients with metastatic prostate cancer ineligible or unwilling to undergo cRP	All patients received SOC (ADT ± ARSI or DOC)	Median (IQR): 42 (24–57) mo.		ND	2-yr CSS: 93% (vs. NLI: HR 0.36, 95% CI:0.14–0.94)	2-yr OS: 93% (vs. NLI: HR 0.28, 95% CI:0.11–0.71)
		RT	26					Median (IQR): 26 (14–51) mo.	ND	ND	2-yr CSS: 100% (vs. NLI: HR 0.33, 95% CI: 0.09–1.20)	2-yr OS: 100% (vs. NLI: HR 0.26, 95% CI: 0.07–0.91)
		NLI	35			For this study, patients with high-volume disease were excluded, leaving only patients with low-volume disease for evaluation		Median (IQR): 24 (12–44) mo.			2-yr CSS: 75%	2-yr OS: 69%

Table 2. Cont.

Author	Year	Comparisons	No. of pts.	Recruitment Year	Country (Institution)	Inclusion Criteria	Treatment after cRP	Follow-Up Duration	Progression-Free	Time to CRPC/CRPC-Free Survival	Cancer-Specific Survival	Overall Survival
Comparative studies between cRP and RP for localized PCa												
Chaloupka et al. [30]	2021	cRP	79	2012–2020	Germany (Ludwig-Maximilians University)	cRP was performed in patients with oligometastasis, defined as <5 bone lesions in the preoperative staging; biopsy-proven PCa, history of RP at one tertiary center and completed follow-up; patients with preoperative ADT and pre-RP RT of the prostate were excluded from further analysis Of 1268 pts, matched cohort of 411 patients were retained after PSM	ND				5-yr CSS: 61%	5-yr OS: 38%
		RP for localized PCa	332				ND				5-yr CSS: 81%	5-yr OS: 57%
Single arm or only including cRP cohort												
Gandaglia et al. [45]	2017	cRP	11	2006–2011	Italy	Patients with oligometastatic PCa	Adjuvant ADT: 10 (91)	Median (IQR): 63 mo. (48–77)	7-yr cPFS: 45%	ND	7-yr CSS: 82%	ND
Heidenreich et al. [32]	2018	cRP	113	ND	Multicenter	Biopsy-proven mPCa who fulfilled the following selection criteria: (1) completely resectable PCa; (2) osseous metastases; (3) absence of gross retroperitoneal LN metastases; (4) absence of bulky pelvic LN metastases >3 cm; (5) no or minimal visceral metastases; (6) ECOG-PS of 0–1; and (7) written informed consent	Neoadjuvant ADT:80 (71), adjuvant ADT: 91 (87)	Median (range): 45.7 mo. (13–96)	Median(range): 72.3 mo. (8–96) 65 pts. remain clinical progression-free at 5yr	ND	ND	3-yr OS: 89.3% 5-yr OS: 80.5%
Xue et al. [44]	2020	cRP + MDT	26	2012–2016	Multicenter (China)	(1) Biopsy-confirmed diagnosis of prostate adenocarcinoma; (2) M1b disease with the presence of 1–5 visible bone metastases (by Tc-99m MDP BS, CT, or MRI); (3) not received RT or chemotherapy in hormone-sensitive phase; (4) adequate organ function; (5) ECOG performance status 0.1; (6) pretreatment total testosterone > 200 ng/dL; and (7) written informed consent	All patients received ADT	Median (range): 43.1 mo. (15–61)	ND	3-yr CRPC-free survival: 75.9% RP + MDT had better CRPC-free survival (HR: 0.41, 95% CI: 0.18–0.95)	3-yr CSS: 91.4% No significant differences between two groups (HR: 0.59, 95% CI: 0.12–2.95)	ND
		cRP only	32					Median (range): 47.6 mo. (18–65)				

Table 2. Cont.

Author	Year	Comparisons	No. of pts.	Recruitment Year	Country (Institution)	Inclusion Criteria	Treatment after cRP	Follow-Up Duration	Progression-Free	Time to CRPC/CRPC-Free Survival	Cancer-Specific Survival	Overall Survival
Mandel et al. [37] (ProMPT trial)	2021	cRP (assessing CTC as prognostic value)	33	2014–2015	Germany (Martini-Klinik Prostate Cancer Center)	(1) Newly diagnosed PCa, with 1–3 bone metastases (positive BS and confirmed by CT or MRI; no PET/CT was used) at the time of diagnosis; (2) asymptomatic patient; (3) absence of visceral metastases; (4) locally resectable tumor (<cT3); (5) PSA at diagnosis <150 mg/dl; and (6) no prior radiation of bone metastases; in addition to cRP, the best systemic therapy (only ADT) was recommended to all patients	All patients were recommended ADT	Median: 39.4 mo.	ND	3-yr CRPC-free survival: 65.6%	ND	3-yr OS: 87.9%
Babst et al. [28]	2021	cRP (assessing the impact of upfront DOC-based doublet therapy)	38	2015–2018	Germany (two centers)	Patients with mHSPC underwent cRP after primary chemohormonal therapy (DOC +ADT)	All patients received ADT continuously	Median (range): 22.6 mo. (5.7–48.6)	ND	Median time to CRPC: 35.9 mo.	ND	ND
Kim et al. [34]	2022	cRP	32	ND	Multicenter (USA, South Korea, Japan)	The major inclusion criterion was biopsy-proven N1M0 or NxM1a/b PCa	All patients received ADT	Median (IQR): 46 (32–53) mo.	ND	ND	ND	5-yr OS: 67% (All patients) 69% (M1 patients)
Takagi et al. [43]	2022	cRP (assessing the feasibility of RARP)	12	2017–2021	Japan (two centers)	Patients with mPCa who had undergone neoadjuvant therapy followed by RARP	Adjuvant ADT: 5 (25)	ND	BCR-free survival: 1-yr: 83.3%/2-yr: 66.7% MFS: 1-yr: 90%/2-yr: 90%	ND	ND	ND

No.: number, Pts.: patients, LT: local therapy, NLT: no local therapy, RT: radiotherapy, EBRT: external beam radiotherapy, BT: brachytherapy, MDT: metastasis-directed therapy, PS: propensity score, PSM: propensity-score matching, ECOG-PS: Eastern Cooperative Oncology Group Performance Status, cRP: cytoreductive radical prostatectomy, CRPC: castration-resistant prostate cancer, SOC: standard of care, RARP: robot-assisted radical prostatectomy, IQR: interquartile range, SD: standard deviation, ADT: androgen deprivation therapy, CAB: combined androgen blockade, ARSI: androgen receptor signaling inhibitor, DOC: docetaxel, NA: not applicable, ND: no data, BCR: biochemical recurrence, CSS: cancer-specific survival, CSM: cancer-specific mortality, OS: overall survival, HR: hazard ratio, CI: confidence interval, PCa: prostate cancer, mPCa: metastatic PCa, CTC: circulating tumor cell, BS: bone scan. * 85 patients underwent cRP.

cRP vs. NLT

In 2014, Culp et al. for the first time showed the OS and CSS benefit of LT for mPCa among 8185 mPCa patients (NLT: n = 7811, cRP: n = 245, brachytherapy [BT]: n = 129) by using the SEER database from 2004 to 2010 [20]. The authors reported that the 5-year OS and CSS were significantly higher in patients undergoing cRP (67.4% and 75.8%, respectively) or BT (52.6% and 61.3%, respectively) compared with those without LT (22.5% and 48.7%, respectively) [20]. After adjusting for the effects of confounders, such as TNM stage and PSA, using multivariable competing risks regression analysis, statistical significance remained (HR for cRP: 0.38 [95% CI: 0.27–0.53], HR for BT: 0.68 [95% CI: 0.49–0.93]) [20]. Thereafter, Antwi et al. and Satkunasivam et al. performed the additional analyses using propensity scores (PS) in 2014 and 2015 [19,26]. Antwi et al. showed that PS-adjusted HR for OS in patients who underwent cRP was 0.22 (95% CI: 0.17–0.28) compared with those without LT [19]. Satkunasivam et al. assessed the same oncologic outcomes in patients 66 years or older (n = 4069) [26]. Owing to the low number of patients who underwent cRP (n = 47), PS-adjusted HR for OS did not reach statistical significance (HR: 0.55 [95% CI: 0.30–1.02]) [26]. In 2017, Parikh et al. published results from the NCDB comprising 6051 patients (NLT: n = 5224, cRP: n = 622, radiotherapy [RT]: n = 205) by adjusting for the effects of confounders such as age, TN stage, and the Charlson comorbidity index (CCI) [25]. The authors showed that the adjusted HR by using the Cox proportional hazard model for OS in patients who underwent cRP was 0.51 (95% CI: 0.45–0.59) and confirmed the OS benefit of cRP even after PS adjustment (HR: 0.27 [95% CI: 0.22–0.33]) [25].

Since 2020, two studies using the SEER database have been published. Jin et al. updated the study period (2010–2014) from the study conducted by Culp et al., comprising 5849 patients (NLT: n = 5628, cRP: n = 159, BT: n = 62) [24]. The authors corroborated previous findings suggesting an OS and CSS benefit by using the Cox proportional hazard models (HR: 0.60 [95% CI: 0.42–0.87], HR: 0.56 [95% CI: 0.37–0.86], respectively) [24]. In addition, a subgroup analysis revealed that patients with bone metastasis or distant LN metastasis were significantly more likely to benefit from definitive local therapy [24]. Despite the limitation of selection bias derived from a population-based study, the detailed analyses adjusting for the effects of confounders revealed an OS and CSS benefit for cRP over NLT.

cRP vs. RT

Jin et al. compared oncologic outcomes by using the SEER database (2004–2015) comprising 19,612 patients (NLT: n = 18,857, cRP: n = 435, RT: n = 320) [23]. The authors confirmed the OS and CSS benefit of LT over NLT even after adjusting for the effects of unmeasured confounders (HR for OS: 0.57 [95% CI 0.50–0.65], HR for CSS: 0.59 [95% CI 0.51–0.68], respectively.) [23]. Furthermore, the authors showed that cRP was associated with significantly better OS and CSS compared with RT after adjusting for the effects of race, age, marital status, TNM stage, GS, and PSA as well as performance status [23]. However, after adjusting for the effects of unmeasured confounders, this statistical significance diminished (HR for OS: 0.63 [95% CI 0.26–1.54] and HR for CSS: 0.47 [95% CI 0.16–1.35], respectively) [23]. Guo et al. created 1:1 PS-matched cohorts (cRP: n = 148, RT: n = 148) based on data from the SEER database (2004–2016) [22]. The authors failed to show the superiority of cRP over RT in terms of OS (HR: 0.73 [95% CI: 0.48–11]) and CSS (HR: 0.77 [95% CI: 0.46–1.30]) [22]. A recently published study using the SEER database (2004–2016) conducted by Stolzenbach et al. comprised 954 patients who underwent cRP and 3326 patients who underwent RT [27]. Despite short follow-up periods (median follow-up was within 2 years), they showed that cRP is associated with significantly better CSS compared with RT after adjusting for age, initial PSA, biopsy GS, and clinical TNM stages using PS and the competing risk regression (HR: 0.82 [95% CI: 0.71–0.94]) [27]. However, the results from the SEER database differ according to the recruitment periods, statistical methods, and follow-up duration, leaving the potential benefits of cRP over RT controversial.

3.2.2. Case-Control Studies

Patient demographics and oncologic outcomes of included studies are shown in Table 2 and Supplementary Table S3.

cRP vs. NLT

Six case-control studies assessing the differential oncologic outcomes were identified. In 2015, Heidenreich et al. assessed the differential oncologic outcomes of cRP ($n = 23$) vs. NLT ($n = 38$) in patients with oligometastatic mPCa (less than three bone metastases) with comparable patient demographics except for baseline PSA [33]. The authors reported significantly better PFS, time to CRPC, and CSS in patients who underwent cRP compared with those who did not undergo LT [33]. In 2017, Poelart et al. reported the preliminary results of the LoMP trial with extremely better oncologic outcomes in terms of 100% of 2-year CSS and OS in patients who underwent cRP ($n = 17$) compared with patients without LT ($n = 29$). On the other hand, Moschini et al. and Steuber et al. showed no differences in CSS or OS between patients who underwent cRP and those who did not [39,42]. In addition, updated results from the LoMP trial comprising 40 patients in each arm (NLT vs. cRP) showed no differences in CRPC-free survival on multivariable analysis [29]. However, most recently, Mistretta et al. demonstrated that NLT was associated with higher rates of progression to mCRPC (HR: 0.40; CI 0.19–0.84 adjusted for the effects of the site of metastasis, HR:0.39; CI 0.19–0.84 adjusted for the effect of PSA) while adjusting only for one confounder [38]. Taken together, there is conflicting evidence on the oncologic benefit of cRP from case-control studies. Notably, these studies included only 17 to 43 patients in the cRP group; therefore, these studies suffered from low statistical power. We initially attempted to perform a meta-analysis to integrate them; however, these studies also suffered different inclusion criteria and unmatched comparators. This suggests the need for well-controlled future trials and for international collaborative multicenter studies with more patients.

cRP vs. RT

Lumen et al. reported comparable oncological outcomes between cRP and RT from the LoMP trial [36]. Comparing cRP ($n = 48$) vs. RT ($n = 26$), the 2-year CSS were 93% vs. 100%, and the 2-year OS were 93% vs. 100%, respectively [36]. Knipper et al. compared the oncologic outcomes of cRP in mHSPC patients with low-volume disease and the results from the STAMPEDE arm H [13,35]. The authors showed comparable 3-year OS and CSS rates for cRP and RT (OS: 91% vs. 81%, CSS: 92% vs. 86%, respectively) [35]. To date, high-quality evidence regarding the differential oncological outcomes between cRP and RT is lacking; nonetheless, the oncological effectiveness of cRP with PLND may be comparable to pelvic RT.

3.2.3. RCT

Up to now, only one RCT, conducted by Dai et al., has been published [31]. The authors conducted an open-label phase-2 RCT to compare the oncologic outcomes between LT ($n = 100$) and NLT ($n = 100$). The LT group comprised 85 (85%) patients who underwent cRP and 11 (11%) patients who underwent RT, whereas 17 patients (17%) eventually received LT in the NLT group. This study showed significantly better OS (HR: 0.44 [95% CI: 0.24–0.81]), radiographic PFS (HR: 0.43 [95% CI: 0.27–0.70]), and PSA-PFS (HR: 0.44 [95% CI: 0.29–0.67]) in patients who underwent LT compared with those who did not during 48 months of median follow-up [31].

3.3. Perioperative Outcomes

3.3.1. Complications

Assessing perioperative outcomes on the basis of different surgical approaches is imperative. Robot-assisted radical prostatectomy (RARP) has recently replaced open and laparoscopic approaches as the standard technique [46,47]. Traditionally, cRP has been performed by using an open approach [33,39,45], while recently, RARP has become the standard procedure even for cRP (Table 3) [29,38,40,41,43].

Table 3. Perioperative outcomes following cRP.

Author	Comparisons	Year	No. of Pts.	Approach of cRP, n (%)	Nerve Sparing	LND, n (%)	LN Removed, n	LN Involvement, n (%)	Estimated Blood Loss, mL	Operation Time, Min	Catheterization, Days	LOS, Days	Postoperative Complication (All), n (%)	Postoperative Complication (CD > 3), n(%)	Rectal Injury, n (%)	PSM, n (%)
Heidenreich et al. [33]	cRP	2015	23	Open RP	ND	All ePLND	ND	13 (57)	Mean (range): 335 (250–600)	Mean (range): 127 (115–145)	Mean (range): 5.6 days (5–12)	Mean (range): 7.8 (6–13)	9 (39)	3 (13)	ND	4 (17)
Poelaert et al. [40] (LoMP trial)	cRP	2017	17	Open: 1 RARP: 16	None	All ePLND	Median (range): 20 (9–47)	12 (71)	Median (range): 250 (100–900)	Median (range): 215 (150–290)	ND	ND	7 (41)	0	0	14 (82)
Moschini et al. [39]	cRP	2017	31	Open RP	ND	All ePLND	Median (IQR): 19 (13–31)	20 (64)	Median (IQR): 400 (250–500)	ND	ND	Median (IQR): 3 (3–5)	30 days: 9 (29) 90 days: 4 (13)	30 days: 2 (6.5) 90 days: 2 (6.5)	0	8 (26)
Steuber et al. [42]	cRP	2017	43	ND	None: 74% Unilateral: 16% Bilateral: 9.3%	ND	Median (IQR): 21 (12–27)	67%	ND	ND	ND	ND	ND	ND	ND	67%
Buelens et al. [29] (LoMP trial)	cRP	2022	40	Open: 2 RARP: 38	None	All ePLND	Median (IQR): 17 (11–21)	31 (78)	Median (IQR): 250 (150–325)	Median (IQR): 205 (165–220)	ND	ND	90 days 20 (50)	2 (5)	0	32 (80)
Sooriakumaran et al. [41] (TRoMbone)	cRP	2022	25	RARP	ND	All ePLND	11 (7–14)	11 (46)	ND	Median (IQR): 185 (165–217)	14 (10–14)	Median (IQR): 1 (1–2)	3 (12.5)	ND	ND	10 (42)
Knipper et al. [35]	cRP	2020	78	Open RP	ND	ND	ND	26 (31)	ND	ND	ND	ND	34 (44)	16 (21)	ND	ND
Dai et al. [31]	cRP	2022	85	Open RP: 68 (80) RARP: 17 (20)	ND	ND	ND	ND	ND	ND	ND	ND	24 (28)	7 (8.2)	1 (1.2)	36 (42)
Chaloupka et al. [30]	cRP	2021	79	Open: 69 (87) RARP:10 (13)	13 (17)	ND	Median (IQR): 10 (6–13)	41 (52)	ND	ND	ND	ND	ND	ND	ND	59 (75)
	RP for localized PCa		332	Open: 116 (35) RARP: 216 (65)	183 (55)	ND	Median (IQR): 11 (6–18)	112 (34)	ND	ND	ND	ND	ND	ND	ND	165 (50)

Table 3. Cont.

Author	Year	Comparisons	No. of Pts.	Approach of CRP, n (%)	Nerve Sparing	LND, n (%)	LN Removed, n	LN Involvement, n (%)	Estimated Blood Loss, mL	Operation Time, Min	Catheterization, Days	LOS, Days	Postoperative Complication (All), n (%)	Postoperative Complication (CD > 3), n(%)	Rectal Injury, n (%)	PSM, n (%)
Gandaglia et al. [41]	2017	cRP	11	Open	ND	All ePLND	Median (IQR): 27 (23–42)	10 (91)	Median (IQR): 750 (600–850)	Median (IQR): 170 (160–380)	ND	Median (IQR): 13 (7–19)	6 (54)	2 (18)	0	8 (73)
Heidenreich et al. [32]	2018	cRP	113	Open: 104 (92) RARP: 9 (8)	ND	None: 1.8% Limited: 8.8% Extended: 89.4%	Median (range): 15.3 (0–57)	70 (62)	ND	Median (range): 145 (95–380)	ND	Median (range): 6.5 (3–21)	38 (34)	11 (9.7)	0	42 (37)
Xue et al. [44]	2020	cRP + MDT	26	Open/LRP	ND	All	ND	10 (39)	ND	ND	ND	ND	ND	ND	ND	3 (12)
		cRP only	32					10 (32)								4 (13)
Mandel et al. [37] (ProMPT trial)	2021	cRP	33	Open: 28 (85) RARP: 5 (15)	ND	ND	ND	24 (73)	ND	ND	ND	ND	ND	ND	ND	24 (73)
Babst et al. [28]	2021	cRP	38	Open: 35 (92) RARP: 3 (7.9)	ND	All	Median (IQR): 18.5 (12–24)	34 (89)	ND	Median (IQR): 196 (157–233)	ND	Median (IQR): 9 (6–10)	within 30 days 5 (13)	within 30 days 4 (11)	0	21 (55)
Kim et al. [34]	2022	cRP	32	ND	ND	ND	ND	20 (62)	Median (IQR): 200 (100–400)	Median (IQR): 225 (198–312)	ND	ND	ND	6%	ND	20 (66)
Takagi et al. [43]	2022	cRP	12	RARP	None	None	ND	ND	Median (IQR): 23 (7–45)	Median (IQR): 85 (70–112) *	ND	ND	0	0	0	1 (8.3)

No.: number, Pts.: patients, MDT: metastasis-directed therapy, RP: radical prostatectomy, PCa: prostate cancer, cRP: cytoreductive radical prostatectomy, RARP: robot-assisted radical prostatectomy, IQR: interquartile range, SD: standard deviation, ADT: androgen deprivation therapy, NA: not applicable, ND: no data, LOS: length of stay, LN: lymph node, LND: lymph node dissection, ePLND: extended pelvic lymph node dissection, PSM: positive surgical margin, focal therapy. * Described as console time.

In total, after combining patients from all studies, there were 155 overall complications reported in 473 patients (33%) and 47 severe complications (CTCAE grade≥ 3) reported in 448 patients (10%) who underwent cRP. Only one rectal injury was reported in 347 patients (0.29%). However, most eligible studies did not report outcome data on cRP for either open or robot-assisted approaches, making meaningful comparisons challenging. The largest multicenter cohort reported by Heidenreich et al. (open: n = 104, RARP: n = 5) showed that the rates of overall and severe complications were 34% and 9.7%, respectively [32].

For open cRP alone, the overall and severe complication rates ranged from 29% to 54% and from 6.5% to 21%, respectively [33,35,39,45]. In comparison, Sooriakumaran et al. reported a 12.5% overall complication rate in patients who underwent cytoreductive RARP (cRARP) [41]; furthermore, Takagi et al., assessing the feasibility of cRARP in 12 patients, reported excellent perioperative outcomes without any complications [43]. Taken together, cRARP seems safer than open cRP, in agreement with the previously demonstrated safety of RARP for localized PCa [48].

3.3.2. Pathologic Outcomes

Of the studies included, 15 provided data on the rates of PSM, ranging from 8.3% to 82% [28–34,37,39–45]. Most studies performed concomitant PLND during cRP; 15 studies provided data on the rates of LN involvement, ranging from 31% to 91% [28–34,37,39–42,44,45]. The wide range of PSM rates suggests the importance of optimal patient selection and the need for adjuvant RT in some patients. Extended PLND should be performed during cRP given the high likelihood of LN involvement.

3.4. Functional Outcomes
3.4.1. Urinary Function
Obstructive Voiding Dysfunction in NLT Patients

Obstructive voiding dysfunction and relevant lower urinary tract symptoms (LUTSs) due to the local progression of PCa are critical clinical issues in the late stages of mPCa [49]. Evaluating the intervention rates for obstructive urinary dysfunction in NLT patients, a retrospective case-control study by Heidenreich et al. showed that 11 of 38 (29%) patients required surgical or percutaneous intervention [33]. The LoMP trial conducted by Poelaert et al. revealed that 11 of 29 (38%) NLT patients required intervention [29]. In addition, Steuber et al. reported that 14 of 40 (35%) NLT patients experienced severe local complications [42]. Notably, Lumen et al. demonstrated that cRP was associated with higher local event-free rates than NLT on multivariable analysis (HR: 0.36 [95% CI: 0.14–0.94]) [36]. Preventing obstructive voiding dysfunction seems to be an essential rationale for undergoing cRP for mPCa patients in the earlier disease stages before disease progression.

Incontinence after cRP

The timing and tools for assessing urinary incontinence after cRP varied across studies (Table 4). Continence rates, defined as pad 0–1/day 1 year after cRP, ranged from 74% to 88% [28,29,35]. Of note, 0 pad achievement rates at 1-year follow-up after cRP ranged from 53% to 92% [28,29,31,32,35]. For example, Knipper et al. showed that 53% who underwent open cRP (n = 78) did not use any pad/day [35]. Furthermore, another large multicenter study conducted by Heidenreich et al. comprising 113 patients (92% of patients underwent open cRP) found a 68% 0 pad rate at 1-year follow-up [32]. In the recent RCT conducted by Dai et al., excellent continence rates, of 92%, at 1 year and 95% at 2 years after cRP were reported, although only 20% of patients underwent cRARP [31]. There are no robust data regarding urinary function following cRARP.

Table 4. Functional outcomes following cRP.

Author	Year	Comparison	No. of Pts.	Approach of cRP, n (%)	Nerve Sparing	Pre-RP Urinary Function, n (%)	Continence during Follow-Up, n (%)	Pre-cRP Erectile Function, n (%)	Erectile Function at Last Follow-Up, n (%)
Heidenreich et al. [33]	2015	cRP	23	Open RP	ND	ND	at last follow-up 0 pads/day: 13 (57) 0–1 pads/day: 21 (91) 2–4 pads/day: 2 (8.7)	ND	ND
Poelaert et al. [40] (LoMP trial)	2017	cRP	17	Open: 1 RARP: 16	None	ND	at 3 mo. Continent and no local symptoms: 12 (71)	ND	ND
		No cRP	29	NA		ND	at 3 mo. Continent and no local symptoms: 13 (45)	ND	ND
Moschini et al. [39]	2017	cRP	31	Open RP	ND	ND	at 90 days 0 pads/day: 24 (77) 1–2 pads/day: 2 (6.5) >2 pads/day: 5 (16)	ND	ND
Buelens et al. [29] (LoMP trial)	2022	cRP	40	Open: 2 RARP: 38	None	ND	Continent (0–1 pads/day) at 1 yr: 31 (79) at last follow-up: 35 (88)	ND	ND
Sooriakumaran et al. [41] (TRoMbone)	2022	cRP	25	RARP	ND	Incontinence: 0	Incontinence at 1 mo: 9 (37.5%) Incontinence at 3 mo: 6 (25%) Incontinence at 6 mo: 4 (17%)	IIEF-5 score (median, IQR): 13.0 (5.5–21.0)	IIEF-5 score at 3 mo. (median, IQR): 5.0 (5.0–6.0)
		No cRP	25	NA		Incontinence: 0	ND	IIEF-5 score (median, IQR): 18.5 (10.0–21.0)	IIEF-5 score at 3 mo. (median, IQR): 5.0 (5.0–12.0)
Knipper et al. [35]	2020	cRP	78	Open RP	ND	ND	at 1 yr 0 pads/day: 20 (53) 0–1 pads/day: 28 (74) 2 pads/day: 2 (5)	ND	ND
Dai et al. [31]	2022	cRP	85	Open RP: 68 (80) RARP: 17 (20)	ND	ND	at 1 yr 0 pads/day: 78 (92) at 2 yrs 0 pads/day: 81 (95)	ND	ND
Chaloupka et al. [30]	2021	cRP	79	Open: 69 (87) RARP: 10 (13)	13 (17)	ICIQ-SF score (mean ± SD): 2.3 ± 4.6	at 25 mo. ICIQ-SF score (mean ± SD): 6.4 ± 5.7 Daily pad usage (mean ± SD): 1.6 ± 2.5 Continence recovery: 66%	IIEF-5 score (mean ± SD): 8.5 ± 10.2 IIEF-5 score > 18: 26.8%	IIEF-5 score (mean ± SD): 1.3 ± 4.2 IIEF-5 score > 18: 2.0%
		RP	332	Open: 116 (35) RARP: 216 (65)	183 (55)	ICIQ-SF score (mean ± SD): 1.1 ± 2.6	at 25 mo. ICIQ-SF score (mean ± SD): 6.4 ± 5.2 Daily pad usage (mean ± SD): 1.2 ± 1.7 Continence recovery: 72%	IIEF-5 score (mean ± SD): 11.3 ± 9.9 IIEF-5 score > 18: 37.2%	IIEF-5 score (mean ± SD): 3.5 ± 6.2 IIEF-5 score > 18: 6.8%

Table 4. *Cont.*

Author	Year	Comparison	No. of Pts.	Approach of cRP, n (%)	Nerve Sparing	Pre-RP Urinary Function, n (%)	Continence during Follow-Up, n (%)	Pre-cRP Erectile Function, n (%)	Erectile Function at Last Follow-Up, n (%)
Gandaglia et al. [45]	2017	cRP	11	Open	ND	ND	at 90 days 0 pads/day: 3 (27)	ND	ND
Heidenreich et al. [32]	2018	cRP	113	Open: 104 (92) RARP: 9 (8)	ND	ND	at 12 mo. 0 pads/day: 68% 1–2 pads/day: 18% >2 pads/day: 14%	ND	ND
Babst et al. [28]	2021	cRP	38	Open: 35 (92) RARP: 3 (7.9)	ND	ND	0–1 pads/day at 1 mo.: 87% at 6 mo.: 92% at 12 mo.: 88%	ND	ND
Takagi et al. [43]	2022	cRP	12	RARP	None	ND	at 24 mo. >2 pads/day: 1 (8.3)	ND	ND

No.: number, Pts.: patients, MDT: metastasis-directed therapy, RP: radical prostatectomy, PCa: prostate cancer, cRP: cytoreductive radical prostatectomy, IQR: interquartile range, SD: standard deviation, ADT: androgen deprivation therapy, NA: not applicable, ND: no data, ICIQ-SF: International Consultation on Incontinence Questionnaire, IIEF: International Index of Erectile Function.

Interestingly, Chaloupka et al. compared the functional outcomes between cRP (open cRP: n = 69, cRARP: n = 13) and RP for localized PCa (open RP: n = 116, RARP: n = 216) [30]. This study revealed comparable continence recovery rates (66% vs. 72%, p = 0.4) as well as International Consultation on Incontinence Questionnaire scores (ICIQ-SF; 6.4 ± 5.7 vs 6.4 ± 5.2 [mean ± SD], p = 1) at 25 months after surgery [30].

3.4.2. Erectile Function

Two studies assessed erectile function before and after cRP using the International Index of Erectile Function (IIEF)-5 score [30,41]. The TroMbone trial revealed comparable IIEF-5 scores between the cRP and NLT groups (Median [IQR]: 5.0 [5.0–6.0] vs. 5.0 [5.0–12.0]) [41]. On the contrary, a study conducted by Chaloupka et al. comparing the functional outcomes between cRP and RP for localized PCa (Open cRP: n = 116, cRARP: n = 216) showed that the IIEF-5 score was significantly lower in the patients who underwent cRP compared with those who underwent RP for localized PCa (mean ± SD: 1.3 ± 4.2 vs. 3.5 ± 6.2, p < 0.001) [30]. The low rates of nerve sparing cRP (cRP: 17% vs. RP for localized PCa: 55%) indeed affect these outcomes [30].

3.4.3. Quality of Life

The TroMbone trial also assessed the patient-reported QOL using the EuroQoL Five Dimensions Five Levels (EQ-5D-5L) questionnaires at baseline and 3 months postrandomization [41]. This study showed a comparative EQ-5D-5L descriptive score at 3 months after randomization between the cRP and NLT groups (median [IQR]: both 1.0 [0.8–1.0]) [41]. Chaloupka et al. compared the general health-related QOL (HRQOL) by global health status (GHS) by using the European Organization for Research and Treatment of Cancer (EORTC) quality-of-life questionnaire (QLQ)-C30 between cRP and RP for the localized PCa group. This study demonstrated no difference in the general HRQOL rates between the two groups at the end of follow-up (44% vs. 56%, p = 0.8) [30]. Interestingly, GHS significantly worsened in localized PCa patients compared with the baseline (−5, p = 0.001), whereas GHS did not significantly change in patients who underwent cRP (+3.2, p = 0.4) [30]. Taken together, cRP seems not to reduce the patient-reported QOL compared with patients with NLT.

4. Conclusions

Population-based studies showed an oncologic benefit to cRP compared with NLT or RT for mPCa, after careful analyses that adjusted for the effects of possible confounders. Nevertheless, these studies suffered from selection bias and lacked relevant data often used for clinical decision-making, such as comorbidity and metastatic burden. Small case-control studies, including only patients with oligometastatic disease, failed to report a clear survival benefit for cRP. Recently, only one RCT, including 85% of cRP patients in the LT group, demonstrated an oncologic benefit of LT in terms of PSA-PFS as well as OS. Perioperative and functional outcomes following cRP seem to be comparable to those of NLT or RP for localized PCa. Taken together, cRP offers promising oncological outcomes, technical feasibility, and acceptable functional outcomes. However, well-designed, adequately powered RCTs with long-term follow-ups are needed to allow a robust and fair comparison of cRP with NLT and RT. Until then, cRP should be considered experimental and assessed only in clinical trials.

Supplementary Materials: The following supporting information can be downloaded at https://www.mdpi.com/article/10.3390/curroncol30020170/s1, Supplementary Figure S1. PRISMA checklist 2009, Supplementary Figure S2. Risk-of-bias assessment of the included RCTs, Supplementary Table S1. Risk-of-bias assessment for NRCTs (ROBINS-I), Supplementary Table S2. Patient characteristics of included population-based studies, Supplementary Table S3. Patient characteristics of included case-control studies.

Author Contributions: T.Y. contributed to the protocol/project development, data collection and management, and manuscript writing/editing. P.R. and T.K. (Tatsushi Kawada) contributed to the data extraction and manuscript writing/editing. K.B., E.L., M.v.D., M.M. and M.C. contributed to the manuscript writing/editing. T.K. (Takahiro Kimura), P.I.K. and A.H. contributed to the manuscript editing. S.F.S. contributed to the supervision, protocol/project development/management, and manuscript editing. All authors have read and agreed to the published version of the manuscript.

Funding: NA (no external funding provided), EUSP Scholarship of the European Association of Urology (PR).

Conflicts of Interest: Takahiro Kimura is a paid consultant/advisor of Astellas, Bayer, Janssen, and Sanofi. Shahrokh F. Shariat has received honoraria from Astellas, AstraZeneca, BMS, Ferring, Ipsen, Janssen, MSD, Olympus, Pfizer, Roche, and Takeda; played a consulting or advisory role with Astellas, AstraZeneca, BMS, Ferring, Ipsen, Janssen, MSD, Olympus, Pfizer, Pierre Fabre, Roche, and Takeda; and was associated with the speakers bureau of Astellas, Astra Zeneca, Bayer, BMS, Ferring, Ipsen, Janssen, MSD, Olympus, Pfizer, Richard Wolf, Roche, and Takeda. The other authors declare no conflict of interest associated with this manuscript.

References

1. Cornford, P.; van den Bergh, R.C.N.; Briers, E.; Van den Broeck, T.; Cumberbatch, M.G.; De Santis, M.; Fanti, S.; Fossati, N.; Gandaglia, G.; Gillessen, S.; et al. EAU-EANM-ESTRO-ESUR-SIOG Guidelines on Prostate Cancer. Part II-2020 Update: Treatment of Relapsing and Metastatic Prostate Cancer. *Eur. Urol.* **2021**, *79*, 263–282. [CrossRef] [PubMed]
2. Armstrong, A.J.; Azad, A.A.; Iguchi, T.; Szmulewitz, R.Z.; Petrylak, D.P.; Holzbeierlein, J.; Villers, A.; Alcaraz, A.; Alekseev, B.; Shore, N.D.; et al. Improved Survival with Enzalutamide in Patients with Metastatic Hormone-Sensitive Prostate Cancer. *J. Clin. Oncol.* **2022**, *40*, 1616–1622. [CrossRef] [PubMed]
3. Chi, K.N.; Chowdhury, S.; Bjartell, A.; Chung, B.H.; Pereira de Santana Gomes, A.J.; Given, R.; Juárez, A.; Merseburger, A.S.; Özgüroğlu, M.; Uemura, H.; et al. Apalutamide in Patients with Metastatic Castration-Sensitive Prostate Cancer: Final Survival Analysis of the Randomized, Double-Blind, Phase III TITAN Study. *J. Clin. Oncol.* **2021**, *39*, 2294–2303. [CrossRef]
4. Fizazi, K.; Foulon, S.; Carles, J.; Roubaud, G.; McDermott, R.; Fléchon, A.; Tombal, B.; Supiot, S.; Berthold, D.; Ronchin, P.; et al. Abiraterone plus prednisone added to androgen deprivation therapy and docetaxel in de novo metastatic castration-sensitive prostate cancer (PEACE-1): A multicentre, open-label, randomised, phase 3 study with a 2 × 2 factorial design. *Lancet* **2022**, *399*, 1695–1707. [CrossRef]
5. Smith, M.R.; Hussain, M.; Saad, F.; Fizazi, K.; Sternberg, C.N.; Crawford, E.D.; Kopyltsov, E.; Park, C.H.; Alekseev, B.; Montesa-Pino, Á.; et al. Darolutamide and Survival in Metastatic, Hormone-Sensitive Prostate Cancer. *N. Engl. J. Med.* **2022**, *386*, 1132–1142. [CrossRef]
6. Fizazi, K.; Tran, N.; Fein, L.; Matsubara, N.; Rodriguez-Antolin, A.; Alekseev, B.Y.; Özgüroğlu, M.; Ye, D.; Feyerabend, S.; Protheroe, A.; et al. Abiraterone acetate plus prednisone in patients with newly diagnosed high-risk metastatic castration-sensitive prostate cancer (LATITUDE): Final overall survival analysis of a randomised, double-blind, phase 3 trial. *Lancet Oncol.* **2019**, *20*, 686–700. [CrossRef]
7. Clarke, N.W.; Ali, A.; Ingleby, F.C.; Hoyle, A.; Amos, C.L.; Attard, G.; Brawley, C.D.; Calvert, J.; Chowdhury, S.; Cook, A.; et al. Addition of docetaxel to hormonal therapy in low-and high-burden metastatic hormone sensitive prostate cancer: Long-term survival results from the STAMPEDE trial. *Ann. Oncol.* **2019**, *30*, 1992–2003. [CrossRef] [PubMed]
8. Davis, I.D.; Martin, A.J.; Zielinski, R.R.; Thomson, A.; Tan, T.H.; Sandhu, S.; Reaume, M.N.; Pook, D.W.; Parnis, F.; North, S.A.; et al. Updated overall survival outcomes in ENZAMET (ANZUP 1304), an international, cooperative group trial of enzalutamide in metastatic hormone-sensitive prostate cancer (mHSPC). *J. Clin. Oncol.* **2022**, *40* (Suppl. S17), LBA5004. [CrossRef]
9. Gravis, G.; Fizazi, K.; Joly, F.; Oudard, S.; Priou, F.; Esterni, B.; Latorzeff, I.; Delva, R.; Krakowski, I.; Laguerre, B.; et al. Androgen-deprivation therapy alone or with docetaxel in non-castrate metastatic prostate cancer (GETUG-AFU 15): A randomised, open-label, phase 3 trial. *Lancet. Oncol.* **2013**, *14*, 149–158. [CrossRef]
10. Kyriakopoulos, C.E.; Chen, Y.H.; Carducci, M.A.; Liu, G.; Jarrard, D.F.; Hahn, N.M.; Shevrin, D.H.; Dreicer, R.; Hussain, M.; Eisenberger, M.; et al. Chemohormonal Therapy in Metastatic Hormone-Sensitive Prostate Cancer: Long-Term Survival Analysis of the Randomized Phase III E3805 CHAARTED Trial. *J. Clin. Oncol.* **2018**, *36*, 1080–1087. [CrossRef]
11. Yanagisawa, T.; Rajwa, P.; Thibault, C.; Gandaglia, G.; Mori, K.; Kawada, T.; Fukuokaya, W.; Shim, S.R.; Mostafaei, H.; Motlagh, R.S.; et al. Androgen Receptor Signaling Inhibitors in Addition to Docetaxel with Androgen Deprivation Therapy for Metastatic Hormone-sensitive Prostate Cancer: A Systematic Review and Meta-analysis. *Eur. Urol.* **2022**, *82*, 584–598. [CrossRef] [PubMed]
12. von Deimling, M.; Rajwa, P.; Tilki, D.; Heidenreich, A.; Pallauf, M.; Bianchi, A.; Yanagisawa, T.; Kawada, T.; Karakiewicz, P.I.; Gontero, P.; et al. The current role of precision surgery in oligometastatic prostate cancer. *ESMO Open.* **2022**, *7*, 100597. [CrossRef] [PubMed]
13. Parker, C.C.; James, N.D.; Brawley, C.D.; Clarke, N.W.; Hoyle, A.P.; Ali, A.; Ritchie, A.W.S.; Attard, G.; Chowdhury, S.; Cross, W.; et al. Radiotherapy to the primary tumour for newly diagnosed, metastatic prostate cancer (STAMPEDE): A randomised controlled phase 3 trial. *Lancet* **2018**, *392*, 2353–2366. [CrossRef] [PubMed]
14. Wang, Y.; Qin, Z.; Wang, Y.; Chen, C.; Wang, Y.; Meng, X.; Song, N. The role of radical prostatectomy for the treatment of metastatic prostate cancer: A systematic review and meta-analysis. *Biosci. Rep.* **2018**, *38*, BSR20171379. [CrossRef] [PubMed]

15. Mao, Y.; Hu, M.; Yang, G.; Gao, E.; Xu, W. Cytoreductive prostatectomy improves survival outcomes in patients with oligometastases: A systematic meta-analysis. *World J. Surg. Oncol.* **2022**, *20*, 255. [CrossRef]
16. Shemshaki, H.; Al-Mamari, S.A.; Geelani, I.A.; Kumar, S. Cytoreductive radical prostatectomy versus systemic therapy and radiation therapy in metastatic prostate cancer: A systematic review and meta-analysis. *Urologia* **2022**, *89*, 16–30. [CrossRef]
17. Christ, S.M.; Pohl, K.; Muehlematter, U.J.; Heesen, P.; Kühnis, A.; Willmann, J.; Ahmadsei, M.; Badra, E.V.; Kroeze, S.G.C.; Mayinger, M.; et al. Imaging-Based Prevalence of Oligometastatic Disease: A Single-Center Cross-Sectional Study. *Int. J. Radiat. Oncol. Biol. Phys.* **2022**, *114*, 596–602. [CrossRef]
18. Liberati, A.; Altman, D.G.; Tetzlaff, J.; Mulrow, C.; Gotzsche, P.C.; Ioannidis, J.P.; Clarke, M.; Devereaux, P.J.; Kleijnen, J.; Moher, D. The PRISMA statement for reporting systematic reviews and meta-analyses of studies that evaluate health care interventions: Explanation and elaboration. *PLoS Med.* **2009**, *6*, e1000100. [CrossRef]
19. Antwi, S.; Everson, T.M. Prognostic impact of definitive local therapy of the primary tumor in men with metastatic prostate cancer at diagnosis: A population-based, propensity score analysis. *Cancer Epidemiol.* **2014**, *38*, 435–441. [CrossRef]
20. Culp, S.H.; Schellhammer, P.F.; Williams, M.B. Might men diagnosed with metastatic prostate cancer benefit from definitive treatment of the primary tumor? A SEER-based study. *Eur. Urol.* **2014**, *65*, 1058–1066. [CrossRef]
21. Gratzke, C.; Engel, J.; Stief, C.G. Role of radical prostatectomy in metastatic prostate cancer: Data from the Munich Cancer Registry. *Eur. Urol.* **2014**, *66*, 602–603. [CrossRef] [PubMed]
22. Guo, X.; Xia, H.; Su, X.; Hou, H.; Zhong, Q.; Wang, J. Comparing the Survival Outcomes of Radical Prostatectomy Versus Radiotherapy for Patients with De Novo Metastasis Prostate Cancer: A Population-Based Study. *Front. Oncol.* **2021**, *11*, 797462. [CrossRef] [PubMed]
23. Jin, K.; Qiu, S.; Jin, H.; Zheng, X.; Zhou, X.; Jin, D.; Li, J.; Yang, L.; Wei, Q. Survival Outcomes for Metastatic Prostate Cancer Patients Treated with Radical Prostatectomy or Radiation Therapy: A SEER-based Study. *Clin. Genitourin. Cancer* **2020**, *18*, e705–e722. [CrossRef]
24. Jin, S.; Wei, J.; Wang, J.; Wang, B.; Wu, J.; Gan, H.; Dai, B.; Qin, X.; Lin, G.; Wei, Y.; et al. Prognostic Value of Local Treatment in Prostate Cancer Patients with Different Metastatic Sites: A Population Based Retrospective Study. *Front. Oncol.* **2020**, *10*, 527952. [CrossRef] [PubMed]
25. Parikh, R.R.; Byun, J.; Goyal, S.; Kim, I.Y. Local Therapy Improves Overall Survival in Patients with Newly Diagnosed Metastatic Prostate Cancer. *Prostate* **2017**, *77*, 559–572. [CrossRef]
26. Satkunasivam, R.; Kim, A.E.; Desai, M.; Nguyen, M.M.; Quinn, D.I.; Ballas, L.; Lewinger, J.P.; Stern, M.C.; Hamilton, A.S.; Aron, M.; et al. Radical Prostatectomy or External Beam Radiation Therapy vs No Local Therapy for Survival Benefit in Metastatic Prostate Cancer: A SEER-Medicare Analysis. *J. Urol.* **2015**, *194*, 378–385. [CrossRef]
27. Stolzenbach, L.F.; Deuker, M.; Collà-Ruvolo, C.; Nocera, L.; Tian, Z.; Maurer, T.; Steuber, T.; Tilki, D.; Briganti, A.; Saad, F.; et al. Radical prostatectomy improves survival in selected metastatic prostate cancer patients: A North American population-based study. *Int. J. Urol.* **2021**, *28*, 834–839. [CrossRef]
28. Babst, C.; Amiel, T.; Maurer, T.; Knipper, S.; Lunger, L.; Tauber, R.; Retz, M.; Herkommer, K.; Eiber, M.; von Amsberg, G.; et al. Cytoreductive radical prostatectomy after chemohormonal therapy in patients with primary metastatic prostate cancer. *Asian J. Urol.* **2022**, *9*, 69–74. [CrossRef]
29. Buelens, S.; Poelaert, F.; Claeys, T.; De Bleser, E.; Dhondt, B.; Verla, W.; Ost, P.; Rappe, B.; De Troyer, B.; Verbaeys, C.; et al. Multicentre, prospective study on local treatment of metastatic prostate cancer (LoMP study). *BJU Int.* **2022**, *129*, 699–707. [CrossRef]
30. Chaloupka, M.; Stoermer, L.; Apfelbeck, M.; Buchner, A.; Wenter, V.; Stief, C.G.; Westhofen, T.; Kretschmer, A. Health-Related Quality of Life following Cytoreductive Radical Prostatectomy in Patients with De-Novo Oligometastatic Prostate Cancer. *Cancers* **2021**, *13*, 5636. [CrossRef]
31. Dai, B.; Zhang, S.; Wan, F.N.; Wang, H.K.; Zhang, J.Y.; Wang, Q.F.; Kong, Y.Y.; Ma, X.J.; Mo, M.; Zhu, Y.; et al. Combination of Androgen Deprivation Therapy with Radical Local Therapy Versus Androgen Deprivation Therapy Alone for Newly Diagnosed Oligometastatic Prostate Cancer: A Phase II Randomized Controlled Trial. *Eur. Urol. Oncol.* **2022**, *5*, 519–525. [CrossRef] [PubMed]
32. Heidenreich, A.; Fossati, N.; Pfister, D.; Suardi, N.; Montorsi, F.; Shariat, S.; Grubmüller, B.; Gandaglia, G.; Briganti, A.; Karnes, R.J. Cytoreductive Radical Prostatectomy in Men with Prostate Cancer and Skeletal Metastases. *Eur. Urol. Oncol.* **2018**, *1*, 46–53. [CrossRef] [PubMed]
33. Heidenreich, A.; Pfister, D.; Porres, D. Cytoreductive radical prostatectomy in patients with prostate cancer and low volume skeletal metastases: Results of a feasibility and case-control study. *J. Urol.* **2015**, *193*, 832–838. [CrossRef] [PubMed]
34. Kim, I.Y.; Mitrofanova, A.; Panja, S.; Sterling, J.; Srivastava, A.; Kim, J.; Kim, S.; Singer, E.A.; Jang, T.L.; Ghodoussipour, S.; et al. Genomic analysis and long-term outcomes of a phase 1 clinical trial on cytoreductive radical prostatectomy. *Prostate Int.* **2022**, *10*, 75–79. [CrossRef] [PubMed]
35. Knipper, S.; Beyer, B.; Mandel, P.; Tennstedt, P.; Tilki, D.; Steuber, T.; Graefen, M. Outcome of patients with newly diagnosed prostate cancer with low metastatic burden treated with radical prostatectomy: A comparison to STAMPEDE arm H. *World J. Urol.* **2020**, *38*, 1459–1464. [CrossRef]
36. Lumen, N.; De Bleser, E.; Buelens, S.; Verla, W.; Poelaert, F.; Claeys, W.; Fonteyne, V.; Verbeke, S.; Villeirs, G.; De Man, K.; et al. The Role of Cytoreductive Radical Prostatectomy in the Treatment of Newly Diagnosed Low-volume Metastatic Prostate Cancer. Results from the Local Treatment of Metastatic Prostate Cancer (LoMP) Registry. *Eur. Urol. Open Sci.* **2021**, *29*, 68–76. [CrossRef]

37. Mandel, P.C.; Huland, H.; Tiebel, A.; Haese, A.; Salomon, G.; Budäus, L.; Tilki, D.; Chun, F.; Heinzer, H.; Graefen, M.; et al. Enumeration and Changes in Circulating Tumor Cells and Their Prognostic Value in Patients Undergoing Cytoreductive Radical Prostatectomy for Oligometastatic Prostate Cancer-Translational Research Results from the Prospective ProMPT trial. *Eur. Urol. Focus.* **2021**, *7*, 55–62. [CrossRef]
38. Mistretta, F.A.; Luzzago, S.; Conti, A.; Verri, E.; Marvaso, G.; Collà Ruvolo, C.; Catellani, M.; Di Trapani, E.; Cozzi, G.; Bianchi, R.; et al. Oligometastatic Prostate Cancer: A Comparison between Multimodality Treatment vs. Androgen Deprivation Therapy Alone. *Cancers* **2022**, *14*, 2313. [CrossRef]
39. Moschini, M.; Morlacco, A.; Kwon, E.; Rangel, L.J.; Karnes, R.J. Treatment of M1a/M1b prostate cancer with or with out radical prostatectomy at diagnosis. *Prostate Cancer Prostatic Dis.* **2017**, *20*, 117–121. [CrossRef]
40. Poelaert, F.; Verbaeys, C.; Rappe, B.; Kimpe, B.; Billiet, I.; Plancke, H.; Decaestecker, K.; Fonteyne, V.; Buelens, S.; Lumen, N. Cytoreductive Prostatectomy for Metastatic Prostate Cancer: First Lessons Learned from the Multicentric Prospective Local Treatment of Metastatic Prostate Cancer (LoMP) Trial. *Urology* **2017**, *106*, 146–152. [CrossRef]
41. Sooriakumaran, P.; Wilson, C.; Rombach, I.; Hassanali, N.; Aning, J.; D Lamb, A.; Cathcart, P.; Eden, C.; Ahmad, I.; Rajan, P.; et al. Feasibility and safety of radical prostatectomy for oligo-metastatic prostate cancer: The Testing Radical prostatectomy in men with prostate cancer and oligo-Metastases to the bone (TRoMbone) trial. *BJU Int.* **2022**, *130*, 43–53. [CrossRef]
42. Steuber, T.; Berg, K.D.; Røder, M.A.; Brasso, K.; Iversen, P.; Huland, H.; Tiebel, A.; Schlomm, T.; Haese, A.; Salomon, G.; et al. Does Cytoreductive Prostatectomy Really Have an Impact on Prognosis in Prostate Cancer Patients with Low-volume Bone Metastasis? Results from a Prospective Case-Control Study. *Eur. Urol. Focus.* **2017**, *3*, 646–649. [CrossRef] [PubMed]
43. Takagi, K.; Kawase, M.; Kato, D.; Kawase, K.; Takai, M.; Iinuma, K.; Nakane, K.; Hagiwara, N.; Yamada, T.; Tomioka, M.; et al. Robot-Assisted Radical Prostatectomy for Potential Cancer Control in Patients with Metastatic Prostate Cancer. *Curr. Oncol.* **2022**, *29*, 2864–2870. [CrossRef] [PubMed]
44. Xue, P.; Wu, Z.; Wang, K.; Gao, G.; Zhuang, M.; Yan, M. Oncological Outcome of Combining Cytoreductive Prostatectomy and Metastasis-Directed Radiotherapy in Patients with Prostate Cancer and Bone Oligometastases: A Retrospective Cohort Study. *Cancer Manag. Res.* **2020**, *12*, 8867–8873. [CrossRef] [PubMed]
45. Gandaglia, G.; Fossati, N.; Stabile, A.; Bandini, M.; Rigatti, P.; Montorsi, F.; Briganti, A. Radical Prostatectomy in Men with Oligometastatic Prostate Cancer: Results of a Single-institution Series with Long-term Follow-up. *Eur. Urol.* **2017**, *72*, 289–292. [CrossRef]
46. Mazzone, E.; Mistretta, F.A.; Knipper, S.; Tian, Z.; Larcher, A.; Widmer, H.; Zorn, K.; Capitanio, U.; Graefen, M.; Montorsi, F.; et al. Contemporary National Assessment of Robot-Assisted Surgery Rates and Total Hospital Charges for Major Surgical Uro-Oncological Procedures in the United States. *J. Endourol.* **2019**, *33*, 438–447. [CrossRef]
47. Ploussard, G.; Grabia, A.; Beauval, J.B.; Barret, E.; Brureau, L.; Dariane, C.; Fiard, G.; Fromont, G.; Gauthé, M.; Mathieu, R.; et al. A 5-Year Contemporary Nationwide Evolution of the Radical Prostatectomy Landscape. *Eur. Urol. Open Sci.* **2021**, *34*, 1–4. [CrossRef]
48. Novara, G.; Ficarra, V.; Rosen, R.C.; Artibani, W.; Costello, A.; Eastham, J.A.; Graefen, M.; Guazzoni, G.; Shariat, S.F.; Stolzenburg, J.U.; et al. Systematic review and meta-analysis of perioperative outcomes and complications after robot-assisted radical prostatectomy. *Eur. Urol.* **2012**, *62*, 431–452. [CrossRef]
49. Won, A.C.; Gurney, H.; Marx, G.; De Souza, P.; Patel, M.I. Primary treatment of the prostate improves local palliation in men who ultimately develop castrate-resistant prostate cancer. *BJU Int.* **2013**, *112*, E250–E255. [CrossRef]

Disclaimer/Publisher's Note: The statements, opinions and data contained in all publications are solely those of the individual author(s) and contributor(s) and not of MDPI and/or the editor(s). MDPI and/or the editor(s) disclaim responsibility for any injury to people or property resulting from any ideas, methods, instructions or products referred to in the content.

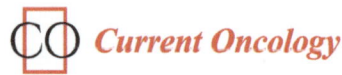 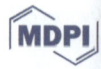

Article

Combining Molecular Subtypes with Multivariable Clinical Models Has the Potential to Improve Prediction of Treatment Outcomes in Prostate Cancer at Diagnosis

Lewis Wardale [1], Ryan Cardenas [1], Vincent J. Gnanapragasam [2,3], Colin S. Cooper [1], Jeremy Clark [1] and Daniel S. Brewer [1,4,*]

[1] Norwich Medical School, University of East Anglia, Norwich Research Park, Norwich NR4 7TJ, UK
[2] Department of Urology, Cambridge University Hospitals NHS Foundation Trust, Cambridge CB2 0QQ, UK
[3] Division of Urology, Department of Surgery, University of Cambridge, Cambridge CB2 0QQ, UK
[4] The Earlham Institute, Norwich Research Park, Norwich NR4 7UZ, UK
* Correspondence: d.brewer@uea.ac.uk

Abstract: Clinical management of prostate cancer is challenging because of its highly variable natural history and so there is a need for improved predictors of outcome in non-metastatic men at the time of diagnosis. In this study we calculated the model score from the leading clinical multivariable model, PREDICT prostate, and the poor prognosis DESNT molecular subtype, in a combined expression and clinical dataset that were taken from malignant tissue at prostatectomy ($n = 359$). Both PREDICT score ($p < 0.0001$, IQR HR = 1.59) and DESNT score ($p < 0.0001$, IQR HR = 2.08) were significant predictors for time to biochemical recurrence. A joint model combining the continuous PREDICT and DESNT score ($p < 0.0001$, IQR HR = 1.53 and 1.79, respectively) produced a significantly improved predictor than either model alone ($p < 0.001$). An increased probability of mortality after diagnosis, as estimated by PREDICT, was characterised by upregulation of cell-cycle related pathways and the downregulation of metabolism and cholesterol biosynthesis. The DESNT molecular subtype has distinct biological characteristics to those associated with the PREDICT model. We conclude that the inclusion of biological information alongside current clinical prognostic tools has the potential to improve the ability to choose the optimal treatment pathway for a patient.

Keywords: prostate cancer; clinical models; predictive models; molecular subtypes; transcriptome; expression; statistical model

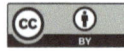

1. Introduction

Prostate cancer is distressingly common (diagnosed in 48,487 of men in UK per year) but not frequently fatal (13% of male cancer deaths) [1]. The progression of prostate cancer is highly heterogeneous [2], and clinical management is challenging [3,4]. It is also estimated, that as many as 50–80% of PSA-detected prostate cancers are clinically irrelevant, that is, even without treatment, they would never have caused any symptoms [5]. This has confounded attempts to develop a consistent and reliable approach to identify aggressive disease. Radical treatment of early prostate cancer, with surgery or radiotherapy, can lead to life changing side-effects of treatment such as impotence or incontinence [6]. There is a need for improved predictors of outcome in non-metastatic men at the time of diagnosis.

One approach is to use the information that is already collected at the point of diagnosis and before treatment, to assess prognosis and the value of treatment. Thurtle et al. (2019) developed an approach, termed 'PREDICT Prostate', that modelled, at the time of diagnosis, prostate cancer specific mortality (PCSM) and non-prostate cancer mortality (NPCM) using separate multivariable Cox models within a competing risks framework [7]. The NPCM model utilises the variables age and comorbidity, while the PCSM model combines age, PSA, Gleason grade, clinical T stage, and proportion of positive biopsy cores at the time of diagnosis. The model shows good discrimination in large validation datasets from the UK (n = 3000; C-index = 0.84; 95% CI: 0.82–0.86) [7], Singapore (n = 2546; C-index = 0.84; 95% CI: 0.80–0.87) [7], Sweden (n = 69,206; C-index = 0.85; 95% CI 0.85–0.86) [8], and the United States of America (n = 171,942; C-index = 0.82; 95% CI 0.81–0.83) [9]. It has been endorsed by the National Institute for Health and Care Excellence (NICE) [10] and is available in a user-friendly web interface (https://prostate.predict.nhs.uk/ (accessed on 1 May 2022)). Another approach to improve prediction of outcome is to use additional novel biomarkers [11].

Within any single cancer disease type, sub-classification using molecular markers can be an important way to accurately determine prognosis, optimise treatment pathways, and help develop targeted drugs. In previous work, we have successfully identified a novel aggressive molecular subtype of human prostate cancer, called DESNT, that can predict outcome after radical surgery (prostatectomy) and is associated with metastasis. This was discovered by applying the Bayesian clustering method Latent Process Decomposition to transcriptome data [12–14]—this takes into account the heterogeneous composition of prostate cancer. Prostatectomy patients with most of their expression assigned to the DESNT type exhibit poor outcomes relative to other patients ($p < 4.28 \times 10^{-5}$; Log-rank test) and has been validated in eight independent transcriptome datasets. Cancers assigned to the DESNT group have an increased risk of developing metastasis (X^2-test, $p = 1.86 \times 10^{-3}$) [13]. The amount of the DESNT signature is an independent prognostic predictor of time to biochemical recurrence (HR = 1.52, 95% CI = [1.36, 1.7], $p = 9.0 \times 10^{-14}$, Cox regression model) [13]. This framework was developed from samples taken at prostatectomy, but we have preliminary data to suggest it's applicability to biopsies [15]. We are in the process of developing a diagnostic lab to utilise the DESNT framework as an accredited clinical test.

In this work we modelled whether adding the poor prognosis DESNT signature to the PREDICT Prostate algorithm has the potential to improve our ability to predict the overall progress of prostate cancer. Transcriptome data from tumour tissue collected at an initial treatment of proctectomy were used as a proxy for the information that could be gathered from cancerous biopsy tissue at the time of diagnosis. Secondary aims are to determine whether the PREDICT Prostate clinical model can predict disease prognosis after surgical treatment of prostate cancer; and find the similarities and differences in the genes and molecular pathways which drive a higher PREDICT score and characterise the DESNT molecular subtype.

2. Materials and Methods

2.1. Datasets and Filtering

Microarray datasets from prostate tissue were processed and normalised as described in Luca et al. (2020) (Table 1). In brief, Affymetrix microarray dataset was normalised using the RMA algorithm [16] or previous normalised values were used. Only probes corresponding to genes measured by all platforms were retained. The CamCap and CancerMap datasets have 40 patients in common and thus 20 of the common samples were excluded at random from each dataset. The ComBat algorithm [17] from the sva R package and quantile transformation, was used to mitigate study-specific effects. The ethical approvals obtained for each dataset are listed in the original publications.

Table 1. Transcriptome datasets used. FF = Fresh Frozen.

Dataset	Primary	Normal	Type	Platform	Citation
MSKCC [18]	131	29	FF	Affymetrix Exon 1.0 ST v2	Taylor et al., 2010
CancerMap [12]	137	17	FF	Affymetrix Exon 1.0 ST v2	Luca et al., 2018
Stephenson [19]	78	11	FF	Affymetrix U133A	Stephenson et al., 2005
CamCap [20]	147	73	FF	Illumina HT12 v4.0 BeadChip	Ross-Adams et al., 2015

The combined dataset was filtered to remove samples that were missing one or more of the clinical variables required for the Prostate PREDICT model (patient's age, T-stage, PSA and the Gleason histological grade group). Only primary tumour tissue from the prostate were included. Duplicate samples were also removed. For the Stephenson dataset only Gleason sum was available, so 44 samples were removed that had a Gleason sum of seven. The resulting dataset consists of 359 samples.

2.2. R Implementation of the Prostate PREDICT Model

The Prostate PREDICT model was originally implemented in the language STRATA [7]. We have translated this to the freely available open-source R statistical programming language [21] and made the code available (https://doi.org/10.5281/zenodo.7248417 accessed on 25 October 2022). Our implementation of the Prostate PREDICT model was extensively verified by comparing the results produced by those of the PREDICT Prostate webpage tool (https://prostate.predict.nhs.uk/tool accessed on 1 May 2022) for a wide variety of inputs. The results were identical, for example, when age = 75, T-stage = 2, PSA = 25 and Gleason score = 4 + 3, the 10-year predicted survival from initial conservative management was 55% via the webpage tool and 0.549 in R. We also examined how the R version PREDICT results vary with clinical variables to ensure that they made logical sense.

As we are interested in reducing radical treatment in prostate cancer the results from the PREDICT model used initial conservative management as the treatment strategy rather than radical treatment. For the datasets used here, comorbidity (the patient had not experienced a hospital admission in the last 2 years for something other than prostate cancer) and detailed biopsy histopathology results were unavailable and so are set to zero, as is done in the online implementation when this information is unavailable. For each sample, the prostate cancer specific mortality probability (PCSM) at ten years after diagnosis (as a percentage) was calculated using as input the associated clinical variables age at diagnosis, PSA at diagnosis, T stage, and prostatectomy Gleason grade group (as a proxy for biopsy Gleason grade group). The non-prostate cancer mortality probability (NPCM, as a percentage) was calculated using age at diagnosis. The PREDICT score, the increase in probability of mortality at 10 years from having prostate cancer, was defined as NPCM-PCSM.

2.3. DESNT Score and Assignment

Latent Process Decomposition (LPD) was applied to the MSKCC dataset [18] to produce the DESNT framework model, exactly as described in Luca et al. (2020) [13]. This model was then applied to the other datasets using the OAS-LPD algorithm, a modified version of the LPD algorithm in which new sample(s) are decomposed into LPD signatures, without retraining the model. Again, as described in Luca et al. (2020). LPD is an unsupervised Bayesian approach which decomposes each sample's expression into signature expression profiles of each molecular subtype. For each sample a score between 0 and 1 is given for each subtype which represents the proportion of a sample's expression that is explained by the signature expression profile for that subtype. Here, the proportion of expression assigned to the DESNT subtype is termed the DESNT score and are the exact scores produced in previous work [13]. If the DESNT score is the largest score across the subtypes, the sample is considered a member of the DESNT subtype.

2.4. Differential Gene Expression Analysis

Differentially expressed genes were identified for each comparison using a moderated t-test implemented in the limma (v 3.52.0) R package [22] with a threshold of Benjamin-Hochberg false discovery rate < 0.05.

2.5. Functional Enrichment Analysis

Functional enrichment analysis was performed using the gProfiler2 (v0.2.1) [23] R package utilising the KEGG, RECTOME, and Gene Ontology database for biological process terms. The gSCS (Set Counts and Sizes) correction method was used to determine significantly enriched pathways and ontology terms with significance $p < 0.05$.

2.6. Statistical Tests

All analyses were performed in R (version 4.1.2) using default parameters unless otherwise stated. Survival analyses were performed using Cox proportional hazards regression models, the log-rank test, and Kaplan–Meier estimator, as implemented in the survival R package with biochemical recurrence after prostatectomy as the end point. Pairwise comparisons of Kaplan–Meier curves using Log-Rank test were performed using the SurvMiner (v 0.4.9), with p-values adjusted using the Benjamini-Hochberg multiple testing correction. All plots were created using ggplot2 (v 3.3.6). All statistical tests performed were two-sided non-parametric tests unless otherwise stated.

3. Results

3.1. Data Overview

We combined transcriptome data from malignant samples taken at an initial treatment of prostatectomy from four studies: the MSKCC [18], CancerMap [12], Stephenson [19] and CamCap [20] studies (Table 1). These were filtered to have results from one primary sample per patient with the required clinical information required for the Prostate PREDICT model ($n = 359$; Table 2). The proportion of expression assigned to the DESNT poor prognosis molecular subtype (DESNT score) were gathered from previous results [13]. For each sample, the prostate cancer specific mortality probability (PCSM) at ten years after diagnosis (as a percentage) was calculated using an implementation of the Prostate PREDICT model in R (see methods), under the assumption of initial conservative management, using as input the associated clinical variables: age at diagnosis, PSA at diagnosis, clinical T stage, and prostatectomy Gleason grade group (as a proxy for biopsy Gleason grade group). The equivalent expected non-prostate cancer mortality (NPCM) was calculated using age at diagnosis. The PREDICT score, the increase in probability of mortality at 10 years caused from having prostate cancer, was defined as NPCM-PCSM.

DESNT scores from our combined dataset had a median value of 0.09 and an interquartile range of 0.32. PREDICT scores had a median value of 5.84 and an interquartile range of 3.24. There was a weak correlation between DESNT score and PREDICT score (Figure 1A; rho = 0.21; $p < 0.05$; Spearmen's correlation). The DESNT score is very variable with respect to the PREDICT score (Figure 1B). The PREDICT score showed a statistically significant increase in samples that were DESNT cancers, i.e., where the proportion assigned to the DESNT subtype was higher than all other subtypes in the framework (Figure 2; $p < 0.001$; Mann–Whitney U test; difference in medians = 1.93).

Table 2. Summary of clinical variables of cohorts. BCR = Biochemical recurrence after prostatectomy as defined by two PSA measurements at values greater than or equal to 0.2 ng/mL. BCR/Follow up is time to biochemical recurrence or last clinical update. T-stage = clinical tumour stage. The PREDICT score, the percentage increase in probability of mortality at 10 years from having prostate cancer, is defined as the non-prostate cancer mortality minus prostate cancer specific mortality at 10 years. DESNT score is the proportion of expression assigned to the DESNT poor prognosis molecular subtype.

Characteristic	CamCap, n = 89 [1]	CancerMap, n = 108 [1]	Stephenson, n = 33 [1]	MSKCC, n = 129 [1]
Age at diagnosis	61 (56, 65)	62 (56, 65)	61 (55, 65)	58 (54, 62)
PSA at diagnosis (ng/mL)	7.9 (6.1, 9.8)	7.9 (5.8, 11.4)	9.8 (6.0, 18.4)	5.9 (4.5, 9.3)
Gleason grade group				
1	12 (13%)	29 (27%)	15 (45%)	40 (31%)
2	52 (58%)	59 (55%)	0 (0%)	53 (41%)
3	16 (18%)	16 (15%)	0 (0%)	21 (16%)
4	8 (9.0%)	1 (0.9%)	10 (30%)	8 (6.2%)
5	1 (1.1%)	3 (2.8%)	8 (24%)	7 (5.4%)
T Stage				
1	48 (54%)	1 (0.9%)	19 (58%)	0 (0%)
2	28 (31%)	58 (54%)	13 (39%)	84 (65%)
3	13 (15%)	49 (45%)	1 (3.0%)	39 (30%)
4	0 (0%)	0 (0%)	0 (0%)	6 (4.7%)
BCR/Follow up (in months)	23 (15, 41)	55 (32, 64)	56 (12, 70)	47 (28, 62)
BCR event				
FALSE	74 (83%)	77 (71%)	16 (48%)	102 (79%)
TRUE	15 (17%)	31 (29%)	17 (52%)	27 (21%)
DESNT Score	0.22 (0.10, 0.37)	0.09 (0.00, 0.31)	0.10 (0.02, 0.34)	0.00 (0.00, 0.18)
PREDICT Score	5.5 (4.7, 7.0)	6.4 (5.0, 8.1)	7.7 (3.6, 10.4)	5.6 (4.2, 7.2)

[1] Median (IQR); n (%)

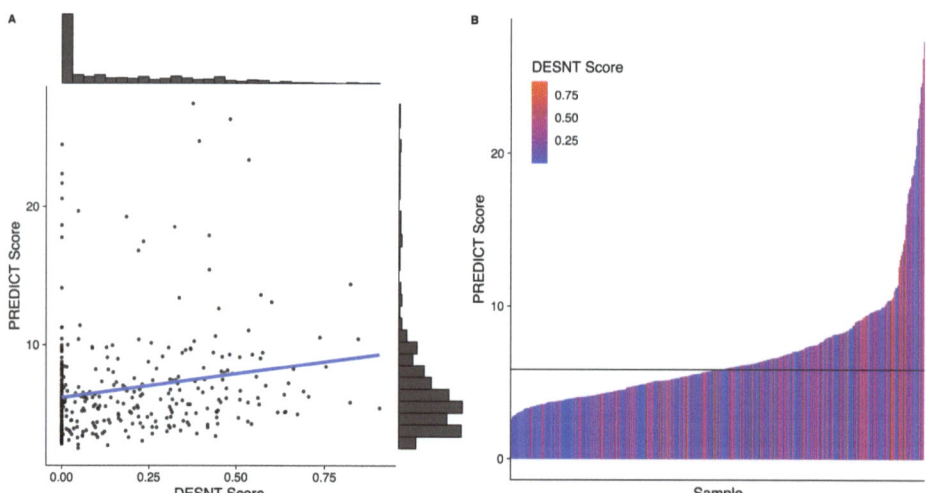

Figure 1. The relationship between Prostate PREDICT score and DESNT score. (**A**) Scatter plot and distribution. (**B**) A waterfall plot showing how the DESNT score varies with PREDICT score. The horizontal line at 5.8 represents the median PREDICT score. The PREDICT score is the percentage increase in probability of mortality at 10 years from having prostate cancer defined as the non-prostate cancer mortality minus prostate cancer specific mortality at 10 years. DESNT score is the proportion of expression that is explained by the signature expression profile of the DESNT molecular subtype.

3.2. Predictive Ability of PREDICT and DESNT Score to Predict Time to Biochemical Recurrence

Both PREDICT score and DESNT score, when applied in separate models, have a significant association with time to biochemical recurrence (PREDICT: $p < 0.0001$, IQR HR = 1.59 [95% CI 1.43–1.76]; DESNT: $p < 0.0001$, IQR HR = 2.08 [95% CI 1.58–2.76]; Cox proportional hazards regression). A joint Cox proportional hazards model built with the two continuous independent variables PREDICT and DESNT score ($p < 0.0001$, IQR HR = 1.53 and 1.79, respectively; Table 3) was significantly better at predicting biochemical recurrence outcome than PREDICT score ($p < 0.001$; likelihood ratio test) or DESNT score ($p < 0.001$) alone. To illustrate this, samples were categorised into DESNT cancers or non-DESNT cancers, and upper PREDICT score or lower PREDICT score (split around the median; Table 4). A Kaplan-Meir plot shows clear delineation between each combination of groups (Figure 3; Log-rank p-value < 0.001). At five years, the estimated proportion that are biochemical recurrence free are 92% (Lower PREDICT score & Not DESNT), 65% (Upper PREDICT score & Not DESNT), 56% (Lower PREDICT score & DESNT), and 38% (Upper PREDICT score & DESNT). Pair-wise, all Kaplan–Meier curves are significantly different ($p < 0.001$; log-rank test; Benjamini-Hochberg adjusted p-values) apart from "Lower PREDICT score & DESNT" vs. "Upper PREDICT score & DESNT" ($p = 0.18$) and "Lower PREDICT score & DESNT" vs. "Upper PREDICT score & Not DESNT" ($p = 0.53$).

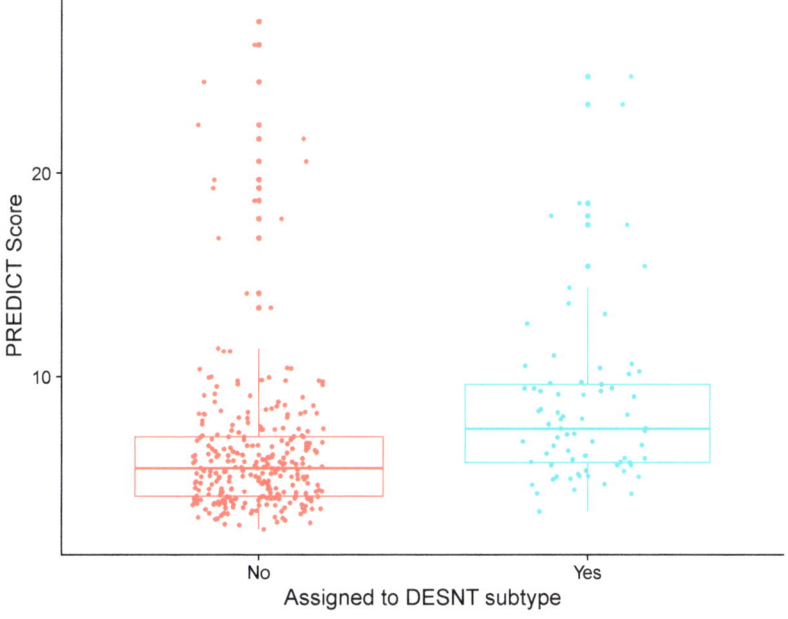

Figure 2. Differences in PREDICT score between prostate cancer samples assigned to DESNT and those not. Samples assigned to DESNT are those where the largest proportion of expression is explained by the expression signature of the DESNT subtype. The PREDICT score is the increase in probability of mortality at 10 years caused by having prostate cancer defined as the non-prostate cancer mortality minus prostate cancer specific mortality at 10 years.

Table 3. Summary of Cox proportional hazard model combining PREDICT score and DESNT score. Endpoint is time to biochemical recurrence.

Variable	IQR Hazard Ratio (HR)	HR Lower 95% CI	HR Upper 95% CI	p-Value
PREDICT Score	1.53	1.37	1.70	<0.0001
DESNT score	1.79	1.34	2.40	<0.0001

Table 4. Discretisation of samples into DESNT vs. non-DESNT (based on the dominant subtype expression signature) and upper and lower PREDICT score (split around the median PREDICT score).

	DESNT	Non-DESNT
Upper PREDICT	53	126
Lower PREDICT	20	160

3.3. Characterisation of the Genes and Biological Processes behind PREDICT and DESNT Scores

To biologically characterise the PREDICT score we compared the expression profiles from samples with the top 25% PREDICT score versus the bottom 25%. We found 451 genes to be significantly differentially expressed (287 downregulated; 164 upregulated; adjusted p-values < 0.05; adapted t-test; Table 5; Table S1). 162 pathways or ontological terms were found to be significantly enriched in upregulated genes and 74 with downregulated genes ($p < 0.05$; Table S2). This corresponded to 63 GO biological process terms, six KEGG pathways, and five Reactome pathways for downregulated genes, and 143 GO biological process terms, four KEGG pathways, and 15 Reactome pathways for downregulated genes (see Table 6 for enriched Reactome pathways).

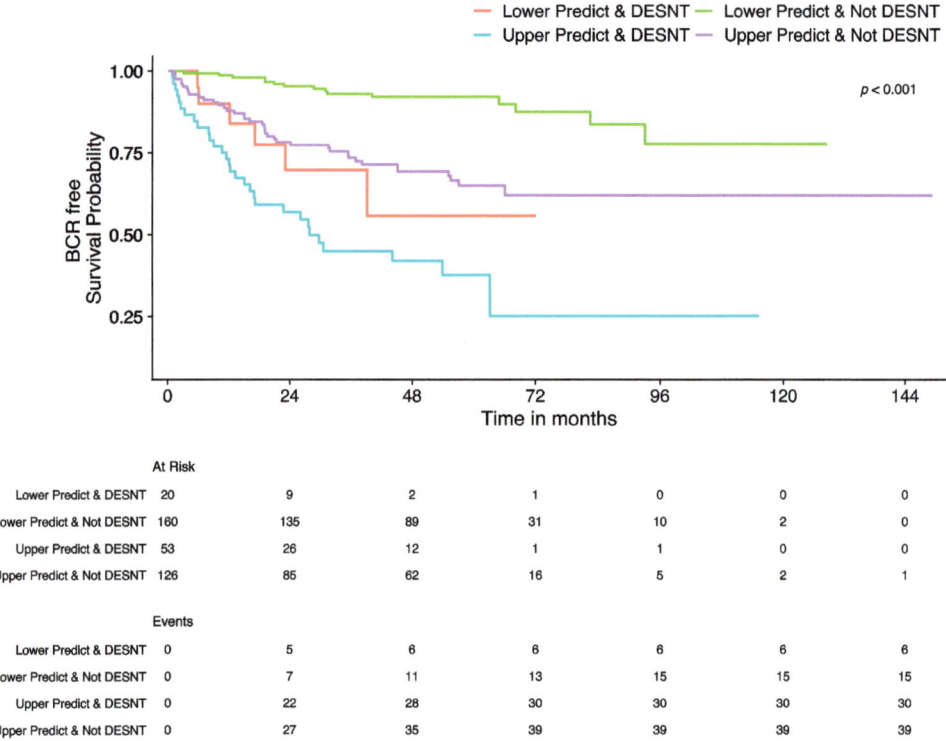

Figure 3. Kaplan–Meier plot showing the survival curves for samples grouped by DESNT and Prostate PREDICT model status. Endpoint is time to biochemical recurrence (BCR). Samples are divided into DESNT vs. non-DESNT and upper PREDICT vs. lower PREDICT (split around the median PREDICT score). The "At Risk" table below the plot shows the number of patients in each group, at the corresponding time point, that have not had a biochemical recurrence event and have longer follow up than that time. The "Events" table shows the cumulative number of biochemical recurrence events observed in a group at that time point.

Table 5. The top ten differentially expressed genes between the samples with the 25% highest PREDICT scores versus the lowest 25% PREDICT scores, ranked by $\log_2$ fold change. p values adjusted for multiple testing correction using the Benjamini-Hochberg algorithm. Whether these genes overlap with the 51 significant differential expressed genes Luca et al. (2020) observed as characteristic of the DESNT subtype and the differentially expressed genes for DESNT found in this study are also shown. Full results in Table S1.

Gene Symbol	$\log_2$ Fold Change	p Value	Adjusted p Value	Overlap with Luca et al. DESNT Genes	Overlap with DESNT DEGs
ANPEP	−1.31	1.54×10^{-8}	1.33×10^{-5}	TRUE	TRUE
CD38	−1.02	1.25×10^{-9}	2.17×10^{-6}	FALSE	TRUE
SLC22A3	−0.95	7.94×10^{-12}	8.28×10^{-8}	FALSE	TRUE
NPY	−0.91	2.84×10^{-4}	1.32×10^{-2}	FALSE	FALSE
MSMB	−0.89	1.22×10^{-5}	1.84×10^{-3}	FALSE	TRUE
MT1G	−0.86	4.51×10^{-7}	1.54×10^{-4}	FALSE	TRUE
MT1M	−0.85	8.34×10^{-6}	1.32×10^{-3}	TRUE	TRUE
COMP	0.84	8.81×10^{-9}	1.02×10^{-5}	FALSE	TRUE
KRT15	−0.77	1.66×10^{-5}	2.25×10^{-3}	FALSE	TRUE
SFRP4	0.76	2.39×10^{-8}	1.66×10^{-5}	FALSE	TRUE

Table 6. Reactome pathways found to be significantly enriched for significantly upregulated or downregulated genes for PREDICT high score samples versus low score samples. Direction = whether pathway is enriched for downregulated or upregulated genes. Full results including KEGG pathway and GO BP terms in Table S2.

Term Name	Direction	p Value	Term Size	Intersection Size	Overlap with DESNT Enriched Terms
Cell Cycle, Mitotic	Up	4.08×10^{-9}	548	28	TRUE
Cell Cycle	Up	2.37×10^{-8}	678	30	TRUE
Mitotic G1 phase and G1/S transition	Up	3.79×10^{-5}	147	12	TRUE
Integrin cell surface interactions	Up	0.002	84	8	FALSE
G1/S-Specific Transcription	Up	0.005	27	5	TRUE
Mitotic Prometaphase	Up	0.006	199	11	TRUE
G1/S Transition	Up	0.006	130	9	TRUE
ECM proteoglycans	Up	0.008	75	7	FALSE
Cell Cycle Checkpoints	Up	0.009	290	13	TRUE
Mitotic Spindle Checkpoint	Up	0.012	109	8	TRUE
M Phase	Up	0.021	407	15	TRUE
Kinesins	Up	0.023	60	6	FALSE
Resolution of Sister Chromatid Cohesion	Up	0.030	123	8	TRUE
Amplification of signal from unattached kinetochores via a MAD2 inhibitory signal	Up	0.032	92	7	TRUE
Amplification of signal from the kinetochores	Up	0.032	92	7	TRUE
Metabolism	Down	0.000	2075	63	FALSE
Cholesterol biosynthesis	Down	0.001	24	6	FALSE
Glutathione conjugation	Down	0.009	34	6	FALSE
Response to metal ions	Down	0.031	14	4	FALSE
Metabolism of lipids	Down	0.046	728	27	FALSE

4507 genes were found to be differentially expressed between DESNT vs. non DESNT samples (1973 downregulated; 2534 upregulated; adjusted p-values < 0.05 adapted t-test; Table 7; Table S3). Of the 51 differential expressed genes Luca et al (2020) observed as characteristic of the DESNT subtype across multiple datasets (49 down-regulated, two up-regulated), all of them were differentially expressed in this analysis and were altered in the same direction (Table S3). A much larger number of genes were identified here as the DESNT characteristic genes reported in Luca et al. are the overlap of differentially expressed genes from multiple different comparisons in independent cohorts. 449 pathways or ontological terms were found to be significantly enriched in upregulated genes and 1391 with downregulated genes (p < 0.05; Table S4). This corresponded to 1288 GO biological process terms, 58 KEGG pathways, and 45 Reactome pathways for downregulated genes, and 373 GO biological process terms nine KEGG pathways, and 67 Reactome pathways for upregulated genes (see Table 8 for the top 10 enriched Reactome pathways).

Of the 451 genes found to be characteristic of PREDICT, the majority (78%) were also found to be differentially expressed in the same direction between DESNT vs. non DESNT samples (Table S1), but only 8% of DESNT differentially expressed genes were found to be differentially expressed in the same direction between PREDICT score high vs. PREDICT score low samples. Only 24 out of 51 characteristic DESNT genes from Luca et al. (2020) were found to characterise PREDICT. 93 out of 236 (40%) enriched pathways/ontology terms were unique to the PREDICT Score (Table S2; 37% GO biological process terms, 80% KEGG pathways and 40% Reactome pathways). Similarly, 1697 out of 1840 (92%) enriched pathways/ontology terms were unique to DESNT (Table S4; 92% GO biological process terms, 97% KEGG pathways and 89% Reactome pathways). Taken together these results are suggestive that DESNT provides additional information to PREDICT based on the underlying biological processes.

Table 7. The top ten differentially expressed genes between the samples classified as DESNT samples versus non-DESNT samples, ranked by $\log_2$ fold change. p values adjusted for multiple testing correction using the Benjamini-Hochberg algorithm. Whether these genes overlap with the 51 significant differential expressed genes Luca et al. (2020) observed as characteristic of the DESNT subtype and the differentially expressed genes for PREDICT score found in this study are also shown. Full results in Table S3.

Gene Symbol	$\log_2$ Fold Change	p Value	Adjusted p Value	Overlap with Luca et al. DESNT Genes	Overlap with PREDICT DEGs
ANPEP	−2.27	4.18×10^{-31}	2.18×10^{-27}	TRUE	TRUE
RLN1	−1.80	4.50×10^{-14}	3.19×10^{-12}	FALSE	FALSE
MT1M	−1.62	1.45×10^{-25}	3.79×10^{-22}	TRUE	TRUE
ALOX15B	−1.44	2.85×10^{-17}	4.95×10^{-15}	FALSE	TRUE
CD38	−1.43	1.99×10^{-23}	1.59×10^{-20}	FALSE	TRUE
MSMB	−1.42	5.48×10^{-14}	3.69×10^{-12}	FALSE	TRUE
MT1G	−1.41	3.30×10^{-19}	1.04×10^{-16}	FALSE	TRUE
F5	1.35	1.06×10^{-19}	3.56×10^{-17}	TRUE	TRUE
LEPREL1	−1.33	1.85×10^{-23}	1.59×10^{-20}	FALSE	TRUE
ACTG2	−1.33	9.88×10^{-23}	6.87×10^{-20}	TRUE	TRUE
ERG	1.31	2.26×10^{-12}	9.90×10^{-11}	FALSE	FALSE

Table 8. The top 10 Reactome pathways found to be uniquely significantly enriched for significantly upregulated or downregulated genes for DESNT sample status, ranked by significance. Direction = whether pathway is enriched for downregulated or upregulated genes. Full results in Table S4.

Term Name	Direction	p Value	Term Size	Intersection Size
Signal Transduction	Down	3.94×10^{-15}	2523	437
Platelet activation, signaling and aggregation	Down	3.91×10^{-11}	258	76
Metabolism of RNA	Up	6.61×10^{-11}	661	173
Translation	Up	1.68×10^{-10}	292	94
Response to elevated platelet cytosolic Ca2+	Down	3.61×10^{-9}	130	46
Signaling by Receptor Tyrosine Kinases	Down	3.99×10^{-9}	502	115
Platelet degranulation	Down	1.27×10^{-8}	125	44
Hemostasis	Down	3.12×10^{-8}	672	140
DNA Replication	Up	3.40×10^{-8}	128	50
Extracellular matrix organization	Down	3.81×10^{-8}	298	77

4. Discussion

In this study we examined four large expression data sets that were taken from primary prostate cancer samples at prostatectomy for men with prostate cancer that had not received any other treatment. This data, along with relevant clinical data, was used as a proxy of the biological information that could be gathered from biopsies at the time of diagnosis. We calculated the model score from the leading clinical multivariable model, PREDICT prostate, and the poor prognosis DESNT molecular subtype. We showed the potential for the PREDICT Prostate clinical model to predict disease prognosis after surgical treatment of prostate cancer. We also found that by combining the DESNT score with the PREDICT score produced a significantly better predictor of outcome following prostatectomy. The return of prostate cancer after prostatectomy is an indication that micrometastases were present at the time of surgery [24]—it is estimated that up to 70% of patients have disseminated tumour cells after prostatectomy [25]. Therefore, poor treatment response at prostatectomy may give an indication of overall disease state. Our findings are important because it suggests that we can make a better-informed decision at the time of diagnosis of whether to perform radical treatment or not if molecular information is included.

For the first time the biological mechanisms behind an increased probability of mortality at ten years after diagnosis caused by prostate cancer (i.e., a higher PREDICT score) has been examined. The top 10 differentially expressed genes are the downregulation of *ANPEP, CD38, SLC22A3, NPY, MSMB, MT1G, MT1M, KRT15, & SFRP4* and upregulation of *COMP*.

ANPEP was the top-ranked downregulated gene in both PREDICT and DESNT analyses. Aminopeptidase N (APN) is the enzyme encoded by *ANPEP* that belongs to a group of widely expressed ectopeptidases [26]. APN is multifunctional for the post-secretory processing of neuropeptides and regulating the access of these molecules to cellular receptors. The role of APN positively associated with intracellular signalling and has been shown to play an important role in metastasis of several malignancies, including prostate cancer through neoangiogenesis [27–29]. Sorenson et al. (2013) observed a significant ($p < 0.001$) downregulation of *ANPEP* expression in prostate cancer in comparison with non- malignant prostate tissue samples [30]. The authors concluded that negative APN immunoreactivity is a prognostic factor for patients harbouring clinically localised prostate cancer for both recurrence-free and cancer-specific survival endpoints.

CD38 has previously been reported as a marker of the luminal cells in human prostate [31]. Using CD38 as a marker, Liu et al. (2016) identified low expression of the gene in a progenitor-like subset of luminal cells within the human prostate that are capable of initiation of human prostate cancer in an in vivo tissue-regeneration assay [32]. They also demonstrated that luminal cells with low CD38 expression are associated with disease progression and poor survival outcome in prostate cancers.

Neuropeptide Y (*NPY*) is a gene involved in various physiological and homeostatic processes such as stress response. Liu et al. (2007) observed lower expression levels of *NPY* that were associated with more aggressive clinical behaviour in prostate cancer [33]. *MT1G* [34], *MSMB* [35], *SLC22A3* [36], *COMP* [37] and *KRT15* [38] have also been associated with aggressive and/or poor clinical outcome in prostate cancer.

Functional enrichment analysis identified many molecular pathways that were upregulated or downregulated in high PREDICT score samples. This included the upregulation of many cell cycle related pathways, a well-known hallmark of cancer [39] and the downregulation of metabolism and cholesterol biosynthesis. Consistent with this result, Rye et al. found robust and consistent downregulation of nearly all genes in the cholesterol synthesis pathway in prostate cancer [40].

In this study we have also shown that the DESNT molecular subtype has shared and distinct biological characteristics to the general aggressive phenotype picked up by the PREDICT prognosis model. A much larger number of differentially expressed genes and enriched pathways were detected. This suggests that samples assigned as DESNT have expression profiles that are more like each other than samples with similar PREDICT scores, and so there is greater statistically power to detect differences. Only 8% of DESNT differentially expressed genes were found to be differentially expressed in the same direction in PREDICT score high samples. There were also many distinct enriched pathways including the downregulation of signalling pathways and extracellular matrix organisation and upregulation of DNA replication and translation. The DESNT signature has a distinctive biological profile, which is further evidence that it is a valid molecular subtype.

This study has several limitations. Firstly, data comes from prostatectomy samples rather than biopsy samples at diagnosis. This confines the characteristics of the cohort and often Gleason score is upgraded at prostatectomy [41], although prostatectomy was the primary treatment closest to diagnosis for these patients and so is a reasonable proxy to use. Secondly, the full power of the PREDICT model could not be utilised as full diagnostic biopsy information was unavailable for these datasets. Thirdly, biochemical recurrence was used as the clinical endpoint whereas metastatic disease or cancer-specific death would be more informative—PREDICT was not developed or calibrated for biochemical relapse as an outcome hence its performance in this setting has not previously been assessed. Finally, compared to the tens of thousands that the PREDICT model has been validated in, the numbers are relatively low, however we have used robust methods to compensate for this and reported confidence intervals throughout. Despite these limitations, the results support the notion of the potential value of including biological measurements along with the clinical variables collected as part of the standard clinical pathway. Future studies where transcriptome data is generated from a large series of biopsies with good quality clinical data with long follow up would be welcomed.

There is a need for improved predictors of outcome in non-metastatic men at the time of diagnosis to allow the optimal treatment pathway to be chosen. The inclusion of biological information, in particular the DESNT poor prognosis molecular subtype, alongside the best-of-breed clinical prognostic tool, PREDICT prostate, has the potential to make this improvement. This combination has the potential to help avoid unnecessary treatments and life-altering side-effects and improve survival in prostate cancer patients.

Supplementary Materials: The following supporting information can be downloaded at: https://www.mdpi.com/article/10.3390/curroncol30010013/s1, Table S1: Significantly differentially expressed genes between the samples with the 25% highest PREDICT scores versus the lowest 25% PREDICT scores; Table S2: KEGG pathways, Reactome pathways, and Gene Ontology biological processes terms found to be significantly enriched for significantly upregulated or downregulated genes for PREDICT high score samples versus low score samples; Table S3: Significantly differentially expressed genes between the samples classified as DESNT samples versus non-DESNT samples; Table S4: KEGG pathways, Reactome pathways, and Gene Ontology biological processes terms found to be significantly enriched for significantly upregulated or downregulated genes for DESNT sample status.

Author Contributions: Conceptualization, D.S.B. and V.J.G.; methodology, D.S.B. and R.C.; software, D.S.B., L.W. and R.C.; formal analysis, D.S.B., L.W. and R.C.; investigation, D.S.B., L.W. and R.C.; resources, D.S.B. and V.J.G.; data curation, D.S.B., L.W. and R.C.; writing—original draft preparation, D.S.B. and L.W.; writing—review and editing, L.W., R.C., V.J.G., C.S.C., J.C. and D.S.B.; visualization, D.S.B. and L.W.; supervision, D.S.B., R.C., J.C. and C.S.C.; project administration, D.S.B., J.C. and C.S.C.; funding acquisition, D.S.B., J.C. and C.S.C. All authors have read and agreed to the published version of the manuscript. All authors critiqued the manuscript for important intellectual content.

Funding: This work was funded by the Bob Champion Cancer Trust, The Masonic Charitable Foundation, The King Family, The Hargrave Foundation and The University of East Anglia. We acknowledge support from Prostate Cancer Research, Movember, Prostate Cancer UK, The Big C Cancer Charity, Cancer Research UK and The Andy Ripley Memorial Fund.

Institutional Review Board Statement: Ethical review and approval were waived for this study due to only publicly available datasets being used. Ethical approval details for each dataset are available in the original publications.

Data Availability Statement: The datasets analysed during the current study are publicly available: MSKCC [18]: https://www.ncbi.nlm.nih.gov/geo/query/acc.cgi?acc=GSE21034 (accessed on 1 May 2016); CancerMap [12]: https://www.ncbi.nlm.nih.gov/geo/query/acc.cgi?acc=GSE94767 (accessed on 1 May 2016); Stephenson [19]: Data available from the corresponding author of this paper. CamCap [20]: https://www.ncbi.nlm.nih.gov/geo/query/acc.cgi?acc=GSE70768 (accessed on 1 May 2016) and https://www.ncbi.nlm.nih.gov/geo/query/acc.cgi?acc=GSE70769 (accessed on 1 May 2016).

Acknowledgments: The authors would like to thank those men with prostate cancer and the subjects who have donated their time and samples to the data sets used in this study. Part of the research presented in this paper was carried out on the High Performance Computing Cluster supported by the Research and Specialist Computing Support service at the University of East Anglia.

Conflicts of Interest: C.S.C. and D.S.B. are co-inventors on a patent application from the University of East Anglia on the detection of DESNT prostate cancer. The funders had no role in the design of the study; in the collection, analyses, or interpretation of data; in the writing of the manuscript; or in the decision to publish the results.

References

1. Cancer Research UK Prostate cancer statistics. Available online: https://www.cancerresearchuk.org/health-professional/cancer-statistics/statistics-by-cancer-type/prostate-cancer (accessed on 17 August 2021).
2. D'Amico, A.V.; Moul, J.; Carroll, P.R.; Sun, L.; Lubeck, D.; Chen, M.-H.; D'Amico, A.V.; Moul, J.; Carroll, P.R.; Sun, L.; et al. Cancer-Specific Mortality After Surgery or Radiation for Patients With Clinically Localized Prostate Cancer Managed During the Prostate-Specific Antigen Era. *J. Clin. Oncol.* **2003**, *21*, 2163–2172. [CrossRef] [PubMed]
3. Attard, G.; Cooper, C.S.; de Bono, J.S. Steroid Hormone Receptors in Prostate Cancer: A Hard Habit to Break? *Cancer Cell* **2009**, *16*, 458–462. [CrossRef] [PubMed]
4. Schiffmann, J.; Wenzel, P.; Salomon, G.; Budäus, L.; Schlomm, T.; Minner, S.; Wittmer, C.; Kraft, S.; Krech, T.; Steurer, S.; et al. Heterogeneity in D'Amico classification-based low-risk prostate cancer: Differences in upgrading and upstaging according to active surveillance eligibility. *Urol. Oncol.* **2015**, *33*, 329.e13–329.e19. [CrossRef]
5. Hamdy, F.C.; Donovan, J.L.; Lane, J.A.; Mason, M.; Metcalfe, C.; Holding, P.; Davis, M.; Peters, T.J.; Turner, E.L.; Martin, R.M.; et al. 10-Year Outcomes after Monitoring, Surgery, or Radiotherapy for Localized Prostate Cancer. *N. Engl. J. Med.* **2016**, *375*, 1415–1424. [CrossRef]
6. Chou, R.; Croswell, J.M.; Dana, T.; Bougatsos, C.; Blazina, I.; Fu, R. Review Annals of Internal Medicine Screening for Prostate Cancer: A Review of the Evidence for the U.S. Preventative Services Task Force. *Ann. Intern. Med.* **2011**, *155*, 762–771. [CrossRef]
7. Thurtle, D.R.; Greenberg, D.C.; Lee, L.S.; Huang, H.H.; Pharoah, P.D.; Gnanapragasam, V.J. Individual prognosis at diagnosis in nonmetastatic prostate cancer: Development and external validation of the PREDICT Prostate multivariable model. *PLoS Med.* **2019**, *16*, e1002758. [CrossRef]
8. Thurtle, D.; Bratt, O.; Stattin, P.; Pharoah, P.; Gnanapragasam, V. Comparative performance and external validation of the multivariable PREDICT Prostate tool for non-metastatic prostate cancer: A study in 69,206 men from Prostate Cancer data Base Sweden (PCBaSe). *BMC Med.* **2020**, *18*, 139. [CrossRef]
9. Lee, C.; Light, A.; Alaa, A.; Thurtle, D.; Schaar, M.V.D.; Gnanapragasam, V.J. Application of a novel machine learning framework for predicting non-metastatic prostate cancer-specific mortality in men using the Surveillance, Epidemiology, and End Results (SEER) database. *Lancet Digit. Health* **2021**, *3*, e158–e165. [CrossRef]
10. NICE. *Prostate Cancer: Diagnosis and Management*; National Institute for Health and Care Excellence: London, UK, 2019.

11. Anceschi, U.; Tuderti, G.; Lugnani, F.; Biava, P.M.; Malossini, G.; Luciani, L.; Cai, T.; Marsiliani, D.; Filianoti, A.; Mattevi, D.; et al. Novel Diagnostic Biomarkers of Prostate Cancer: An Update. *Curr. Med. Chem.* **2019**, *26*, 1045–1058. [CrossRef]
12. Luca, B.; Brewer, D.S.; Edwards, D.R.; Edwards, S.; Whitaker, H.C.; Merson, S.; Dennis, N.; Cooper, R.A.; Hazell, S.; Warren, A.Y.; et al. DESNT: A Poor Prognosis Category of Human Prostate Cancer. *Eur. Urol. Focus* **2018**, *4*, 842–850. [CrossRef]
13. Luca, B.; Moulton, V.; Ellis, C.; Edwards, D.R.; Campbell, C.; Cooper, R.A.; Clark, J.; Brewer, D.S.; Cooper, C.S. A novel stratification framework for predicting outcome in patients with prostate cancer. *Br. J. Cancer* **2020**, *122*, 1467–1476. [CrossRef] [PubMed]
14. Luca, B.-A.; Moulton, V.; Ellis, C.; Connell, S.P.; Brewer, D.S.; Cooper, C.S. Convergence of Prognostic Gene Signatures Suggests Underlying Mechanisms of Human Prostate Cancer Progression. *Genes* **2020**, *11*, 802. [CrossRef] [PubMed]
15. Ellis, C. Using Latent Process Decomposition to Classify Prostate and Colorectal Cancers. Ph.D. Thesis, University of East Anglia, School of Computing Sciences, Norwich, UK, 2021.
16. Irizarry, R.A.; Hobbs, B.; Collin, F.; Beazer-Barclay, Y.D.; Antonellis, K.J.; Scherf, U.; Speed, T.P. Exploration, normalization, and summaries of high density oligonucleotide array probe level data. *Biostatistics* **2003**, *4*, 249–264. [CrossRef]
17. Johnson, W.E.; Li, C.; Rabinovic, A. Adjusting batch effects in microarray expression data using empirical Bayes methods. *Biostat. Oxf. Engl.* **2007**, *8*, 118–127. [CrossRef]
18. Taylor, B.S.; Schultz, N.; Hieronymus, H.; Gopalan, A.; Xiao, Y.; Carver, B.S.; Arora, V.K.; Kaushik, P.; Cerami, E.; Reva, B.; et al. Integrative Genomic Profiling of Human Prostate Cancer. *Cancer Cell* **2010**, *18*, 11–22. [CrossRef] [PubMed]
19. Stephenson, A.J.; Smith, A.; Kattan, M.W.; Satagopan, J.; Reuter, V.E.; Scardino, P.T.; Gerald, W.L. Integration of gene expression profiling and clinical variables to predict prostate carcinoma recurrence after radical prostatectomy. *Cancer* **2005**, *104*, 290–298. [CrossRef]
20. Ross-Adams, H.; Lamb, A.D.D.; Dunning, M.J.J.; Halim, S.; Lindberg, J.; Massie, C.M.M.; Egevad, L.A.A.; Russell, R.; Ramos-Montoya, A.; Vowler, S.L.L.; et al. Integration of copy number and transcriptomics provides risk stratification in prostate cancer: A discovery and validation cohort study. *EBioMedicine* **2015**, *2*, 1133–1144. [CrossRef]
21. R Core Team. R: A Language and Environment for Statistical Computing. Available online: https://www.r-project.org/ (accessed on 7 April 2020).
22. Ritchie, M.E.; Phipson, B.; Wu, D.; Hu, Y.; Law, C.W.; Shi, W.; Smyth, G.K. limma powers differential expression analyses for RNA-sequencing and microarray studies. *Nucleic Acids Res.* **2015**, *43*, e47. [CrossRef]
23. Kolberg, L.; Raudvere, U.; Kuzmin, I.; Vilo, J.; Peterson, H. gprofiler2—An R package for gene list functional enrichment analysis and namespace conversion toolset g:Profiler. *F1000Research* **2020**, *9*, ELIXIR-709. [CrossRef]
24. Msaouel, P.; Pissimissis, N.; Halapas, A.; Koutsilieris, M. Mechanisms of bone metastasis in prostate cancer: Clinical implications. *Best Pract. Res. Clin. Endocrinol. Metab.* **2008**, *22*, 341–355. [CrossRef]
25. Morgan, T.M.; Lange, P.H.; Porter, M.P.; Lin, D.W.; Ellis, W.J.; Gallaher, I.S.; Vessella, R.L. Disseminated Tumor Cells in Prostate Cancer Patients after Radical Prostatectomy and without Evidence of Disease Predicts Biochemical Recurrence. *Clin. Cancer Res.* **2009**, *15*, 677–683. [CrossRef] [PubMed]
26. Carl-McGrath, S.; Lendeckel, U.; Ebert, M.; Röcken, C. Ectopeptidases in tumour biology: A review. *Histol. Histopathol.* **2006**, *21*, 1339–1353. [CrossRef] [PubMed]
27. Menrad, A.; Speicher, D.; Wacker, J.; Herlyn, M. Biochemical and functional characterization of aminopeptidase N expressed by human melanoma cells. *Cancer Res.* **1993**, *53*, 1450–1455. [PubMed]
28. Ishii, K.; Usui, S.; Sugimura, Y.; Yoshida, S.; Hioki, T.; Tatematsu, M.; Yamamoto, H.; Hirano, K. Aminopeptidase N regulated by zinc in human prostate participates in tumor cell invasion. *Int. J. Cancer* **2001**, *92*, 49–54. [CrossRef]
29. Hashida, H.; Takabayashi, A.; Kanai, M.; Adachi, M.; Kondo, K.; Kohno, N.; Yamaoka, Y.; Miyake, M. Aminopeptidase N is involved in cell motility and angiogenesis: Its clinical significance in human colon cancer. *Gastroenterology* **2002**, *122*, 376–386. [CrossRef]
30. Sørensen, K.D.; Abildgaard, M.O.; Haldrup, C.; Ulhøi, B.P.; Kristensen, H.; Strand, S.; Parker, C.; Høyer, S.; Borre, M.; Ørntoft, T.F. Prognostic significance of aberrantly silenced ANPEP expression in prostate cancer. *Br. J. Cancer* **2013**, *108*, 420–428. [CrossRef]
31. Kramer, G.; Steiner, G.; Fodinger, D.; Fiebiger, E.; Rappersberger, C.; Binder, S.; Hofbauer, J.; Marberger, M. High Expression of a CD38-Like Molecule in Normal Prostatic Epithelium and its Differential Loss in Benign and Malignant Disease. *J. Urol.* **1995**, *154*, 1636–1641. [CrossRef]
32. Liu, X.; Grogan, T.R.; Hieronymus, H.; Hashimoto, T.; Mottahedeh, J.; Cheng, D.; Zhang, L.; Huang, K.; Stoyanova, T.; Park, J.W.; et al. Low CD38 Identifies Progenitor-like Inflammation-Associated Luminal Cells that Can Initiate Human Prostate Cancer and Predict Poor Outcome. *Cell Rep.* **2016**, *17*, 2596–2606. [CrossRef]
33. Liu, A.; Furusato, B.; Ravindranath, L.; Chen, Y.; Srikantan, V.; McLeod, D.G.; Petrovics, G.; Srivastava, S. Quantitative analysis of a panel of gene expression in prostate cancer–with emphasis on NPY expression analysis. *J. Zhejiang Univ. Sci. B* **2007**, *8*, 853–859. [CrossRef]
34. Henrique, R.; Jerónimo, C.; Hoque, M.O.; Nomoto, S.; Carvalho, A.L.; Costa, V.L.; Oliveira, J.; Teixeira, M.R.; Lopes, C.; Sidransky, D. MT1G hypermethylation is associated with higher tumor stage in prostate cancer. *Cancer Epidemiol Biomark. Prev.* **2005**, *14*, 1274–1278. [CrossRef]

55. Bergström, S.H.; Järemo, H.; Nilsson, M.; Adamo, H.H.; Bergh, A. Prostate tumors downregulate microseminoprotein-beta (MSMB) in the surrounding benign prostate epithelium and this response is associated with tumor aggressiveness. *Prostate* **2018**, *78*, 257–265. [CrossRef] [PubMed]
56. Chen, L.; Hong, C.; Chen, E.C.; Yee, S.W.; Xu, L.; Almof, E.U.; Wen, C.; Fujii, K.; Johns, S.J.; Stryke, D.; et al. Genetic and Epigenetic Regulation of the Organic Cation Transporter 3, SLC22A3. *Pharm. J.* **2013**, *13*, 110–120. [CrossRef] [PubMed]
57. Englund, E.; Canesin, G.; Papadakos, K.S.; Vishnu, N.; Persson, E.; Reitsma, B.; Anand, A.; Jacobsson, L.; Helczynski, L.; Mulder, H.; et al. Cartilage oligomeric matrix protein promotes prostate cancer progression by enhancing invasion and disrupting intracellular calcium homeostasis. *Oncotarget* **2017**, *8*, 98298–98311. [CrossRef]
58. Zhong, P.; Shu, R.; Wu, H.; Liu, Z.; Shen, X.; Hu, Y. Low KRT15 expression is associated with poor prognosis in patients with breast invasive carcinoma. *Exp. Ther. Med.* **2021**, *21*, 305. [CrossRef]
59. Hanahan, D. Hallmarks of Cancer: New Dimensions. *Cancer Discov.* **2022**, *12*, 31–46. [CrossRef] [PubMed]
60. Rye, M.B.; Bertilsson, H.; Andersen, M.K.; Rise, K.; Bathen, T.F.; Drabløs, F.; Tessem, M.-B. Cholesterol synthesis pathway genes in prostate cancer are transcriptionally downregulated when tissue confounding is minimized. *BMC Cancer* **2018**, *18*, 478. [CrossRef]
61. Corcoran, N.M.; Hong, M.K.H.; Casey, R.G.; Hurtado-Coll, A.; Peters, J.; Harewood, L.; Goldenberg, S.L.; Hovens, C.M.; Costello, A.J.; Gleave, M.E. Upgrade in Gleason score between prostate biopsies and pathology following radical prostatectomy significantly impacts upon the risk of biochemical recurrence. *BJU Int.* **2011**, *108*, E202–E210. [CrossRef]

Disclaimer/Publisher's Note: The statements, opinions and data contained in all publications are solely those of the individual author(s) and contributor(s) and not of MDPI and/or the editor(s). MDPI and/or the editor(s) disclaim responsibility for any injury to people or property resulting from any ideas, methods, instructions or products referred to in the content.

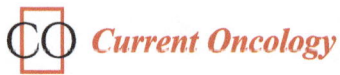

Article

Intraoperative 3D-US-mpMRI Elastic Fusion Imaging-Guided Robotic Radical Prostatectomy: A Pilot Study

Marco Oderda [1,*], Giorgio Calleris [1], Daniele D'Agate [1], Marco Falcone [1], Riccardo Faletti [2], Marco Gatti [2], Giancarlo Marra [1], Alessandro Marquis [1] and Paolo Gontero [1]

[1] Department of Surgical Sciences-Urology, Città della Salute e della Scienza di Torino, Molinette Hospital, University of Turin, 10126 Torino, Italy
[2] Department of Radiology, Città della Salute e della Scienza di Torino, Molinette Hospital, University of Turin, 10126 Torino, Italy
* Correspondence: marco.oderda@unito.it; Tel.: +39-3479383465

Abstract: Introduction: When performing a nerve-sparing (NS) robotic radical prostatectomy (RARP) cancer location based on multiparametric MRI (mpMRI) is essential, as well as the location of positive biopsy cores outside mpMRI targets. The aim of this pilot study was to assess the feasibility of intraoperative 3D-TRUS-mpMRI elastic fusion imaging to guide RARP and to evaluate its impact on the surgical strategy. Methods: We prospectively enrolled 11 patients with organ-confined mpMRI visible prostate cancer (PCa), histologically confirmed at transperineal fusion biopsy using Koelis Trinity. Before surgery, the 3D model of the prostate generated at biopsy was updated, showing both mpMRI lesions and positive biopsy cores, and was displayed on the Da Vinci robotic console using TilePro™ function. Results: Intraoperative 3D modeling was feasible in all patients (median of 6 min). The use of 3D models led to a major change in surgical strategy in six cases (54%), allowing bilateral instead of monolateral NS, or monolateral NS instead of non-NS, to be performed. At pathologic examination, no positive surgical margins (PSMs) were reported. Bilateral PCa presence was detected in one (9%), four (36%), and nine (81%) patients after mpMRI, biopsy, and RARP respectively. Extracapsular extension was found in two patients (18%) even if it was not suspected at MRI. Conclusions: Intraoperative 3D-TRUS-mpMRI modeling with Koelis Trinity is feasible and reliable, helping the surgeon to maximize functional outcomes without increasing the risk of positive surgical margins. The location of positive biopsy cores must be registered in 3D models, given the rates of bilateral involvement not seen at mpMRI.

Keywords: elastic fusion; intraoperative; robotic radical prostatectomy; 3D; ultrasound

1. Introduction

Robot-assisted radical prostatectomy (RARP) has become the standard surgical treatment for organ-confined prostate cancer (PCa), with the aim to maximize functional recovery while maintaining oncological radicality. When feasible, a nerve-sparing (NS) approach should follow the capsular profile of the prostate to obtain the preservation of neurovascular bundles (NVBs) without incurring in positive surgical margins (PSMs) [1]. To date, the reported prevalence of PSM after RARP is approximately 9% for organ-confined disease and up to 37% for pT3 cancers, and NS surgery has been associated with an increased risk of side-specific PSM, even in low-risk cancers [2].

Currently, multiparametric magnetic resonance imaging (mpMRI) provides essential data concerning cancer location and capsular involvement and might change the extent of NS surgery in more than one out of three patients [3]. However, a non-negligible proportion of cancer foci within the gland remains unseen at mpMRI [4]. Moreover, it is still difficult for surgeons to translate mpMRI findings into real-time appreciation of tumor volume and location during RARP.

To overcome these issues, three-dimensional (3D) imaging reconstruction techniques have been proposed, including 3D printing, virtual reality, and augmented reality [5–7]. Indeed, 3D visualization could facilitate RARP in terms of training, surgical planning, and intraoperative guidance. However, reconstruction of 3D models is usually based on preoperative mpMRI, and therefore does not consider cancer foci not seen at mpMRI but detected with systematic sampling.

The Koelis Trinity system creates a precise 3D model of the prostate, integrating mpMRI sequences and real-time 3D ultrasound (US) with a unique elastic fusion technology that shows not only mpMRI-visible lesions, but also all positive biopsy core locations [8]. The same system can be used to perform the diagnostic fusion biopsy and to guide the execution of RARP with an intraoperative acquisition of 3D-US images to be fused with the previously generated 3D model of the prostate. The aim of this pilot study was to assess the feasibility of the intraoperative 3D-US-mpMRI elastic fusion imaging to guide RARP and to evaluate its impact on the surgical strategy to decide an NS approach.

2. Materials and Methods

This was a pilot study enrolling 11 consecutive patients addressed to RARP for clinically localized PCa. All patients had undergone diagnostic 1.5 T or 3 T mpMRI and subsequent fusion biopsy. mpMRIs were reviewed by experienced radiologists (M.G. and R.F.) and suspicious lesions were scored according to the PIRADS v2.1 classification. Fusion biopsies were performed transperineally with Koelis Trinity system (Koelis, Meylan, France), which creates a precise and highly detailed 3D map of the prostate integrating 3D-US, multimodal elastic fusion, and organ-based tracking. During the examination, a 3D transrectal US (TRUS) probe creates a 3D reference model of the prostate which is fused with mpMRI sequences showing suspicious lesions. New images are taken to register the location of the biopsy needle at each biopsy. Thanks to the organ-based technology, the device follows the position of the prostate and not that of the probe, automatically compensating for patient movement and prostate deformation. After biopsy, the 3D model of the prostate was updated with histological findings, highlighting all the biopsy cores found as PCa. On the day of RARP, all patients underwent intraoperative second-look elastic fusion imaging with Koelis Trinity; a new 3D-TRUS acquisition was performed during the initial steps of surgery (before bladder detachment), allowing for retrieval of the previous MRI and biopsy information in the current exam and the 3D model of the prostate. The output was displayed on the Da Vinci robotic console using the TilePro™ function, providing guidance during surgery (Figure 1).

RARPs were performed using a four-arm Da Vinci Xi Surgical System (Intuitive Surgical, Sunnyvale, CA, USA) by one experienced surgeon (P.G., >1000 cases), while intraoperative TRUS and fusion imaging procedures required an additional operator experienced in fusion biopsy with Koelis Trinity (M.O., >500 cases). The NS approach was defined as bilateral, unilateral, or non-NS, while the extent of NVBs preservation was defined on side-based level as intrafascial or interfascial [9].

The endpoints of the study were to evaluate the feasibility of intraoperative 3D-US-mpMRI modeling and its impact on surgical strategy as compared to the preoperative planning decided during weekly staff meetings. The pathological findings were compared to MRI and biopsy data. The study was conducted according to the Declaration of Helsinki. Ethics committee approval was waived due to non-invasive and non-interventional nature of this study. All involved patients signed an informed consent form for photo and video acquisition for clinical research purposes. Statistical analyses were performed with SPSS version 26.0 (IBM Corp, Armonk, NY, USA). The entire procedure did not lead to any additional costs so long we used the system utilized to routinely perform prostate fusion biopsies.

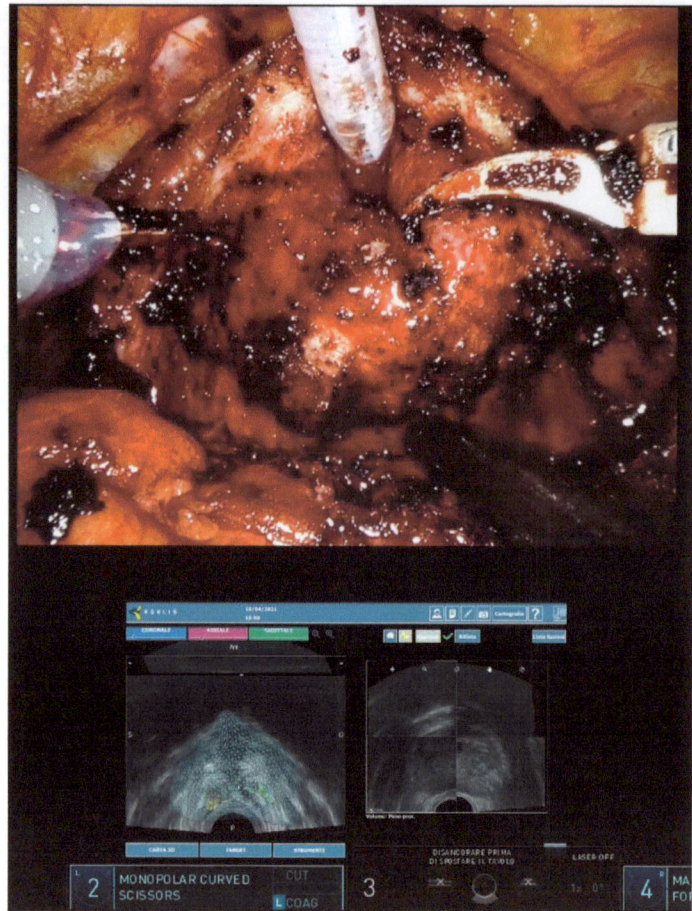

Figure 1. The 3D model is visualised live on the Da Vinci robotic console using the TilePro™ function providing guidance during surgery.

3. Results

Intraoperative 3D modeling with Koelis Trinity was feasible in all patients, requiring a very limited amount of time to be performed, with a median of 6 min per patient (range 5–10). Patients' characteristics are shown in Table 1, including data on MRI, fusion biopsy and radical prostatectomy.

Table 1. Patients' characteristics.

	Baseline Data
Age, years, mean ± SD	68.9 ± 7.4
PSA, ng/dl, mean ± SD	7.5 ± 2.1
Positive DRE, n (%)	4 (36%)
Previous negative biopsies, n (%)	4 (36%)
Prostate volume, cc, mean ± SD	44 ± 13.2

Table 1. *Cont.*

MRI data	
Target number, n (%)	
- Single	8 (73%)
- Multiple	3 (27%)
Target location, n (%)	
- Monolateral	10 (91%)
- Bilateral	1 (9%)
PIRADS score, n (%)	
- 3	1 (9%)
- 4	9 (82%)
- 5	1 (9%)
Lesion diameter, mm, mean ± SD	8.8 ± 3.5
Extracapsular extension suspicion, n (%)	0 (0%)
Fusion biopsy results	
Biopsy cores taken, n, median (range)	
- Targeted	3 (3–6)
- Systematic	12 (8–20)
Cancer detection within MRI target, n (%)	11 (100%)
Cancer detection outside MRI target, n (%)	6 (54%)
Lesion location, n (%)	
- Monolateral	7 (64%)
- Bilateral	4 (36%)
ISUP grade, n (%)	
- 1	2 (18%)
- 2	5 (45%)
- 3	1 (9%)
- 4	3 (27%)
ISUP upgrade due to systematic cores, n (%)	0 (0%)
Radical prostatectomy findings	
Pathological stage, n (%)	
- pT2	9 (81%)
- pT3a	2 (27%)
Positive surgical margins	0 (0%)
Cancer detection within MRI target, n (%)	11 (100%)
Cancer detection outside MRI target, n (%)	9 (82%)
ISUP grade, n (%)	
- 1	0 (0%)
- 2	7 (63%)
- 3	1 (9%)
- 4	3 (27%)
Lesion location, n (%)	
- Monolateral	2 (18%)
- Bilateral	9 (82%)

DRE: digital rectal examination.

As compared to preoperative surgical planning, the use of 3D models led to a major change in surgical strategy in six cases (54%), where a bilateral NS was performed instead of a monolateral NS, or a monolateral NS was performed instead of non-NS (Table 2).

Table 2. Impact of 3D modeling on surgical planning and comparison between clinical and pathological findings.

	Biopsy ISUP Grade	Clinical Stage at MRI	Preoperative NS Planning	Intraoperative NS Execution	Pathological Stage	Pathological ISUP Grade
Case 1	2	cT2a	Monolateral NS	Bilateral NS	pT2aR0	2
Case 2	2	cT2a	Monolateral NS	Bilateral NS	pT2cR0	2
Case 3	4	cT2a	Non-NS	Non-NS	pT2bR0	4
Case 4	4	cT2a	Non-NS	Monolateral NS	pT2cR0	4
Case 5	2	cT2a	Monolateral NS	Bilateral NS	pT2cR0	2
Case 6	4	cT2a	Monolateral NS	Monolateral NS	pT3aR0	4
Case 7	1	cT2a	Bilateral NS	Bilateral NS	pT2cR0	2
Case 8	2	cT2a	Monolateral NS	Bilateral NS	pT2cR0	2
Case 9	2	cT2a	Monolateral NS	Monolateral NS	pT3aR0	2
Case 10	1	cT2a	Bilateral NS	Bilateral NS	pT2cR0	2
Case 11	3	cT2c	Monolateral NS	Bilateral NS	pT2cR0	3

In three cases (27%), an intrafascial NS was performed instead of an interfascial NS, thanks to the virtual localization of positive cancer cores. No change of management was reported in four patients (36%). At pathologic examination, no PSMs were reported.

All MRI targets were confirmed as PCa both at fusion biopsy and RARP. Bilateral PCa presence was detected in one patient (9%) at MRI, four patients (36%) after fusion biopsy, and nine patients (81%) after RARP. The maximum International Society of Urological Pathology (ISUP) grade at biopsy always corresponded to MRI-visible lesions. Upgrade from biopsy to RARP was detected in two patients only, from ISUP 1 to 2. Extracapsular extension was found in two patients (18%) even if it was not suspected at MRI; in both cases, the location of extracapsular extension was the same as the index lesion.

4. Discussion

The use of US to provide intraoperative visualization of prostatic anatomy and NVBs has been explored since 2006, when Ukimura et al. published a series of 77 patients who underwent TRUS during laparoscopic radical prostatectomy to identify NVBs, to define the prostate apex contour and to evaluate the location of hypoechoic cancer nodules [10]. In their series, the use of intraoperative TRUS monitoring allowed for precise dissection tailored to the specific prostate contour anatomy, leading to a 20% decrease in PSMs [11]. More recently, the feasibility of a robotically manipulated TRUS for real-time monitoring of the prostate and periprostatic anatomy during RARP was assessed by Hung et al., showing that it can provide valuable anatomic information with the aim to maximize functional preservation [12].

While TRUS is useful in identifying real-time anatomical landmarks of the prostate, in the last few years, it has been completely replaced by mpMRI for the detection of cancer foci [13]. The integration of mpMRI and TRUS images has led to the fusion imaging that now guides most biopsies performed in the diagnostic work-up of PCa. Ukimura and Gill were the first to apply a fusion system between real-time TRUS and preoperative mpMRI during laparoscopic radical prostatectomy [14]. More recently, they developed a 3D surgical navigation model based on 3D-TRUS-guided prostate biopsies. Five key anatomic structures (prostate, image-visible biopsy-proven "index" cancer lesion, neurovascular bundles, urethra, and recorded biopsy trajectories) were image-fused and displayed onto the TilePro function of the robotic console. In their experience, the 3D model facilitated careful surgical dissection in the vicinity of the biopsy-proven index lesion, achieving negative PSMs in 90% of patients [7].

In line these authors, we believe that the potential of both 3D-TRUS and mpMRI must be exploited to build a successful, real-time 3D model of the prostate. On the strength of our experience on fusion biopsy [8], we decided to use the only available fusion system that integrates 3D-TRUS and mpMRI images, which is able to track the location of all the biopsy cores. This way, we obtained intraoperative models carrying data on the location of both mpMRI-visible and mpMRI-invisible cancer foci, detected with the systematic sampling.

In the present study, we demonstrated the feasibility of intraoperative 3D modeling with Koelis Trinity. The 3D reconstruction of the prostate was quickly obtained using the "second look" function, an option that allows for the retrieval of the 3D model constructed during the diagnostic biopsy and the location of all the biopsy cores found to be positive for PCa. We used the 3D-TRUS probe to achieve prostate volume during the first steps of surgery, before bladder detachment, to avoid image disturbances. With the transrectal probe in place, we were also able to generate several 3D models during surgery, tracking the position of the robotic instruments in relation to the location of cancer foci and identifying the exact area of the suspected pseudocapsule bulging (if any). The 3D-US-mpMRI-assisted approached allowed us to perform a nerve-sparing technique, watching out for an extra-capsular extension in the exact area of risk and eventually allowing us to modify the plan of dissection. This maneuver becomes more difficult with the progress of RARP; with the development of the space between the prostate and rectum after incision of Denonvilliers' fascia, carbon dioxide posterior to the prostate interferes with visualization. As noted by Ukimura et al., however, by this late stage of the procedure we have usually already acquired all the relevant information regarding the anatomy of the prostate and the location of cancer foci [11]. The 3D models generated by Koelis Trinity were visible at the robotic console using the TilePro™ function and were judged very helpful by the surgeon (P.G.) to visualize the location of cancer foci, especially when deciding to perform NS surgery. The guidance of 3D models led to more NS surgeries being performed, and more intrafascial approaches, as compared to what was initially planned during preoperative staff meetings, without increasing PSMs.

During this pilot study, the visualization of 3D models at the robotic console was beside the intraoperative view, without any alignment to the organ. The creation of a dedicated software able to achieve a real-time alignment of images represents the next challenge to develop automated and reliable augmented reality (AR). AR technologies have been recently proposed by Schiavina et al. [5] and Porpiglia et al. [6] with promising results to tailor the surgical dissection to the index lesions. Both models, however, were uniquely based on mpMRI images and therefore did not consider possible mpMRI-invisible locations detected by systematic sampling. Furthermore, in both cases the alignment of 3D model during surgery was manually performed by a professional, introducing a dangerously subjective element.

The comparison between pathologic and mpMRI findings in our study deserves special comment. On one hand, all lesions detected by mpMRI were confirmed to be PCa at fusion biopsy and RARP. On the other hand, however, the correlation between mpMRI findings and location of all cancerous areas in the prostate was imperfect, with a significant proportion of PCa foci found in regions other than those detected at mpMRI, even if clinically significant. Of note, the number of patients with bilateral PCa increased from one at mpMRI to four after fusion biopsy (thanks to systematic cores) and to nine after RARP. This finding is quite alarming and highlights once again the importance of a 3D model that tracks the location of positive biopsy cores. Several reports have shown the risk of finding mpMRI-invisible cancer foci. In 2019, a study performed on 185 candidates for hemiablation showed that only 33.5% of patients had unilateral cancer on final histopathology after radical prostatectomy. Significant cancer on biopsy and mpMRI-negative lobes was found in 38.9% of 185 lobes [15]. All these things considered, it would seem that mpMRI sometimes sees only the "tip of the iceberg". In our series, the lesions detected by mpMRI were the ones with the highest grade at biopsy, and an upgrade from the biopsy to the final specimen was noted only in a minority of cases. Finally, two of our patients were diagnosed as pT3 in spite of a negative mpMRI, which can sometimes miss the initial signs of extracapsular extension. The use of 3D modeling, however, allowed us to perform more conservative surgeries without increasing our PSM rates.

We acknowledge that this is only a pilot study and further studies must be on a larger series of patients to validate these preliminary results. Furthermore, the accuracy of the 3D reconstruction should be assessed, probably with the intraoperative use of fiducials. The ultimate goal is represented by the automated alignment of the 3D model on the organ seen at the robotic console.

5. Conclusions

Intraoperative 3D-TRUS-mpMRI modeling with Koelis Trinity is feasible, reliable and cheap, helping surgeons to maximize functional outcomes without increasing the risk of positive surgical margins. The potential of 3D-US together with mpMRI data allows for the generation of a model that provides information on the prostate anatomy, the location of mpMRI visible cancers, and also positive systematic biopsies. The registration of biopsy cores is particularly important, given the rates of bilateral cancer involvement not seen at mpMRI.

Author Contributions: Conception and design, M.O.; acquisition of data, A.M., G.C., and M.G.; analysis and interpretation of data, M.O. and R.F.; drafting of the manuscript, M.O., G.C., and D.D.; critical revision of the manuscript for important intellectual content, A.M., R.F., G.M., and M.F.; statistical analysis, M.O.; obtaining funding, (N/A); administrative, technical, or material support, (N/A); supervision, P.G. All authors have read and agreed to the published version of the manuscript.

Funding: This research received no external funding.

Institutional Review Board Statement: Ethics committee approval was waived due to non-invasive and non-interventional nature of this study.

Informed Consent Statement: All involved patients signed an informed consent to photo and video acquisition for clinical research purposes.

Data Availability Statement: The data presented in this study are available on request from the corresponding author.

Conflicts of Interest: Marco Oderda has worked as a consultant for Koelis™.

Abbreviations

3D = three-dimensional; TRUS = transrectal ultrasound; mpMRI = multi-parametric magnetic resonance imaging; NS = nerve-sparing; RARP = robotic radical prostatectomy; PCa = prostate cancer; PSMs = positive surgical margins; NVB = neuro-vascular bundle.

References

1. Walz, J.; Epstein, J.I.; Ganzer, R.; Graefen, M.; Guazzoni, G.; Kaouk, J.; Menon, M.; Mottrie, A.; Myers, R.P.; Patel, V.; et al. A Critical Analysis of the Current Knowledge of Surgical Anatomy of the Prostate Related to Optimisation of Cancer Control and Preservation of Continence and Erection in Candidates for Radical Prostatectomy: An Update. *Eur. Urol.* **2016**, *70*, 301–311. [CrossRef]
2. Yossepowitch, O.; Briganti, A.; Eastham, J.A.; Epstein, J.; Graefen, M.; Montironi, R.; Touijer, K. Positive Surgical Margins After Radical Prostatectomy: A Systematic Review and Contemporary Update. *Eur. Urol.* **2014**, *65*, 303–313. [CrossRef]
3. Marenco, J.; Orczyk, C.; Collins, T.; Moore, C.; Emberton, M. Role of MRI in planning radical prostatectomy: What is the added value? *World J. Urol.* **2019**, *37*, 1289–1292. [CrossRef] [PubMed]
4. Bonekamp, D.; Schelb, P.; Wiesenfarth, M.; Kuder, T.A.; Deister, F.; Stenzinger, A.; Nyarangi-Dix, J.; Röthke, M.; Hohenfellner, M.; Schlemmer, H.-P.; et al. Histopathological to multiparametric MRI spatial mapping of extended systematic sextant and MR/TRUS-fusion-targeted biopsy of the prostate. *Eur. Radiol.* **2019**, *29*, 1820–1830. [CrossRef] [PubMed]

5. Schiavina, R.; Bianchi, L.; Lodi, S.; Cercenelli, L.; Chessa, F.; Bortolani, B.; Gaudiano, C.; Casablanca, C.; Droghetti, M.; Porreca, A.; et al. Real-time Augmented Reality Three-dimensional Guided Robotic Radical Prostatectomy: Preliminary Experience and Evaluation of the Impact on Surgical Planning. *Eur. Urol. Focus* **2020**, *7*, 1260–1267. [CrossRef]
6. Porpiglia, F.; Checcucci, E.; Amparore, D.; Manfredi, M.; Massa, F.; Piazzolla, P.; Manfrin, D.; Piana, A.; Tota, D.; Bollito, E.; et al. Three-dimensional Elastic Augmented-reality Robot-assisted Radical Prostatectomy Using Hyperaccuracy Three-dimensional Reconstruction Technology: A Step Further in the Identification of Capsular Involvement. *Eur. Urol.* **2019**, *76*, 505–514. [CrossRef]
7. Ukimura, O.; Aron, M.; Nakamoto, M.; Shoji, S.; Abreu, A.L.D.C.; Matsugasumi, T.; Berger, A.; Desai, M.; Gill, I.S. Three-dimensional surgical navigation model with TilePro display during robot-assisted radical prostatectomy. *J. Endourol.* **2014**, *28*, 625–630. [CrossRef]
8. Oderda, M.; Marra, G.; Albisinni, S.; Altobelli, E.; Baco, E.; Beatrici, V.; Cantiani, A.; Carbone, A.; Ciccariello, M.; Descotes, J.-L.; et al. Accuracy of elastic fusion biopsy in daily practice: Results of a multicenter study of 2115 patients. *Int. J. Urol. Off. J. Jpn. Urol. Assoc.* **2018**, *25*, 990–997. [CrossRef] [PubMed]
9. Walz, J.; Burnett, A.L.; Costello, A.J.; Eastham, J.A.; Graefen, M.; Guillonneau, B.; Menon, M.; Montorsi, F.; Myers, R.P.; Rocco, B.; et al. A critical analysis of the current knowledge of surgical anatomy related to optimization of cancer control and preservation of continence and erection in candidates for radical prostatectomy. *Eur. Urol.* **2010**, *57*, 179–192. [CrossRef] [PubMed]
10. Ukimura, O.; Gill, I.S. Real-time transrectal ultrasound guidance during nerve sparing laparoscopic radical prostatectomy: Pictorial essay. *J. Urol.* **2006**, *175*, 1311–1319. [CrossRef] [PubMed]
11. Ukimura, O.; Magi-Galluzzi, C.; Gill, I.S. Real-time transrectal ultrasound guidance during laparoscopic radical prostatectomy: Impact on surgical margins. *J. Urol.* **2006**, *175*, 1304–1310. [CrossRef] [PubMed]
12. Hung, A.J.; Abreu, A.L.D.C.; Shoji, S.; Goh, A.C.; Berger, A.K.; Desai, M.M.; Aron, M.; Gill, I.S.; Ukimura, O. Robotic transrectal ultrasonography during robot-assisted radical prostatectomy. *Eur. Urol.* **2012**, *62*, 341–348. [CrossRef]
13. Mottet, N.; van den Bergh, R.C.; Briers, E.; Van den Broeck, T.; Cumberbatch, M.G.; De Santis, M.; Fanti, S.; Fossati, N.; Gandaglia, G.; Gillessen, S.; et al. EAU-EANM-ESTRO-ESUR-SIOG Guidelines on Prostate Cancer-2020 Update. Part 1: Screening, Diagnosis, and Local Treatment with Curative Intent. *Eur. Urol.* **2021**, *79*, 243–262. [CrossRef]
14. Ukimura, O.; Ahlering, T.E.; Gill, I.S. Transrectal ultrasound-guided, energy-free, nerve-sparing laparoscopic radical prostatectomy. *J. Endourol.* **2008**, *22*, 1993–1995. [CrossRef]
15. Choi, Y.H.; Yu, J.W.; Kang, M.Y.; Sung, H.H.; Jeong, B.C.; Seo, S.I.; Jeon, S.S.; Lee, H.M.; Jeon, H.G. Combination of multiparametric magnetic resonance imaging and transrectal ultrasound-guided prostate biopsies is not enough for identifying patients eligible for hemiablative focal therapy for prostate cancer. *World J. Urol.* **2019**, *37*, 2129–2135. [CrossRef]

Disclaimer/Publisher's Note: The statements, opinions and data contained in all publications are solely those of the individual author(s) and contributor(s) and not of MDPI and/or the editor(s). MDPI and/or the editor(s) disclaim responsibility for any injury to people or property resulting from any ideas, methods, instructions or products referred to in the content.

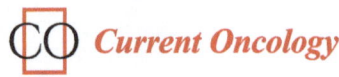

Article

Development of a Prediction Model for Positive Surgical Margin in Robot-Assisted Laparoscopic Radical Prostatectomy

Ying Hao [1,2], Qing Zhang [2], Junke Hang [2,3], Linfeng Xu [2], Shiwei Zhang [2] and Hongqian Guo [1,2,3,*]

1. Department of Urology, Nanjing Drum Tower Hospital Clinical College of Jiangsu University, Nanjing 210008, China
2. Institute of Urology, Nanjing University, Nanjing 210008, China
3. Department of Urology, Nanjing Drum Tower Hospital Clinical College of Nanjing Medical University, Nanjing 210008, China
* Correspondence: dr.ghq@nju.edu.cn; Tel.: +86-83106666

Abstract: A positive surgical margin (PSM) is reported to have some connection to the occurrence of biochemical recurrence and tumor metastasis in prostate cancer after the operation. There are no clinically usable models and the study is to predict the probability of PSM after robot-assisted laparoscopic radical prostatectomy (RALP) based on preoperative examinations. It is a retrospective cohort from a single center. The Lasso method was applied for variable screening; logistic regression was employed to establish the final model; the strengthened bootstrap method was adopted for model internal verification; the nomogram and web calculator were used to visualize the model. All the statistical analyses were based on the R-4.1.2. The main outcome was a pathologically confirmed PSM. There were 151 PSMs in the 903 patients, for an overall positive rate of 151/903 = 16.7%; 0.727 was the adjusted C statistic, and the Brier value was 0.126. Hence, we have developed and validated a predictive model for PSM after RALP for prostate cancer that can be used in clinical practice. In the meantime, we observed that the International Society of Urological Pathology (ISUP) score, Prostate Imaging Reporting and Data System (PI-RADS) score, and Prostate-Specific Antigen (PSA) were the independent risk factors for PSM.

Keywords: prediction model; positive surgical margin (PSM); robot-assisted laparoscopic radical prostatectomy (RALP)

1. Introduction

According to the 2020 global cancer statistics released by the International Agency for Research on Cancer (IARC), there were more than 1.4 million newly diagnosed cases of prostate cancer worldwide in 2020, accounting for 7.3% of new cancers, ranking third after breast cancer and lung cancer [1]. In China, the incidence of prostate cancer has steadily increased since 2015, owing to the continuous westernization of diet structure and lifestyle, as well as population aging [2–4]. However, compared with other types of cancer, prostate cancer is relatively inactive, and most patients have access to surgery with positive therapeutic effects. Consequently, the mortality rate of prostate cancer is much lower than the morbidity rate. Even in relatively advanced cases, neoadjuvant treatment does not preclude the possibility of achieving local benefits [5,6] to obtain the opportunity for surgery. Therefore, radical prostatectomy (whether laparoscopic or robot-assisted) remains the first line treatment option for prostate cancer [7,8]. However, the effect of surgery varies greatly from one patient to the other, and there is still a phenomenon of biochemical recurrence or even tumor metastasis in 27–53% of patients after surgery, which, in extreme cases, can even be fatal to the patient [9]. Multiple studies have demonstrated that a positive surgical margin (PSM) has been in relationship to the phenomenon of biochemical recurrence and tumor metastasis in prostate cancer after the operation [10–12]. Some studies have also indicated that different surgical methods, surgical pathways, and resection levels had an impact on the surgical margin. For example, robot-assisted laparoscopic radical prostatectomy (RALP) with Retzius preservation (or the posterior approach) has a more favorable prognosis regarding urinary incontinence but carries a greater risk of developing a PSM [13]. Nerve-sparing increases the risk of ipsilateral PSM [14]. The new anatomical tip dissection adopting the pubic prostatectomy collar opening technique may have a beneficial effect on the operative cutting edge if surgery is performed [15]. As a consequence of this, preoperative surgical margin judgment is a crucial part of the planning process for surgical procedures.

Currently, some studies on the related predictive factors of surgical margins of prostate cancer have been discovered. The following factors have been identified as independent predictors of PSM: preoperative PSA, biopsy Gleason score, percentage of positive biopsy needles, biopsy nerve infiltration, pathological Gleason score, pathological stage, lymph node positivity, the extracapsular extension of the tumor, and seminal vesicle infiltration [16–18]. Previously, some similar prediction models were established, but the models included a few factors or were only based on MR, or the score was relatively rough and not precise enough [19–21]. There has been no research done to help visualize the complicated model, which makes it inconvenient for both clinical and application work. As a result, we hope to obtain a more comprehensive and detailed model to compensate for the shortcomings of previous models. Moreover, we will illustrate the model using a nomogram. A web calculator will also be provided to make the model easier to use.

2. Materials and Methods

2.1. Study Design and Data Sources

We conducted a retrospective cohort study on a large population of patients with prostate cancer using patient data obtained from the Doctor's Work System of Nanjing Drum Tower Hospital. We included prostate cancer patients who underwent RALP in Nanjing Drum Tower Hospital from January 2018 to December 2021, and excluded patients who received preoperative neoadjuvant treatment, patients with a history of prostate-related surgery, patients who experienced prostate biopsy in an external hospital, and cases with important data missing. To rule out the possibility of metastasis, all patients underwent preoperative imaging examinations. Patients whose Gleason score $\geq 3+4$ underwent lymphadenectomy. To make full use of the data, all of it was applied to establish the derived data set, and the enhanced bootstrap method was employed to conduct internal data verification.

2.2. Outcome

The outcome was a positive postoperative pathological margin. A positive margin is the extension of a cancer cell within the ink section of a RALP specimen [22]. The result of PSM will be determined after a staining procedure performed by an experienced pathologist. To ensure the authenticity of the data, the pathologist was not aware of the predictors' results when measuring the outcome.

2.3. Predictors

Based on previous research findings, we examined the factors that influence the surgical margin [16–18] and added some new variables. All predictors were measured by a qualified physician before surgery. To ensure the authenticity of the data, clinicians and test physicians were unaware of the outcomes when measuring the predictors, and each predictor was measured independently without mutual interference. Following are the details of the predictors.

Age: The patient's age at the time of surgery.

BMI: The patient's BMI at the time of hospitalization.

Prostate volume (V): The volume of the prostate measured at the time of the B-ultrasound-fused magnetic resonance prostate biopsy.

Percent of positive needles (PPN): The ratio of the total number of needles to the number of needles that reached tumor cells.

International Society of Urological Pathology (ISUP) score: According to the consensus of the classification meeting of the Society of Urological Pathology, the ISUP score was provided by prostate biopsy pathology [23].

Percent of Tumor (PT): The sum of the tumor fractions per needle in the tissue obtained through a prostate biopsy multiplied by 100.

Prostate Imaging Reporting and Data System (PI-RADS) score: It was provided by the suspicious nodule from the preoperative 3.0T MRI. The film was read and the results were given by a professional imaging doctor.

Tumor location (TL): The location of the suspicious nodule from the preoperative 3.0T MRI of the patients before surgery, which was read by a professional in medical imaging. It was grouped according to the peripheral zone (P), transitional zone (T), mixed (M), and Negative (prostate cancer is not currently being considered).

Maximal tumor diameter (D): The maximal diameter of the suspicious nodule that can be quantified in the preoperative 3.0T MRI of the patients.

The number of tumors (NT): The number of suspicious nodules on the preoperative 3.0T MRI of the patients.

Clinical staging of the tumor provided by MRI (T-MRI): It was evaluated on the basis of the preoperative 3.0T MRI and the pathological results of the prostate biopsy. It was categorized according to the latest eighth edition of tumor-staging criteria issued by the Joint Commission on Cancer (AJCC) [24]. Stages less than or equal to T2a are divided into group 1; T2b into group 2; the patients with staging greater than or equal to T2c were divided into group 3.

Prostate-Specific Antigen (PSA): PSA is valued before the patient's prostate biopsy (at the time of the initial diagnosis), with some missing data replaced by preoperative PSA values.

PSA density (PSAD): The portion of PSA in the prostate volume.

Inflammation index (II): Neutrophil count * platelet count/lymphocyte count. The information was obtained from the patient's preoperative routine blood test in order to evaluate preoperative inflammation.

Time from biopsy to surgery (t): The time between the prostate biopsy and the RALP. It was considered that the biopsy might cause local inflammation and edema of the prostate, which may affect the surgical margin.

Operator: The operator performing RALP for the patients. It was grouped according to the experience of RALP.

Others: Other risk factors, which predominantly include but are not limited to nerve involvement by biopsy, patients with EPE or SVI, and patients with substantial clinical manifestations.

2.4. Sample Size

The sample size is determined by the amount of data available. Because the percentage of missing data was small (21/903 = 2.3%) and the type of missing data was significant after eliminating the missing data, a total of 882 complete data were obtained.

2.5. Statistical Analysis Method

The potential predictors were determined through literature searches and discussions with experts at Nanjing Drum Tower Hospital. First, logistic regression was used for univariate analysis. After that, the variables were screened using the Lasso method. The Lasso method is a kind of compression estimation [25]. As the number of predictive variables in this study was more than the number of positive samples (according to the standard of EPV $\geq$ 10:1), collinearity was suspected among the predictive variables. It is necessary to use the Lasso method for screening variables to increase penalty terms, control collinearity, and avoid over-fitting to a certain extent. Based on the optimal lambda value nine prediction factors including age, PPN, ISUP, PT, D, PI-RADS, TL, T-MRI, and PSA were screened out for the establishment of the final logistic regression model. Since no treatment was performed on the patient, the interaction terms were not taken into account during the modeling process. Finally, the enhanced bootstrap method was used for internal verification. The nomogram was used to calculate the probability of each individual's prediction. To detail the assessment of the effect of model predictions, we will report model accuracy (C-statistic), model calibration (calibration map), and others (Brier score).

Since there was no standard probabilistic risk stratification as a point of reference, we divided the PSM risk of patients into four groups with low risk, low–medium risk, medium–high risk, and high risk by using the statistical concept and quartile.

3. Results

3.1. Study Population

In total, 903 patients met our inclusion criteria and 882 samples were used for modeling after excluding 21 with missing data. Figure 1 is a flowchart of sample inclusion and exclusion.

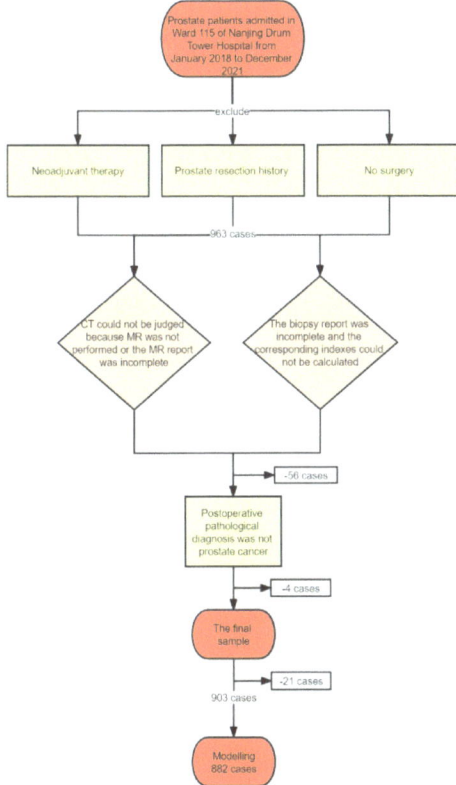

Figure 1. Inclusion and exclusion flowchart.

Table 1 indicates the baseline characteristics of overall and positive- and negative-margin patients. It is demonstrated that the age of the patients is concentrated in the range of 65 to 75 years, and as a whole, the majority of patients are in an early clinical stage, which is manifested as low histological score (ISUP) and MRI score (PI-RADS). At the same time, significant differences in age, PPN, ISUP, PT, PI-RADS, TL, D, T-MRI, PSA, PSAD, and Others can be observed between the margin-positive and margin-negative groups.

Table 1. Baseline characteristics of patients with prostate cancer. Values are numbers (percentages) of patients.

	Level	Overall	NSM	PSM	p	Test	SMD
n		903	752	151			
age (median [IQR])		70.00 [66.00, 75.00]	70.00 [65.00, 74.00]	71.00 [66.00, 77.00]	0.014	nonnorm	0.240
BMI (mean (SD))		24.60 (2.95)	24.60 (2.93)	24.58 (3.06)	0.922		0.009
V (median [IQR])		32.40 [24.70, 44.90]	33.05 [24.78, 45.92]	31.10 [24.20, 39.20]	0.095	nonnorm	0.139
PPN (median [IQR])		0.36 [0.21, 0.50]	0.34 [0.19, 0.50]	0.44 [0.29, 0.67]	<0.001	nonnorm	0.559
ISUP (%)	1	235 (26.0)	218 (29.0)	17 (11.3)	<0.001		0.587
	2	264 (29.2)	230 (30.6)	34 (22.5)			
	3	230 (25.5)	179 (23.8)	51 (33.8)			
	4	164 (18.2)	118 (15.7)	46 (30.5)			
	5	10 (1.1)	7 (0.9)	3 (2.0)			
PT (median [IQR])		14.29 [6.25, 25.94]	12.50 [5.53, 23.47]	24.29 [12.32, 37.71]	<0.001	nonnorm	0.669
PI-RADS (%)	3	193 (21.4)	180 (23.9)	13 (8.6)	<0.001		0.673
	4	355 (39.3)	311 (41.4)	44 (29.1)			
	5	318 (35.2)	227 (30.2)	91 (60.3)			
	N	37 (4.1)	34 (4.5)	3 (2.0)			
TL (%)	M	236 (26.1)	185 (24.6)	51 (33.8)	0.056		0.246
	N	32 (3.5)	28 (3.7)	4 (2.6)			
	p	354 (39.2)	307 (40.8)	47 (31.1)			
	T	281 (31.1)	232 (30.9)	49 (32.5)			
D (median [IQR])		1.30 [0.90, 1.90]	1.30 [0.90, 1.80]	1.70 [1.20, 2.40]	<0.001	nonnorm	0.545
NT (%)	0	37 (4.1)	33 (4.4)	4 (2.6)	0.520		0.154
	1	546 (60.5)	458 (60.9)	88 (58.3)			
	2	263 (29.1)	217 (28.9)	46 (30.5)			
	3	51 (5.6)	40 (5.3)	11 (7.3)			
	4	6 (0.7)	4 (0.5)	2 (1.3)			
T-MRI (%)	1	483 (53.5)	428 (56.9)	55 (36.4)	<0.001	exact	0.426
	2	75 (8.3)	55 (7.3)	20 (13.2)			
	3	345 (38.2)	269 (35.8)	76 (50.3)			
PSA (median [IQR])		8.94 [6.40, 13.61]	8.57 [6.11, 12.10]	14.90 [8.02, 23.77]	<0.001	nonnorm	0.561
PSAD (median [IQR])		0.27 [0.18, 0.44]	0.26 [0.17, 0.40]	0.42 [0.27, 0.80]	<0.001	nonnorm	0.570
II (median [IQR])		376.68 [276.07, 519.53]	382.54 [274.14, 515.20]	366.61 [282.82, 541.58]	0.965	nonnorm	0.022
margin (%)	0	752 (83.3)	752 (100.0)	0 (0.0)	<0.001		NaN
	1	151 (16.7)	0 (0.0)	151 (100.0)			
t (median [IQR])		14.00 [10.00, 18.00]	14.00 [10.00, 18.00]	13.00 [10.00, 18.00]	0.571	nonnorm	0.019
Operator (%)	1	416 (46.1)	339 (45.1)	77 (51.0)	0.397		0.122
	2	409 (45.3)	346 (46.0)	63 (41.7)			
	3	78 (8.6)	67 (8.9)	11 (7.3)			
Others (%)	0	858 (95.0)	722 (96.0)	136 (90.1)	0.004		0.235
	1	45 (5.0)	30 (4.0)	15 (9.9)			

V: Prostate volume; PPN: Percent of positive needles; ISUP, International Society of Urological Pathology; PT: Percent of Tumor; PI-RADS, Prostate Imaging Reporting and Data System; TL: Tumor location; D: Maximal tumor diameter; NT: Number of tumors; T-MRI: Clinical staging of the tumor provided by MRI. Stages less than or equal to T2a are divided into group 1; T2b into group 2; the patients with staging greater than or equal to T2c were divided into group 3; PSA: Prostate-Specific Antigen; II: Inflammation index; t: Time from biopsy to surgery; Others: Other risk factors.

For the new predictors worthy of concern, the median of PPN is 0.34 in the NSM group and 0.44 in the PSM group, which was distinguished by substantial differences. The same difference appeared in the PT factor, with a median PT of 12.5 in the NSM group and 24.29 in the PSM group. Since tumors are often irregular in shape and their volumes are not easy to measure, we introduced the concept of the longest diameter. We were surprised to find a significant distribution, with a median of 1.3 for D in the NSM group and up to 1.7 in the PSM group. PSAD based on PSA performed similarly to PSA, possibly because the prostate volumes did not show distinctions between the two groups. However, the performance of NT, II, T, and Others was not satisfactory.

3.2. Modeling

There were only 151 events, and yet we considered 17 predictors. To satisfy the requirement that a factor must be assigned to at least 10 events, we began with univariate analysis. Table 2 shows the estimated values, standard errors, and p-values of the regression coefficients for univariate analysis. Finally, 10 factors including age, PPN, ISUP, PT, D, PI-RADS, PSA, PSAD, TL, and Others were selected for subsequent screening. Because clinical staging is a relatively important parameter for prostate cancer, we included it in subsequent screening, although it was not significant in univariate analysis.

Table 2. Regression coefficients for univariate analysis.

Coefficients:	Univariate Analysis		
	Estimate	Std. Error	Pr (>|z|)
age	0.039	0.014	0.006 ***
BMI	−0.019	0.031	0.546
V	−0.007	0.005	0.159
PPN	2.266	0.4.5	2.13×10^{-8} ***
ISUP-2	0.573	0.315	0.069 *
ISUP-3	1.270	0.299	2.13×10^{-5} ***
ISUP-4	1.480	0.311	1.90×10^{-6} ***
ISUP-5	1.681	0.735	0.022 **
PT	0.040	0.006	1.8×10^{-11} ***
D	0.693	0.115	1.67×10^{-9} ***
PI-RADS-4	0.551	0.322	0.087 *
PI-RADS-5	1.544	0.306	4.5×10^{-7} ***
PI-RADS-N	−0.313	0.779	0.688
NT-1	0.417	0.543	0.443
NT-2	0.515	0.555	0.354
NT-3	0.819	0.630	0.193
NT-4	1.705	1.055	0.106
PSA	0.026	0.009	0.006 ***
PSAD	1.263	0.220	9.59×10^{-9} ***
T-MRI-2	0.070	0.373	0.852
T-MRI-3	0.235	0.246	0.342
TL-N	−1.484	0.745	0.046 **
TL-p	−0.607	0.231	0.009 ***
TL-T	−0.127	0.224	0.574
II	0.0002	0.000	0.692
t	−0.001	0.004	0.796
Others-1	0.860	0.345	0.013 **
Operator 100–200 cases	−0.220	0.191	0.248
Operator <100 cases	−0.387	0.363	0.286

* $p < 0.1$; ** $p < 0.05$; *** $p < 0.01$, Univariate analysis was based on the logistic model.

After screening by the Lasso method, we obtained the final prediction factors and the final prediction model. Table 3 demonstrates the regression coefficient estimates, OR, 95% CI, and p-values for the final prediction model. Nomograms, as depicted in Figure 2, will be used to visualize models for the convenience of clinicians.

Table 3. The prediction model.

Coefficients	Estimate	OR	95% Confidence Interval		Pr (>|z|)
age	0.020	1.020	0.991	1.051	0.180
PPN	0.696	2.006	0.424	9.500	0.381
ISUP-2	0.260	1.297	0.673	2.502	0.438
ISUP-3	0.630	1.877	0.968	3.636	0.063 *
ISUP-4	0.846	2.329	1.172	4.630	0.016 **
ISUP-5	1.243	3.466	0.742	16.202	0.115
PT	0.017	1.017	0.993	1.043	0.169
D	0.076	1.079	0.747	1.559	0.687
PI-RADS-4	0.349	1.417	0.727	2.762	0.306
PI-RADS-5	0.699	2.012	0.979	4.135	0.058 *
PI-RADS-N	−1.358	0.257	0.013	4.907	0.367
PSA	0.026	1.026	1.008	1.045	0.006 ***
T-MRI2	0.070	1.072	0.516	2.228	0.852
T-MRI3	0.235	1.264	0.780	2.050	0.342
TL-N	1.357	3.883	0.211	71.321	0.361
TL-*p*	−0.360	0.697	0.408	1.193	0.189
TL-T	0.430	1.537	0.908	2.604	0.110
Intercept	−5.203	0.005			0.00001 ***

Observations: 882.000, Log Likelihood: −337.820, Akaike Inf. Crit: 711.639, * $p < 0.1$; ** $p < 0.05$; *** $p < 0.01$, OR and 95% CI were calculated by SPSS 22.

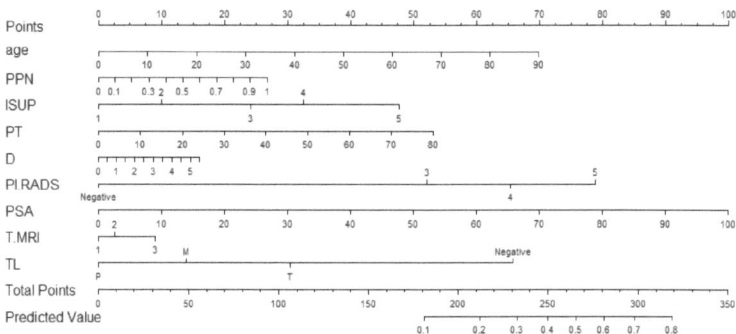

Figure 2. The nomogram.

To make it easier for using, we also provide a web calculator. This is the website for the calculator. https://doctor-h.shinyapps.io/dynnomapp/ (accessed on 23 November 2022).

As shown in Figure 2, If a patient was 70 years old, the ratio of positive needles was 0.5, the histological grade was 3, and the total tumor ratio was 30. The longest diameter of the suspicious nodule was 1.53, the suspicious nodule score was 4, the PSA was 7.55, the location of the suspicious nodule was a transitional zone, and the clinical stages were 2c and above. With a total score of 385 and a PSM probability of 0.276, they belonged to the low-risk group with PSM.

The discrimination of the final model was calculated by the C statistic (this was the model discrimination index, and the greater the value, the better the discrimination). The C statistic upon the model establishment was 0.764 (0.722, 0.806), and the C statistic after internal verification and adjustment was 0.727. Moreover, the degree of calibration is shown as the Brier value (a measure of the model's degree of calibration, with a lower value indicating a better degree of calibration, generally less than 0.25), which is 0.118 after modeling and 0.126 after adjustments by internal validation. The calibration curve is shown in Figure 3. It could be observed that the model had a suitable replacement in the low-risk and medium-risk groups, and a generally acceptable fit in the medium-risk and high-risk groups, which would overestimate the result to some extent.

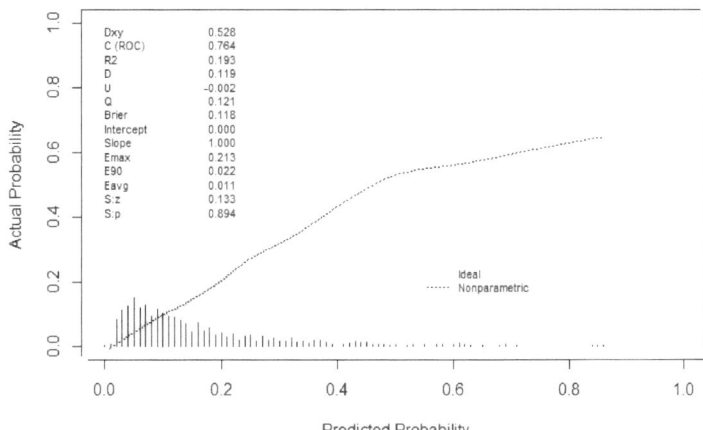

Figure 3. The calibration curve. Both the C statistic and Brier value in the figure are precalibration values. The C statistic after internal verification and adjustment was 0.727. The Brier value was 0.126 after internal validation adjustments. Both of them are acceptable.

Pathology information is provided as Appendix A (Table A1).

4. Discussion

We have developed and validated models to predict the risk of PSMs after RALP in patients with prostate cancer. This algorithm combines the influencing factors mentioned in previous studies with new variables associated with an increased risk of PSM. These included age, PPN, ISUP, PT, D, PI-RADS, TL, T-MRI, and PSA. The final model has been generated (Table 3). The model performed comparably in the validation and development data sets, and we deemed it clinically available.

The widely accepted view that prostate cancer is an age-related disease has been confirmed by numerous studies. As early as 2010, the American Cancer Society suggested that men with an average risk should receive information about the uncertainty, risk, and potential benefits of prostate cancer screening from age 50, while men in high-risk groups should receive this information before age 50. Based on the information, the patient decides whether to accept the examination [26]. Age has also been found to be an independent predictor of shorter prostate cancer-specific survival in men diagnosed with metastatic prostate cancer, even in an era of more effective treatment [27]. Now, we have also discovered and reported that age is a predictor of PSM after RALP in patients with prostate cancer. Some researchers have pointed out a male-specific association between the accumulation of DNA damage related to mutation and aging and the prostate cancer biomarker poly (ADP-ribose)-polymerase (PARP) [28]. This may be one of the reasons and corresponding research can be conducted to investigate it.

ISUP is the grading standard of prostate cancer for judging the malignancy and the prognosis of tumors established by the International Society of Urological Pathology, which is generally accepted to be the case that, the larger the subgroup, the worse the prognosis will be [29]. Such trends are also present in our model, with higher subgroups suggesting a higher risk of PSMs.

PI-RADS is an overall score of suspected prostate cancer nodules based on multi-parameter magnetic resonance imaging (mpMRI) proposed by the American Radiological Society (ACR) and the European Society of Urological Surgery (ESUR). The second edition published in 2016 is the latest standard for mpMRI imaging and reporting [30]. However, due to distinct equipment and the reporter's experience, there may still be bias. Overall, the PI-RADS score was consistent with the direction of risk for PSM. Upon examining the regression model, we discovered that a PI-RADS score of 5 had a significant impact on the outcomes.

Tumor location was grouped according to previous studies [18]. The location of the tumor within the transitional zone was associated with an increased risk of PSM.

Compared with other studies using postoperative pathological staging [16], we prefer to use clinical staging (T-MRI) because it is available preoperatively. The criteria for T-MRI were by the AJCC cancer-staging 8th edition [24]. As a result, a higher T-MRI implies a higher risk of PSM. This may also explain the relevance of neoadjuvant therapy in patients with locally advanced stages, as the tumor may shrink to reduce T-MRI after neoadjuvant therapy. Surgical treatment at this time can reduce the risk of PSM.

PSA, as an essential biomarker of prostate cancer, has been widely used for the screening of various prostate cancers. Hereby, we reported that the probability of a high PSA level is relatively high in patients with a high risk of PSM.

In addition, the new indicators contain an intriguing element. The proportion of positive biopsy needles (PPN) can be approximated as a random sample, so a higher PPN means a larger tumor with a higher likelihood of cutting the tumor. This is in line with our observation that the risk of PSM rises as PPN levels rise. This phenomenon is also similar to the results reported in other studies [17]. Percentage of Tumor (PT) is a new concept we proposed based on PPN. We present this concept, because there may be a large number of positive needles in a biopsy but a small amount of tumor per needle. We expected it to perform better than PPN, but the result was not ideal. Although p (0.169) for PT was less than PPN (0.381), indicating that PT was more likely to influence the results of PSM than PPN, its regression coefficient (0.017) was less than PPN (0.696), indicating that PT contributed less to the results than PPN. A larger sample size may then be required to verify the relevance of the PT. The tumor maximum diameter (D) is a new measurement we brought forward. The majority of the tumors are irregular and their volume is difficult to measure, which is the primary motivation for proposing this index. To date, no investigator has included it as a predictor of PSM. In the subgroup comparison, we obtained that D's distribution in the PSM group and the NSM group was significantly different, but after being included in the regression model, D's contribution was not optimistic. However, we can still find the influence of the change of D on the risk of PSM. This may be an approximation of the tumor's volume. Similarly, a larger sample size may subsequently be required to verify the importance of D.

The predictive factors included in this study are all indicators in the preoperative necessary examinations for clinical patients, which were easily acquired and explained in clinical work. For junior doctors who still lack clinical experience, this model can be regarded as a tool for their rapid adaptation to clinical work. Meanwhile, the inclusion of more predictors makes PSM more specific and predictable. If it extends from prostate cancer to other systems, it is reasonable to believe that similar research can be conducted to improve the therapeutic value of surgery for cancer in general.

The methods and standards for the derivation and validation of prediction models are presented in the 2015 TRIPOD Statement by the BMJ [31]. Its advantage is to make the research logic and process more rigorous, to make the report content more comprehensive and standardized, and to make different prediction models comparable. Currently, no study has pointed out any glaring flaws in the TRIPOD statement. The key advantages of the prediction model established in this study include: it covered the entire contents of the preoperative examination of prostate cancer, and these variables are easy to measure. The greatest advantage lies in the visualization of the model, which transforms abstract variables into practical evaluation tools. The limitations of this study include the possibility of bias due to insufficient valid data and information bias: First, because the rate of PSM is comparatively low (16.7%), which implies that inadequate relative sample size may cause some deviations from the results. In this instance, univariate analysis was considered to pre screen factors. Although this approach has been questioned by statisticians, there seems to be no better solution to solve similar dilemmas. Second, most patients included in this study are in the early clinical stage. This may allow the study model to perform effectively in early-stage patients and may perform poorly in the overall patient population. Eventually, additional validation studies may be required to cover a larger patient population.

Modeling and validation are currently performed on the same set of practices and individuals, while an independent validation study would be a more rigorous test that should be performed. We consequently expect other researchers interested in this research to apply data from different institutions and even divergent races to verify this model.

5. Conclusions

In conclusion, we have developed and validated a predictive model for PSM after RALP for prostate cancer that can be used in clinical practice. Simultaneously, we found that the ISUP score, PI-RADS score, and PSA were the independent risk factors for PSM. In this model, previous studies' factors were referred to, and some new factors were proposed to predict more comprehensively. This is probably the most relatively comprehensive and operable prediction model in this field. Although it still has certain limitations, the discrimination and calibration performance of the model are acceptable overall.

Author Contributions: Y.H.: methodology, software, validation, formal analysis, investigation, data curation, writing—original draft, visualization. Q.Z.: conceptualization, Resources, writing—review and editing. J.H.: investigation, data curation. L.X.: conceptualization, resources. S.Z.: conceptualization. H.G.: resources, supervision, project administration, funding acquisition. All authors have read and agreed to the published version of the manuscript.

Funding: This research was funded by the Chinesisch-Deutsches Mobilitätsprogramm, grant number M-0670.

Institutional Review Board Statement: Not applicable.

Informed Consent Statement: Informed consent was obtained from all subjects involved in the study.

Data Availability Statement: Not applicable.

Conflicts of Interest: The authors declare no conflict of interest. The funders had no role in the design of the study; in the collection, analyses, or interpretation of data; in the writing of the manuscript; or in the decision to publish the results.

Appendix A

Table A1. Pathology Information.

		NSM	PSM	p
n		752	151	
ML (%)	Apex	0	45 (33.1)	0.143
	Periphery	0	42 (30.9)	
	Base	0	23 (16.9)	
	Apex + Periphery	0	12 (8.8)	
	Base + Periphery	0	6 (4.4)	
	Base + Apex	0	4 (2.9)	
	Apex + Base + Periphery	0	3 (2.2)	
	Periphery + Spermaduct	0	1 (0.7)	
Gleason (%)	3 + 3	105 (14.0)	3 (2.0)	<0.001
	3 + 4	394 (52.4)	71 (47.0)	
	3 + 5	1 (0.1)	0 (0.0)	
	4 + 3	194 (25.8)	51 (33.8)	
	4 + 4	41 (5.5)	16 (10.6)	
	4 + 5	14 (1.9)	9 (6.0)	
	5 + 3	2 (0.3)	1 (0.7)	
	5 + 4	1 (0.1)	0 (0.0)	

Table A1. Cont.

		NSM	PSM	p
N (%)	1	396 (52.7)	100 (66.2)	0.1
	2	220 (29.3)	28 (18.5)	
	3	61 (8.1)	10 (6.6)	
	m	75 (9.9)	13 (8.6)	
TL (%)	M	160 (21.3)	47 (31.1)	<0.001
	p	380 (50.5)	40 (26.5)	
	T	212 (28.2)	64 (42.4)	
EPE (%)	0	504 (67.0)	45 (29.8)	<0.001
	1	248 (33.0)	106 (70.2)	
SVI (%)	0	720 (95.7)	123 (81.5)	<0.001
	1	32 (4.3)	28 (18.5)	
VI (%)	0	730 (97.1)	139 (92.1)	0.006
	1	22 (2.9)	12 (7.9)	
NI(%)	0	332 (44.1)	25 (16.6)	<0.001
	1	420 (55.9)	126 (83.4)	
Lymph node (%)	0	288 (38.3)	86 (57.0)	
	1	11 (1.5)	9 (6.0)	
	2	453 (60.2)	56 (37.1)	
pT (%)	T2	503 (66.9)	43 (28.5)	<0.001
	T3a	217 (28.9)	79 (52.3)	
	T3b	32 (4.3)	27 (17.9)	
	T4	0 (0.0)	2 (1.3)	

ML: Margin location; N: Number of the tumor; TL: Tumor location; VI: Vascular invasion; NI: Invasion of nerve; SVI: Seminal vesicle invasion.

References

1. Sung, H.; Ferlay, J.; Siegel, R.L.; Laversanne, M.; Soerjomataram, I.; Jemal, A.; Bray, F. Global Cancer Statistics 2020: GLOBOCAN Estimates of Incidence and Mortality Worldwide for 36 Cancers in 185 Countries. *CA Cancer J. Clin.* **2021**, *71*, 209–249. [CrossRef] [PubMed]
2. Zheng, R.; Zhang, S.; Zeng, H.; Wang, S.; Sun, K.; Chen, R.; Li, L.; Wei, W.; He, J. Cancer incidence and mortality in China, 2016. *J. Natl. Cancer Cent.* **2022**, *2*, 1–9. [CrossRef]
3. Feng, R.-M.; Zong, Y.-N.; Cao, S.-M.; Xu, R.-H. Current cancer situation in China: Good or sbad news from the 2018 Global Cancer Statistics? *Cancer Commun. Lond. Engl.* **2019**, *39*, 22. [CrossRef] [PubMed]
4. Xia, C.; Dong, X.; Li, H.; Cao, M.; Sun, D.; He, S.; Yang, F.; Yan, X.; Zhang, S.; Li, N.; et al. Cancer statistics in China and United States, 2022: Profiles, trends, and determinants. *Chin. Med. J. (Engl.)* **2022**, *135*, 584–590. [CrossRef] [PubMed]
5. Liu, W.; Yao, Y.; Liu, X.; Liu, Y.; Zhang, G.-M. Neoadjuvant hormone therapy for patients with high-risk prostate cancer: A systematic review and meta-analysis. *Asian J. Androl.* **2021**, *23*, 429–436. [CrossRef]
6. McKay, R.R.; Berchuck, J.; Kwak, L.; Xie, W.; Silver, R.; Bubley, G.J.; Chang, P.K.; Wagner, A.; Zhang, Z.; Kibel, A.S.; et al. Outcomes of Post-Neoadjuvant Intense Hormone Therapy and Surgery for High Risk Localized Prostate Cancer: Results of a Pooled Analysis of Contemporary Clinical Trials. *J. Urol.* **2021**, *205*, 1689–1697. [CrossRef]
7. Costello, A.J. Considering the role of radical prostatectomy in 21st century prostate cancer care. *Nat. Rev. Urol.* **2020**, *17*, 177–188. [CrossRef]
8. Sooriakumaran, P.; Karnes, J.; Stief, C.; Copsey, B.; Montorsi, F.; Hammerer, P.; Beyer, B.; Moschini, M.; Gratzke, C.; Steuber, T.; et al. A Multi-institutional Analysis of Perioperative Outcomes in 106 Men Who Underwent Radical Prostatectomy for Distant Metastatic Prostate Cancer at Presentation. *Eur. Urol.* **2016**, *69*, 788–794. [CrossRef]
9. Van den Broeck, T.; van den Bergh, R.C.N.; Briers, E.; Cornford, P.; Cumberbatch, M.; Tilki, D.; De Santis, M.; Fanti, S.; Fossati, N.; Gillessen, S.; et al. Biochemical Recurrence in Prostate Cancer: The European Association of Urology Prostate Cancer Guidelines Panel Recommendations. *Eur. Urol. Focus* **2020**, *6*, 231–234. [CrossRef]
10. Morizane, S.; Yumioka, T.; Makishima, K.; Tsounapi, P.; Iwamoto, H.; Hikita, K.; Honda, M.; Umekita, Y.; Takenaka, A. Impact of positive surgical margin status in predicting early biochemical recurrence after robot-assisted radical prostatectomy. *Int. J. Clin Oncol.* **2021**, *26*, 1961–1967. [CrossRef]
11. Martini, A.; Gandaglia, G.; Fossati, N.; Scuderi, S.; Bravi, C.A.; Mazzone, E.; Stabile, A.; Scarcella, S.; Robesti, D.; Barletta, F.; et al. Defining Clinically Meaningful Positive Surgical Margins in Patients Undergoing Radical Prostatectomy for Localised Prostate Cancer. *Eur. Urol. Oncol.* **2021**, *4*, 42–48. [CrossRef]
12. Lee, W.; Lim, B.; Kyung, Y.S.; Kim, C.-S. Impact of positive surgical margin on biochemical recurrence in localized prostate cancer *Prostate Int.* **2021**, *9*, 151–156. [CrossRef] [PubMed]

13. Rosenberg, J.E.; Jung, J.H.; Edgerton, Z.; Lee, H.; Lee, S.; Bakker, C.J.; Dahm, P. Retzius-sparing versus standard robotic-assisted laparoscopic prostatectomy for the treatment of clinically localized prostate cancer. *Cochrane Database Syst. Rev.* **2020**, *8*, CD013641. [CrossRef] [PubMed]
14. Soeterik, T.F.W.; van Melick, H.H.E.; Dijksman, L.M.; Stomps, S.; Witjes, J.A.; van Basten, J.P.A. Nerve Sparing during Robot-Assisted Radical Prostatectomy Increases the Risk of Ipsilateral Positive Surgical Margins. *J. Urol.* **2020**, *204*, 91–95. [CrossRef]
15. Koga, F.; Ito, M.; Kataoka, M.; Fukushima, H.; Nakanishi, Y.; Takemura, K.; Suzuki, H.; Sakamoto, K.; Kobayashi, S.; Tobisu, K.-I. Novel anatomical apical dissection utilizing puboprostatic "open-collar" technique: Impact on apical surgical margin and early continence recovery. *PLoS ONE* **2021**, *16*, e0249991. [CrossRef] [PubMed]
16. Kang, S.G.; Schatloff, O.; Haidar, A.M.; Samavedi, S.; Palmer, K.J.; Cheon, J.; Patel, V.R. Overall rate, location, and predictive factors for positive surgical margins after robot-assisted laparoscopic radical prostatectomy for high-risk prostate cancer. *Asian J. Androl.* **2016**, *18*, 123–128. [CrossRef]
17. Tuliao, P.H.; Koo, K.C.; Komninos, C.; Chang, C.H.; Choi, Y.D.; Chung, B.H.; Hong, S.J.; Rha, K.H. Number of positive preoperative biopsy cores is a predictor of positive surgical margins (PSM) in small prostates after robot-assisted radical prostatectomy (RARP). *BJU Int.* **2015**, *116*, 897–904. [CrossRef]
18. Li, Y.; Fu, Y.; Li, W.; Xu, L.; Zhang, Q.; Gao, J.; Li, D.; Li, X.; Qiu, X.; Guo, H. Tumour location determined by preoperative MRI is an independent predictor for positive surgical margin status after Retzius-sparing robot-assisted radical prostatectomy. *BJU Int.* **2020**, *126*, 152–158. [CrossRef] [PubMed]
19. Tian, X.-J.; Wang, Z.-L.; Li, G.; Cao, S.-J.; Cui, H.-R.; Li, Z.-H.; Liu, Z.; Li, B.-L.; Ma, L.-L.; Zhuang, S.-R.; et al. Development and validation of a preoperative nomogram for predicting positive surgical margins after laparoscopic radical prostatectomy. *Chin. Med. J. (Engl.)* **2019**, *132*, 928–934. [CrossRef]
20. Park, M.Y.; Park, K.J.; Kim, M.; Kim, J.K. Preoperative MRI-based estimation of risk for positive resection margin after radical prostatectomy in patients with prostate cancer: Development and validation of a simple scoring system. *Eur. Radiol.* **2021**, *31*, 4898–4907. [CrossRef]
21. Xu, B.; Luo, C.; Zhang, Q.; Jin, J. Preoperative characteristics of the P.R.O.S.T.A.T.E. scores: A novel predictive tool for the risk of positive surgical margin after radical prostatectomy. *J. Cancer Res. Clin. Oncol.* **2017**, *143*, 687–692. [CrossRef] [PubMed]
22. Wettstein, M.S.; Saba, K.; Umbehr, M.H.; Murtola, T.J.; Fankhauser, C.D.; Adank, J.-P.; Hofmann, M.; Sulser, T.; Hermanns, T.; Moch, H.; et al. Prognostic Role of Preoperative Serum Lipid Levels in Patients Undergoing Radical Prostatectomy for Clinically Localized Prostate Cancer. *Prostate* **2017**, *77*, 549–556. [CrossRef]
23. Epstein, J.I.; Amin, M.B.; Reuter, V.E.; Humphrey, P.A. Contemporary Gleason Grading of Prostatic Carcinoma: An Update With Discussion on Practical Issues to Implement the 2014 International Society of Urological Pathology (ISUP) Consensus Conference on Gleason Grading of Prostatic Carcinoma. *Am. J. Surg. Pathol.* **2017**, *41*, e1–e7. [CrossRef]
24. Amin, M.B.; Greene, F.L.; Edge, S.B.; Compton, C.C.; Gershenwald, J.E.; Brookland, R.K.; Meyer, L.; Gress, D.M.; Byrd, D.R.; Winchester, D.P. The Eighth Edition AJCC Cancer Staging Manual: Continuing to build a bridge from a population-based to a more "personalized" approach to cancer staging. *CA Cancer J. Clin.* **2017**, *67*, 93–99. [CrossRef]
25. Zhang, Z.; Tian, Y.; Bai, L.; Xiahou, J.; Hancock, E. High-order covariate interacted Lasso for feature selection. *Pattern Recognit. Lett.* **2017**, *87*, 139–146. [CrossRef]
26. Wolf, A.M.D.; Wender, R.C.; Etzioni, R.B.; Thompson, I.M.; D'Amico, A.V.; Volk, R.J.; Brooks, D.D.; Dash, C.; Guessous, I.; Andrews, K.; et al. American Cancer Society guideline for the early detection of prostate cancer: Update 2010. *CA Cancer J. Clin.* **2010**, *60*, 70–98. [CrossRef] [PubMed]
27. Bernard, B.; Burnett, C.; Sweeney, C.J.; Rider, J.R.; Sridhar, S.S. Impact of age at diagnosis of de novo metastatic prostate cancer on survival. *Cancer* **2020**, *126*, 986–993. [CrossRef]
28. Deniz, M.; Zengerling, F.; Gundelach, T.; Moreno-Villanueva, M.; Bürkle, A.; Janni, W.; Bolenz, C.; Kostezka, S.; Marienfeld, R.; Benckendorff, J.; et al. Age-related activity of Poly (ADP-Ribose) Polymerase (PARP) in men with localized prostate cancer. *Mech. Ageing Dev.* **2021**, *196*, 111494. [CrossRef] [PubMed]
29. Epstein, J.I.; Egevad, L.; Amin, M.B.; Delahunt, B.; Srigley, J.R.; Humphrey, P.A. Grading Committee The 2014 International Society of Urological Pathology (ISUP) Consensus Conference on Gleason Grading of Prostatic Carcinoma: Definition of Grading Patterns and Proposal for a New Grading System. *Am. J. Surg. Pathol.* **2016**, *40*, 244–252. [CrossRef] [PubMed]
30. Weinreb, J.C.; Barentsz, J.O.; Choyke, P.L.; Cornud, F.; Haider, M.A.; Macura, K.J.; Margolis, D.; Schnall, M.D.; Shtern, F.; Tempany, C.M.; et al. PI-RADS Prostate Imaging—Reporting and Data System: 2015, Version 2. *Eur. Urol.* **2016**, *69*, 16–40. [CrossRef]
31. Collins, G.S.; Reitsma, J.B.; Altman, D.G.; Moons, K.G.M. Transparent reporting of a multivariable prediction model for individual prognosis or diagnosis (TRIPOD): The TRIPOD statement. *BMJ* **2015**, *350*, g7594. [CrossRef] [PubMed]

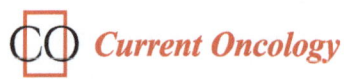

Brief Report

Single-Center Comparison of [^{64}Cu]-DOTAGA-PSMA and [^{18}F]-PSMA PET–CT for Imaging Prostate Cancer

Siroos Mirzaei [1,*], Rainer Lipp [2], Shahin Zandieh [3] and Asha Leisser [1]

[1] Department of Nuclear Medicine with PET-Center, Clinic Ottakring (Wilhelminenspital), 1160 Vienna, Austria; AshaLeisser@gesundheitsverbund.at
[2] Department of Internal Medicine, Medical University of Graz, 8036 Graz, Austria; RainerLipp@gesundheitsverbund.at
[3] Department of Radiology and Nuclear Medicine, Hanusch Hospital, 1160 Vienna, Austria; Shahin.Zandieh@gesundheitsverbund.at
* Correspondence: siroos.mirzaei@gesundheitsverbund.at

Abstract: Introduction: the diagnostic performance of [^{64}Cu]-DOTAGA-PSMA PET–CT imaging was compared retrospectively to [^{18}F]-PSMA PET–CT in prostate cancer patients with recurrent disease and in the primary staging of selected patients with advanced local and possible metastatic disease. Methods: We retrospectively selected a total of 100 patients, who were consecutively examined in our department, with biochemical recurrence after radical prostatectomy or who had progressive local and possible metastatic disease in the last 3 months prior to this investigation. All patients were examined with a dedicated PET–CT scanner (Biograph; Siemens Healthineers). A total of 250 MBq (3.5 MBq per kg bodyweight, range 230–290 MBq) of [^{64}Cu]-DOTAGA-PSMA or [^{18}-F] PSMA was applied intravenously. PET images were performed 1 h post-injection (skull base to mid-thigh). The maximum standardized uptake values (SUVmax) of PSMA-positive lesions and the mean standardized uptake value (SUVmean) of the right liver lobe were measured. Results: All but 9/50 of the patients (18%; PSA range: 0.01–0.7 µg/L) studied with [^{64}Cu]-DOTAGA-PSMA and 6/50 of the ones (12%; PSA range: 0.01–4.2) studied with [^{18}F]-PSMA had at least one positive PSMA lesion shown by PET–CT. The total number of lesions was higher with [^{64}Cu]-DOTAGA-PSMA (209 vs. 191); however, the median number of lesions was one for [^{64}Cu]-DOTAGA-PSMA and two for [^{18}F]-PSMA. Interestingly, the median SUVmean of the right liver lobe was slightly higher for [^{18}F]-PSMA (11.8 vs. 8.9). Conclusions: [^{64}Cu]-DOTAGA-PSMA and [^{18}F]-PSMA have comparable detection rates for the assessment of residual disease in patients with recurrent or primary progressive prostate cancer. The uptake in the liver is moderately different, and therefore at least the SUVs of the lesions in both studies would not be comparable.

Keywords: [^{64}Cu]/[^{18}F] PSMA; oncology; prostate cancer; PSMA positron emission; tomography/computed tomography (PET–CT); prostate-specific membrane; antigen (PSMA)

Citation: Mirzaei, S.; Lipp, R.; Zandieh, S.; Leisser, A. Single-Center Comparison of [^{64}Cu]-DOTAGA-PSMA and [^{18}F]-PSMA PET–CT for Imaging Prostate Cancer. *Curr. Oncol.* **2021**, *28*, 4167–4173. https://doi.org/10.3390/curroncol28050353

Received: 23 August 2021
Accepted: 13 October 2021
Published: 15 October 2021

Publisher's Note: MDPI stays neutral with regard to jurisdictional claims in published maps and institutional affiliations.

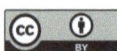

Copyright: © 2021 by the authors. Licensee MDPI, Basel, Switzerland. This article is an open access article distributed under the terms and conditions of the Creative Commons Attribution (CC BY) license (https://creativecommons.org/licenses/by/4.0/).

1. Introduction

Prostate cancer (PCa) is one of the most commonly diagnosed malignancies in men with a total of 1,414,259 new cases and an estimated 375,000 deaths worldwide in 2020 [1]. The treatment management of PCa depends on the site and extent of disease (local/nodal vs. systemic disease) [2]. Even though several novel pharmacologic drugs have been introduced to the therapeutic armamentarium against metastatic PCa, advanced disease still represents a fatal condition for these patients [3]. For proper staging, imaging modalities such as CT, multiparametric MRI and bone scans are recommended in patients with intermediate risk and localized or locally advanced high-risk PCa [2]. In cases of biochemical recurrence (BCR) after radical prostatectomy or radiation therapy, functional PET–CT imaging using radiolabeled choline or prostate-specific membrane antigen (PSMA) ligands have been introduced [4]. PSMA is a transmembrane protein that is expressed in normal and neoplastic prostate tissue, with a structure composed of a 707-amino-acid external portion, a 19-amino-acid internal portion and a 24-amino-acid transmembrane portion [5]. In light of its specificity, PSMA has been selected as the biological target of a number of radiolabeled small molecules, such as [^{68}Ga]-PSMA-11, [^{18}F]-DCFPyL and [^{18}F]-PSMA-1007 [6]. PSMA ligands can not only be coupled to diagnostic radionuclides such as [^{68}Ga], [^{18}F] and [^{64}Cu], but also to therapeutic radionuclides (e.g., [^{177}Lu], and [^{225}Ac]), allowing a theranostic approach to PC diagnosis and treatment [7]. Previous studies have shown a high diagnostic performance of [^{68}Ga]-labeled urea-based PSMA in the detection of lymph node metastases in BCR patients [8]. Additionally, PSMA ligands in molecular PET imaging provide a higher tumor detection rate as compared to choline ligands in patients with BCR, especially in cases of very low PSA levels [9].

PSMA-PET has become a highly accurate staging tool in multiple settings in clinical routine, although its exact uses in clinical practice remain to be determined. We use it in our department for staging treatment-naïve locally advanced disease as well as recurrent and metastatic disease. To overcome the logistical difficulties of obtaining a [^{68}Ga] generator, [^{64}Cu]-PSMA and [^{18}F]-PSMA have been introduced. [^{64}Cu] possesses a relatively long half-life (t1/2) of 12.7 h, allowing imaging of smaller molecules, larger, slower clearing proteins and nanoparticles. Uniquely, it decays by three processes, namely, positron (17.8%, Emax = 0.65 MeV), electron capture (43.8%) and beta decay (38.4%, Emax = 0.57 MeV), and can thus be used for both treatment and imaging [10]. Its lower positron range compared to the commonly used [^{68}Ga] grants a better spatial resolution. The high diagnostic potential of [^{64}Cu]-PSMA PET–CT imaging has been clinically investigated in the past, and different chelators to [^{64}Cu] are used (11). DOTA and NODAGA chelators form stable complexes with Cu and have been clinically used [11]. Another PSMA ligand which was introduced recently is ^{64}Cu-PSMA-BCH, which was shown to have a high stability in vivo with a lower uptake in the liver than ^{64}Cu-PSMA-617 [12]. PSMA I&T labeled with ^{64}Cu also showed the feasibility of PET imaging through in vitro and in vivo studies [13]. In patients with low PSA values, a better performance was observed for ^{64}Cu-PSMA-617 PET/CT compared to ^{18}F-choline PET/CT in restaging after BCR [14].

In contrast, [^{18}F] has been well established as a diagnostic radionuclide due to its physical and nuclear characteristics: a high positron decay ratio (97%), a relatively short half-life (109.7 min) and low positron energy (Emax = 0.63 MeV) [15].

The aim of our study is to evaluate the uptake behavior of [^{64}Cu]-DOTAGA-PSMA with DOTAGA as a possible stable chelator compared to [^{18}F]-PSMA PET–CT in a routine clinical setting in PCa patients.

2. Methods

We selected retrospectively a total number of 100 patients (50 examined with [^{64}Cu]-DOTAGA-PSMA and 50 with [^{18}F]-PSMA PET–CT), who were consecutively examined in our department, with biochemical recurrence after radical prostatectomy or had progressive local disease in the last 3 months and were scheduled for either radiation or systemic therapy. Routinely, we perform, due to logistic reasons, [^{64}Cu]-DOTAGA-PSMA one day per week and [^{18}F]-PSMA PET–CT one day per week. All patients were examined with a dedicated PET–CT scanner (Biograph; Siemens Healthineers) in compliance with the 1964 Declaration of Helsinki and the responsible regulatory bodies in Austria. Formal consent was obtained from all patients prior to examination. A total of 250 MBq (3.5 MBq per kg bodyweight, range 230–290 MBq) of [^{64}Cu]-DOTAGA PSMA or [^{18}-F] PSMA was applied intravenously. PET images were performed 1 h post-injection (skull base to mid-thigh). The SUVmax of the suspected lesions and the SUVmean of the right liver lobe were measured.

Statistical Analysis

For the two patient cohorts the median values of age, PSA value at time of PET–CT the SUVmean of the right liver lobe and the SUVmax of the lesion with the highest uptake as well as the total number of lesions are presented in Table 1.

Table 1. Patient characteristic of the two groups. Ranges are given in parenthesis.

	Median Age in y	Median PSA in ng/dL	Median SUVmean of the Liver	Total Number of Lesions	Median SUVmax of the Hottest Lesions
[^{64}Cu]-DOTAGA-PSMA	74 (51–90)	5.59 (0.01–969)	8.9 (5.5–14.9)	209 (0–15)	10.5 (1.8–65.0)
[^{18}F]-PSMA	73 (57–92)	4.5 (0.01–220)	11.8 (1.8–21.2)	191 (0–15)	9.2 (3.3–109)

Additionally, we performed a Student's *t*-test to identify significant differences between the two patient cohorts.

3. Results

Patient baseline characteristics are listed in Table 1. The two patient cohorts were comparable, as we found no significant differences with regard to age range, PSA values at the time of examination and the SUVmax of the hottest lesion (Table 2). In Figures 1 and 2 we show one representable patient case for each cohort.

Table 2. Results of a Student's *t*-test for outlining potential significant differences between the two patient cohorts that were either examined with [^{64}Cu]-DOTAGA-PSMA PET–CT or [^{18}F]-PSMA PET–CT.

	Age in y	Total Number of Lesions	PSA Value in ng/dL	SUVmax Hottest Lesion	SUVmean Liver
p-value	0.3	0.8	0.1	0.7	0.000002 *

Statistically significant *p*-values < 0.05 are marked with (*).

In total, 209 lesions were detected with [^{64}Cu]-DOTAGA-PSMA, whereas 191 lesions were with [^{18}F]-PSMA. All but 9/50 (18%) of the patients (PSA range 0.01–0.7) studied with [^{64}Cu]-DOTAGA PSMA and 6/50 (12%) of the ones (PSA range 0.01–4.2) studied with [^{18}F]-PSMA had no lesions shown by PET–CT. We did not find significant differences in median PSA values between the two groups ($p = 0.1$) or any association between prostate uptake and the number of positive lesions in PSMA PET.

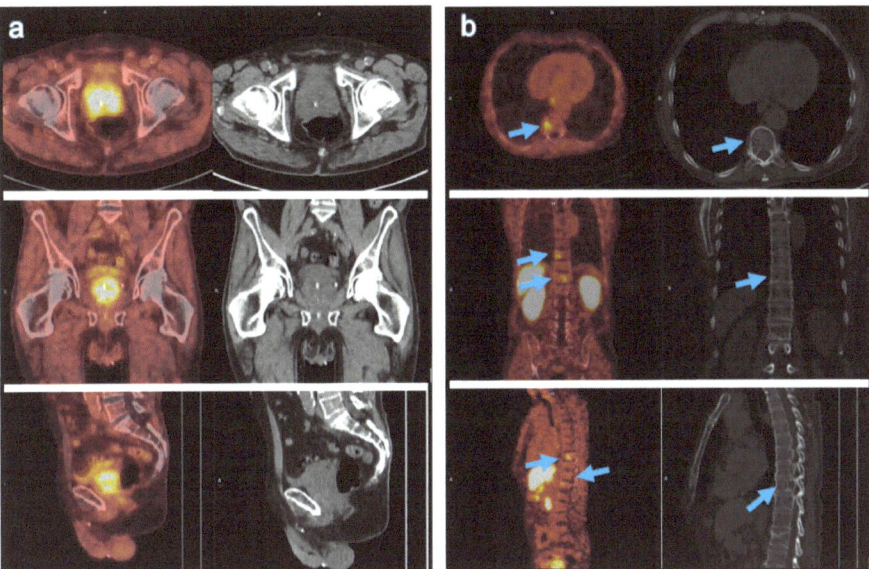

Figure 1. Primary staging of a treatment-naïve, 75-year-old patient with PCa which has metastasized to the bone, using [^{64}Cu]-DOTAGA-PSMA PET–CT. The PSA value at the time of PET–CT was 47 µg/L. (**a**) The PSMA-positive primary tumor (SUVmax apical: 9.5; left base: 8.0). (**b**) The PSMA-positive bone metastases in T10 and T12 (respective SUVmax: 5.3 and 4.6); the arrow in the correlating low-dose CT images point to the metastasis in T10.

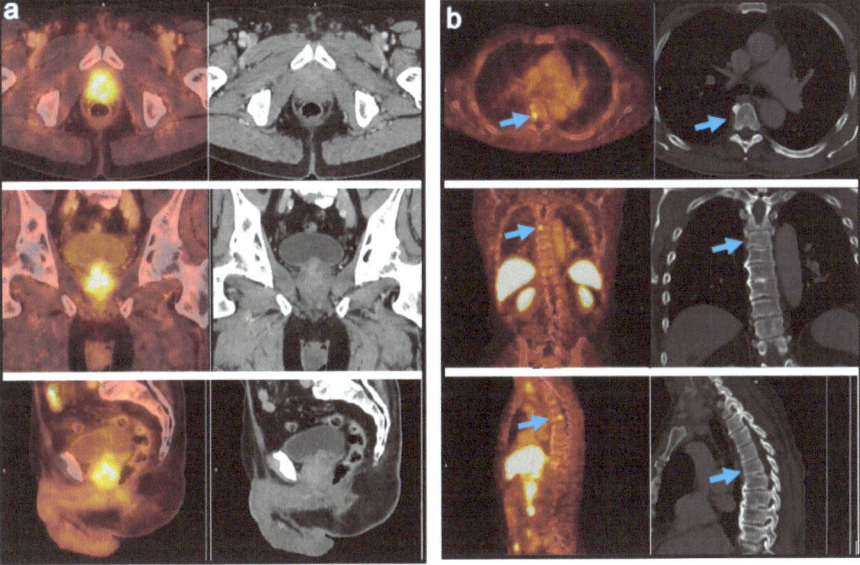

Figure 2. Primary staging of a treatment-naïve, 70-year-old patient with PCa metastasizing to the 5th and 9th thoracic vertebrae, using [^{18}F]-PSMA PET–CT. The PSA value at the time of examination was 7.8 µg/L. (**a**) The PSMA-positive primary tumor (SUVmax 6.4). (**b**) The PSMA-positive bone metastasis in T5 (SUVmax 3.7).

4. Discussion

The results in this study in regard to negative findings are superior to our previous study with [^{64}Cu]-NODAG-PSMA, where 20.8% of the patients did not show any lesions in PET scans [11]. However, the previous study was performed on a stand-alone PET scan (without CT), and therefore this comparison is of limited significance.

The total number of lesions was higher with [^{64}Cu]-DOTAGA-PSMA (209 vs. 191); however, the median value of lesions was one for [^{64}Cu]-DOTAGA-PSMA and two for [^{18}F]-PSMA, and thus failed to be statistically significant ($p = 0.07$). Interestingly, the median value of SUVmean of the right liver lobe was significantly higher with [^{18}F]-PSMA ($p < 0.05$). We measure and mention this parameter in our PET reports in order to compare different studies at different time points, or if they are performed with different radiopharmaceuticals.

In our study, we found comparable results between [^{64}Cu]-DOTAGA-PSMA and [^{18}F]-PSMA in our patients. The performance of both radiopharmaceuticals were comparable and better than our previously published results with [^{64}Cu]-NODAG-PSMA PET, with the limitation that the latter was performed on a stand-alone PET scanner [11]. This suggests in vivo stability of [^{64}Cu]-DOTAGA-PSMA as it could be shown for [^{64}Cu]-NODAGA-PSMA in our previous study [11]. Additionally, as mentioned elsewhere, [^{64}Cu] as a radionuclide for PSMA shows more favorable physical characteristics, such as a longer half-life of 12.7 h and a small positron range with increased spatial resolution [16]. Interestingly, in a study, ^{64}Cu-PSMA-617-PET was demonstrated to be feasible for imaging prostate cancer for both the primary tumor site and metastases, whereas later imaging 2–22 h post-injection showed no additional, clinically relevant benefit compared to the early scans [17].

It was not the aim of this study to look for any impact of Gleason score (GS) on PET results; however, in a previous publication we could not find any correlation between GS and PSMA-PET [11]. Furthermore, downregulation of PSMA expression due to androgen deprivation therapy (ADT) might have an influence on size reduction in tumors [18], and some of our patients were under ADT treatment. Additionally, there are published limitations of [^{68}Ga]-PSMA with a very low expression of PSMA in dedifferentiated tumors, the absence of a relationship between [^{68}Ga]-PSMA uptake and Gleason score in addition to the downregulation of PSMA expression by ADT [18]. The introduction of copper as a ligand in primary staging and in recurrent disease demonstrates an excellent resolution of the detected lesions with a very high lesion-to-background contrast. Grubmüller et al investigated the diagnostic potential of [^{64}Cu]-PSMA-617 PET/CT in primary staging or as PSMA radioligand therapy in 29 PCa patients [19]. The preliminary results of this study highlighted the high potential of [^{64}Cu]-PSMA ligands in patients with recurrent disease and in the primary staging of selected patients with progressive local disease. Our results with [^{64}Cu]-DOTAGA-PSMA compared to [^{18}F]-PSMA PET–CT demonstrate a similar high detection rate of recurrent disease and a high stability in vivo for [^{64}Cu]-DOTAGA-PSMA.

The limitations of this study are the retrospective nature, lack of intra-individual comparison, that the histopathology of all lesions was not obtainable in our patients and that only the number of lesions were analyzed. However, PCa was proven by biopsy or histopathology.

5. Conclusions

[^{64}Cu]-DOTAGA-PSMA and [^{18}F]-PSMA have comparable detection rates for the assessment of residual disease in patients with recurrent or primary progressive PCa. The uptake in the liver is moderately different, and therefore the SUV of the lesions in both studies would not be comparable.

Author Contributions: Conceptualization, S.M.; methodology, S.M.; validation, S.M.; formal analysis S.M., A.L., R.L. and S.Z.; investigation, S.M. and A.L.; resources, S.M. and A.L.; data curation, S.M. and A.L.; writing—original draft, S.M. and A.L.; writing—review and editing, A.L. and R.L.; supervision,

S.M.; project administration, S.M.; funding acquisition, A.L. All authors have read and agreed to the published version of the manuscript.

Funding: This research received no external funding.

Institutional Review Board Statement: All patients were examined with a dedicated PET-CT scanner (Biograph, Siemens, Healthineers) in compliance with the 1964 Declaration of Helsinki and the responsible regulatory bodies in Austria.

Informed Consent Statement: Formal consent was obtained from all patients prior to examination.

Data Availability Statement: The above-mentioned data were acquired from our in-house PET–CT center. No other publicly archived dataset was analyzed.

Conflicts of Interest: The authors declare no conflict of interest.

References

1. Sung, H.; Ferlay, J.; Siegel, R.L.; Laversanne, M.; Soerjomataram, I.; Jemal, A.; Bray, F. Global cancer statistics 2020: GLOBOCAN estimates of incidence and mortality worldwide for 36 cancers in 185 countries. *CA Cancer J. Clin.* **2021**, *71*, 209–249. [CrossRef] [PubMed]
2. Heidenreich, A.; Bastian, P.J.; Bellmunt, J.; Bolla, M.; Joniau, S.; van der Kwast, T.; Mason, M.; Matveev, V.; Wiegel, T.; Zattoni, F.; et al. EAU guidelines on prostate cancer. part 1: Screening, diagnosis, and local treatment with curative intent-update 2013. *Eur. Urol.* **2014**, *65*, 124–137. [CrossRef] [PubMed]
3. Swami, U.; McFarland, T.R.; Nussenzveig, R.; Agarwal, N. Advanced Prostate Cancer: Treatment Advances and Future Directions. *Trends Cancer* **2020**, *6*, 702–715. [CrossRef] [PubMed]
4. von Eyben, F.E.; Picchio, M.; von Eyben, R.; Rhee, H.; Bauman, G. 68Ga-Labeled Prostate-specific Membrane Antigen Ligand Positron Emission Tomography/Computed Tomography for Prostate Cancer: A Systematic Review and Meta-analysis. *Eur. Urol. Focus* **2018**, *4*, 686–693. [CrossRef] [PubMed]
5. Chang, S.S. Overview of prostate-specific membrane antigen. *Rev. Urol.* **2004**, *6*, S13–S18. [PubMed]
6. Pastorino, S.; Riondato, M.; Uccelli, L.; Giovacchini, G.; Giovannini, E.; Duce, V.; Ciarmiello, A. Toward the Discovery and Development of PSMA Targeted Inhibitors for Nuclear Medicine Applications. *Curr. Radiopharm.* **2020**, *13*, 63–79. [CrossRef] [PubMed]
7. Lütje, S.; Heskamp, S.; Cornelissen, A.S.; Poeppel, T.D.; van den Broek, S.A.; Rosenbaum-Krumme, S.; Bockisch, A.; Gotthardt, M.; Rijpkema, M.; Boerman, O.C. PSMA Ligands for Radionuclide Imaging and Therapy of Prostate Cancer: Clinical Status. *Theranostics* **2015**, *5*, 1388–1401. [CrossRef] [PubMed]
8. Rauscher, I.; Maurer, T.; Beer, A.J.; Graner, F.P.; Haller, B.; Weirich, G.; Doherty, A.; Gschwend, J.E.; Schwaiger, M.; Eiber, M. Value of 68Ga-PSMA HBED-CC PET for the Assessment of Lymph Node Metastases in Prostate Cancer Patients with Biochemical Recurrence: Comparison with Histopathology After Salvage Lymphadenectomy. *J. Nucl. Med.* **2016**, *57*, 1713–1719. [CrossRef] [PubMed]
9. Morigi, J.J.; Stricker, P.D.; van Leeuwen, P.J.; Tang, R.; Ho, B.; Nguyen, Q.; Hruby, G.; Fogarty, G.; Jagavkar, R.; Kneebone, A.; et al. Prospective Comparison of 18F-Fluoromethylcholine Versus 68Ga-PSMA PET/CT in Prostate Cancer Patients Who Have Rising PSA After Curative Treatment and Are Being Considered for Targeted Therapy. *J. Nucl. Med.* **2015**, *56*, 1185–1190. [CrossRef] [PubMed]
10. Williams, H.A.; Robinson, S.; Julyan, P.; Zweit, J.; Hastings, D. A comparison of PET imaging characteristics of various copper radioisotopes. *Eur. J. Nucl. Med. Mol. Imaging* **2005**, *32*, 1473–1480. [CrossRef] [PubMed]
11. Sevcenco, S.; Klingler, H.C.; Eredics, K.; Friedl, A.; Schneeweiss, J.; Knoll, P.; Kunit, T.; Lusuardi, L.; Mirzaei, S. Application of Cu-64 NODAGA-PSMA PET in Prostate Cancer. *Adv. Ther.* **2018**, *35*, 779–784. [CrossRef]
12. Liu, T.; Liu, C.; Zhang, Z.; Zhang, N.; Guo, X.; Xia, L.; Jiang, J.; Xie, Q.; Yan, K.; Rowe, S.P.; et al. 64Cu-PSMA-BCH: A new radiotracer for delayed PET imaging of prostate cancer. *Eur. J. Nucl. Med. Mol. Imaging* **2021**. [CrossRef] [PubMed]
13. Lee, C.H.; Lim, I.; Woo, S.K.; Kim, K.I.; Lee, K.C.; Song, K.; Choi, C.W.; Lim, S.M. The Feasibility of 64CU-PSMA I&T PET for Prostate Cancer. *Cancer Biother. Radiopharm.* **2021**. [CrossRef]
14. Cantiello, F.; Crocerossa, F.; Russo, G.I.; Gangemi, V.; Ferro, M.; Vartolomei, M.D.; Lucarelli, G.; Mirabelli, M.; Scafuro, C.; Ucciero, G.; et al. Comparison Between 64Cu-PSMA-617 PET/CT and 18F-Choline PET/CT Imaging in Early Diagnosis of Prostate Cancer Biochemical Recurrence. *Clin. Genitourin. Cancer* **2018**, *16*, 385–391. [CrossRef] [PubMed]
15. Jacobson, O.; Kiesewetter, D.O.; Chen, X. Fluorine-18 radiochemistry, labeling strategies and synthetic routes. *Bioconjug. Chem.* **2015**, *26*, 1–18. [CrossRef] [PubMed]
16. Evangelista, L.; Luigi, M.; Cascini, G.L. New issues for copper-64: From precursor to innovative PET tracers in clinical oncology. *Curr. Radiopharm.* **2013**, *6*, 117–123. [CrossRef] [PubMed]
17. Hoberück, S.; Wunderlich, G.; Michler, E.; Hölscher, T.; Walther, M.; Seppelt, D.; Platzek, I.; Zöphel, K.; Kotzerke, J. Dual-time-point 64 Cu-PSMA-617-PET/CT in patients suffering from prostate cancer. *J. Labelled Comp. Radiopharm.* **2019**, *62*, 523–532. [CrossRef] [PubMed]

18. Afshar-Oromieh, A.; Avtzi, E.; Giesel, F.L.; Holland-Letz, T.; Linhart, H.G.; Eder, M.; Eisenhut, M.; Boxler, S.; Hadaschik, B.A.; Kratochwil, C.; et al. The diagnostic value of PET/CT imaging with the (68)Ga-labelled PSMA ligand HBED-CC in the diagnosis of recurrent prostate cancer. *Eur. J. Nucl. Med. Mol. Imaging* **2015**, *42*, 197–209. [CrossRef] [PubMed]
19. Grubmüller, B.; Baum, R.P.; Capasso, E.; Singh, A.; Ahmadi, Y.; Knoll, P.; Floth, A.; Righi, S.; Zandieh, S.; Meleddu, C.; et al 64Cu-PSMA-617 PET/CT imaging of prostate adenocarcinoma: First in-human. *Cancer Biother. Radiopharm.* **2016**, *31*, 277–286. [CrossRef] [PubMed]

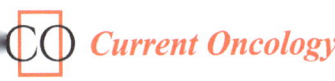

Communication

Nondetectable Prostate Carcinoma (pT0) after Radical Prostatectomy: A Narrative Review

Nikolaos Kalampokis [1], Nikolaos Grivas [2,3,*], Markos Karavitakis [3,4], Ioannis Leotsakos [3,5], Ioannis Katafigiotis [3,5], Marcio Covas Moschovas [6], Henk van der Poel [2] and European Association of Urology (EAU) Young Academic Urologists (YAU) Robotic Urology Working Group [†]

[1] Department of Urology, G. Hatzikosta General Hospital, 45001 Ioannina, Greece; kalampokas88@gmail.com
[2] Department of Urology, The Netherlands Cancer Institute-Antoni van Leeuwenhoek Hospital, 1066 CX Amsterdam, The Netherlands; h.vd.poel@nki.nl
[3] Department of Urology, Lefkos Stavros Hospital, 11528 Athens, Greece; markoskaravitakis@yahoo.gr (M.K.); ioannisdleotsakos@gmail.com (I.L.); katafigiotis.giannis@gmail.com (I.K.)
[4] Department of Urology, University General Hospital of Heraklion, University of Crete, Medical School, 14122 Heraklion, Greece
[5] Department of Urology, Medical School, National & Kapodistrian University of Athens, 14122 Athens, Greece
[6] Department of Urology, Advent Health Global Robotics Institute, Celebration, FL 34747, USA; marcio.moschovas.md@adventhealth.com
* Correspondence: nikolaosgrivas@hotmail.com; Tel.: +31-205121543; Fax: +31-205122459
† The European Association of Urology (EAU) Young Academic Urologists (YAU) Robotic Urology Working Group are listed in the author contributions.

Abstract: (1) Background: Following radical prostatectomy (RP), the absence of a demonstrable tumor on the specimen of a previously histologically proven malignancy is known as the pT0 stage. The aim of our present study is to perform a narrative review of current literature in order to determine the frequency and oncological outcomes in patients with pT0 disease. (2) Methods: A narrative review of all available literature was performed. (3) Results: The incidence of pT0 ranges between 0.07% and 1.3%. Predictors of the pT0 stage are only a single biopsy core with low-grade cancer, a cancer length not exceeding 2 mm and a high prostate volume. Biochemical recurrence ranges between 0 and 11%. (4) Conclusions: The absence of malignancy in the RP specimen despite a previous positive biopsy is a rare and unpredictable finding. Although the prognosis is considered to be excellent in most of the cases, a continued close follow-up is warranted.

Keywords: prostate cancer; prostatectomy; vanishing cancer

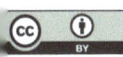

1. Introduction

Over the past decades, the implementation of a widely accepted screening program for the early detection of prostate cancer has resulted in even more patients being diagnosed with low-grade, small in size malignancies. Following radical prostatectomy (RP), the absence of a demonstrable tumor on the specimen of a previously histologically proven malignancy is known as the pT0 stage. Although this is a well-known phenomenon for individuals receiving neoadjuvant hormonal therapy (NHT), the incidence of pT0 among patients who are directly treated with RP without prior androgen deprivation therapy (ADT) is <2% [1–4].

The aim of our present study is to perform a review of current literature in order to determine the frequency and oncological outcomes in patients with pT0 disease, as well as possible factors serving as predictors of the pT0 stage in candidates for RP.

2. Materials and Methods

Medline Epub Ahead of Print, In-Process and Other Non-Indexed Citations, Ovid MEDLINE(R) Daily and Ovid MEDLINE(R) 1946 to 30 November 2021 were systematically searched to detect all relevant studies based on the following literature search strategy (undetectable OR pT0 OR vanishing) AND (prostatectomy). After excluding citations in abstract form, and non-English citations, titles/abstracts of full papers were screened Review articles, editorial letters and comments were excluded. Two review authors (NK and NG) independently scanned the titles, abstracts or both of every record retrieved, to determine which studies should be further assessed and extracted all data. Disagreements were resolved through consensus or after consultation with a third review author (MK). A total of 679 unique abstracts were identified by the search and 215 were selected for full-text screening. After full-text screening, 23 studies met the inclusion criteria (Figure 1).

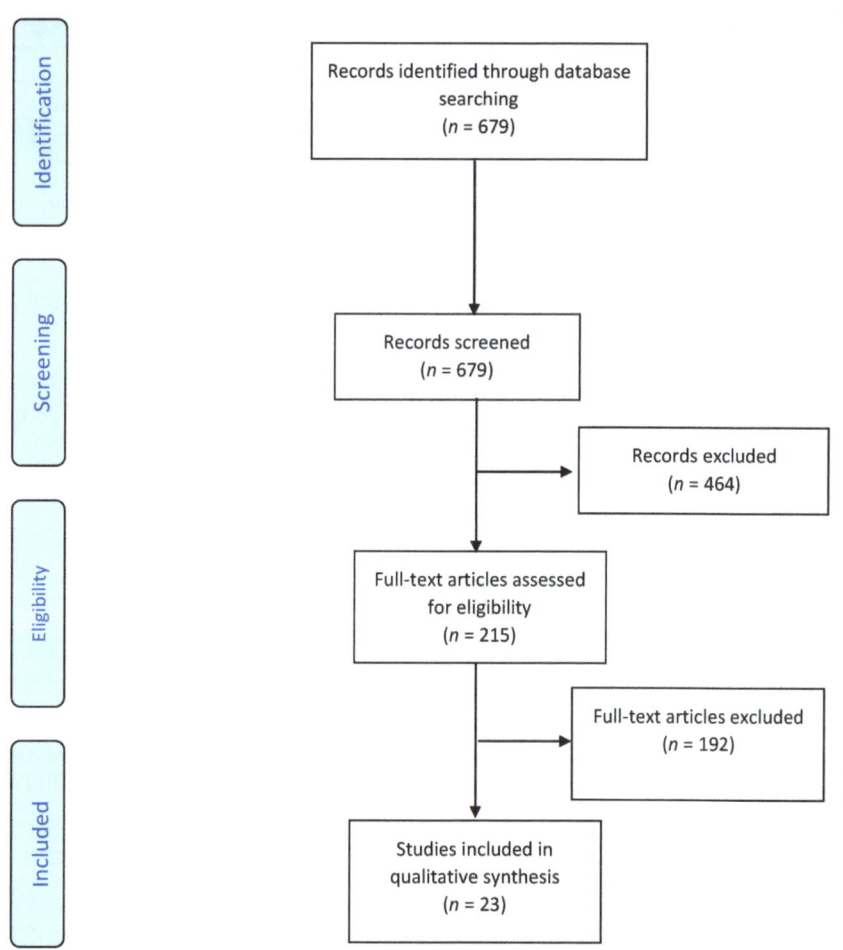

Figure 1. Preferred Reporting Items for Systematic Reviews and Meta-analysis.

3. Results

3.1. Frequency and Possible Causes of Cancer Absence in Prostatectomy Specimen

The first cases of pT0 disease were reported by Goldstein et al. back in 1995 and they were described as the vanishing cancer phenomenon [2]. The authors re-evaluated the data of 13 patients (11 with minimal and two with no cancer in the prostatectomy specimen, and they concluded that even after meticulous histopathologic examination, cancer may be impossible to be found in every RP specimen.

In three consecutive studies, a group of pathologists reported their experience with patients diagnosed and treated for prostate cancer in the Johns Hopkins Hospital over a period of 9 years (1997–2005) [4–6]. According to them, there was an increase in the number of patients diagnosed with pT0 by almost five times (from 0.07% in 1997 to 0.34% in 2005).

In 2004, Bostwick et al. found that 38 out of 6843 patients, who were treated with RP at their institution during a 30-year period, had no sign of malignancy in the surgical specimen [3]. Interestingly, they reported a decrease of the vanishing cancer incidence by more than 10 times, while at the time of publication, the current incidence was estimated at approximately 0.2%.

More recently, a pooled analysis by Gross et al. included more than 18,000 patients and reported a pT0 rate equal to 0.4% (CI: 0.3–0.5%) [7]. Similarly, in 2019, Knipper et al. performed a large population-based analysis using the SEER database and reported a pT0 rate of 0.2% [8].

As regards the association of the pT0 stage with specific racial characteristics, three large studies conducted in French and German institutions reported an incidence ranging from 0.4% to 0.8% [9–11], while a study of 702 Asian patients showed a rate of pT0 staging equal to 1.3% [12].

So far, several mechanisms have been proposed in an effort to explain the absence of detectable malignancy in the RP specimen. According to Descazeaud et al. the most plausible explanation would be that of a high-volume prostate, which would make it difficult for a pathologist to detect small in size tumors [9]. Another possible explanation would be that specimen mix-up and several techniques have been established so far with an aim to avoid such a case of malpractice [4]. Other explanations would be (1) the initial core biopsy was positive for an entity mimicking prostate cancer (e.g., high-grade prostate intraepithelial neoplasia); (2) the tumor was entirely removed during a transurethral resection (TURP); or (3) pre-operative ADT resulted in downstaging of the disease [13].

3.2. Possible Pre-Operative Predictors of pT0 Stage

So far, there have been several studies trying to confirm the existence of pre-operative factors that could help us predict which of the patients would be more likely to receive the diagnosis of pT0 disease following RP.

A large single-institution study by Descazeaud et al. was probably the first one trying to create a predictive model for the pT0 stage [9]. According to the authors, the simultaneous existence of only one biopsy core with low-grade cancer, a cancer length on biopsy not exceeding 2 mm and a prostate larger than 60 g in weight was found to have a specificity of 99% and a sensitivity of 82% in predicting pT0 on radical prostatectomy. Interestingly, the negative predictive value of their model was found to be equal to 99%, which means that it would be almost impossible for a patient not sharing all the aforementioned characteristics to be diagnosed with pT0.

Working towards the same goal, Bream at al. examined a North American population and concluded that patients with co-existence of a PSA level below 7.5 ng/mL, a Gleason score of 6, a clinical T1c stage and a single biopsy core with cancer occupying less than 1% of tissue could be probably better served with active surveillance instead of RP, unless a repeat biopsy yields more concerning findings [14].

In 2011, Capitanio et al. conducted a study, which included patients diagnosed with T1a and T1b disease after being operated on for benign prostatic hyperplasia, and according to them pT0 cancer was, as expected, associated with lower prostate specific antigen (PSA) levels [15]. Similarly, Moreira et al. after examining patients regardless of pre-operative treatment, showed that a lower Gleason score and PSA levels as well as any pre-operative treatment in the form of ADT or radiotherapy, were found to be independent predictors of the pT0 stage with an accuracy equal to 75% [16].

In 2018, Chung et al. conducted a study, which included patients undergoing RP after being diagnosed with incidental prostate cancer (T1a–1b) [17]. Among the 95 patients of the study, there were 28 individuals with absence of malignancy in the prostatectomy specimen (pT0). It is worth mentioning that according to their findings, patients with incidental cancer who have both an invisible lesion on multiparametric magnetic resonance imaging (MRI) and PSA density lower than 0.08 following TURP could be safely considered for active surveillance instead of radical prostatectomy.

Finally, a SEER-based analysis by Knipper et al. produced a model with only three variables reaching independent predictor status, namely the number of positive biopsy cores, the number of biopsies taken and the Gleason score [8]. Nevertheless, according to them, the extremely low prevalence of the under examination clinical entity (0.2% according to the authors) could not guarantee that a model with accuracy equal to 79% would be of any usefulness in everyday clinical practice.

Data from these older studies show that the vast majority of men with pT0 had low-risk PCa which, today, should be offered active surveillance. Risk stratification of patients is of the utmost importance in order to avoid over-treatment and its possible side effects.

3.3. pT0 Stage following Hormonal Therapy

Among others, several studies have dealt with the correlation between NHT and pT0 following RP. The main goal of neoadjuvant is to reduce positive surgical margins and rates of disease recurrence. Hormonal pre-treatment is already known to cause a reduction of the tumor size [18] by causing a variety of regressive changes, thus leaving scattered malignant cells behind [19,20] and making the post-treatment detection of the tumor extremely difficult. Nevertheless, it has been shown that even if the initial pathologic evaluation failed to detect the presence of tumors, an extensive re-evaluation would identify malignant cells in more than 60% of those cases.

In 2000, Kollermann et al. compared the effect of PSA-monitored prolonged neoadjuvant endocrine treatment (PPNET) on the number of post-operative pT0 reports, when compared to the standard 3-month treatment schedule [21]. According to their findings, a patient receiving prolonged hormonal treatment (mean duration = 9 months) was three times more likely to receive a diagnosis of the pT0 stage, which indirectly implies that the 3-month schedule does not exploit the full potential of neoadjuvant treatment.

3.4. pT0 Diagnosis: Follow-Up and Oncological Outcomes

A summary of oncological outcomes of patients with the pT0 stage are presented in Table 1. In one of the first studies dealing with the prognosis of the pT0 stage, a research team from Berlin analyzed a group of 174 patients receiving pre-operative ADT and found that 21% of them were staged as pT0 after RP [13]. When the aforementioned patients were matched for a Gleason score with patients diagnosed as pT2–3, there was no difference in PSA free survival rate, which according to the authors means that biochemical progression does occur despite possible downstaging to pT0 after prolonged NHT.

In 2003, Herkommer et al. presented a study on the incidence of pT0 on a nation-wide basis (Germany). Among 3609 patients undergoing RP, there were 28 individuals who were staged as pT0 (0.8%) [10]. All patients, irrespective of stage, had undetectable PSA levels within 4 weeks after operation. Moreover, none of them had biochemical or clinical progression of their disease during follow-up (mean period: 62 months). During the same year, an article published by Kollermann et al. tried to shed some light on the hypothesis that in pT0 cases following prolonged NHT, the biochemical relapse is not only extremely rare but also derives from systemic disease recurrence [22]. Based on their findings, both hypotheses were disproved. In total, 18.4% (7 out of 38) of the pT0 patients had a median time to PSA relapse equal to 14 months, while localization studies showed at least a local source of PSA production for six out of seven patients. More specifically, in half of the cases local recurrence was malignant in nature.

In 2004, in a large single-institution retrospective study collecting data over a period of 30 years, none of the 38 patients with the pT0 stage had either biochemical or clinical recurrence over a mean follow-up period of 9.6 years [3]. Similarly, a smaller study showed no recurrence but the sample size was too small (11 patients with pT0) and the mean follow-up period was only 30 months [9].

In 2009, Bessede et al. released their findings of a multi-center study on 7693 patients who underwent radical prostatectomy without hormonal pretreatment [11]. They found 30 cases of the pT0 stage, which were separated into nonsignificant, intermediate and significant risk subgroups based on pre-operative clinical and histopathological characteristics. According to the authors, none of those patients had a disease recurrence at 82-month follow-up, which according to them is translated into an excellent prognosis for pT0 patients irrespective of pre-treatment criteria (i.e., clinical stage, PSA value, Gleason score on biopsy). On the other hand, Gurski et al. concluded that the recurrence rate of their pT0 patients was clinically significant since 26% (six of 23) of them developed biochemical recurrence during follow-up [23]. A possible explanation for their findings could be a long follow-up period, which was described by them as "adequate" without giving further details of the exact duration.

More than 20,000 patients who underwent RP between 1987 and 2012 at the Mayo Clinic were included in a retrospective study conducted by Moreira and his colleagues [16]. Seven of the 62 patients (11%) who were diagnosed as pT0 developed recurrence after a median follow-up of 10.9 years. Moreover, when patients of the pT0 group were matched with patients of the non-pT0 group, they were reported to have a statistically significant better recurrence-free survival rate ($p = 0.008$). Interestingly, all of the patients experiencing recurrence had received pre-operative treatment and potential explanations for that finding include the fact that more aggressive tumors are traditionally selected to receive neoadjuvant treatment and the masking effects of previous treatments on cancer cells.

Finally, a large population-based study [8] showed that at a 9-year follow-up the cancer specific survival rate for pT0 patients was equal to 99.5% and almost identical to that of the non-pT0 group (98.8%). However, according to the authors the very low prevalence of the pT0 disease could not guarantee any meaningful statistical comparison.

Table 1. Oncological outcomes of patients with pT0 stage.

Study	pT0 Cases (*n*)	Follow-Up Duration	Outcome
Gurski et al. [23]	23	Reported as adequate	26% developed biochemical recurrence
Knipper et al. [8]	358	9 years	3 cancer specific deaths (99.5% cancer-specific survival)
Chung et al. [17]	28	68.37 months (median)	No clinical or biochemical recurrence
Moreira et al. [16]	62	10.9 years (median)	11% with disease recurrence 1.6% with systemic progression
Bream et al. [14]	4	3 months–10 years	No clinical or biochemical recurrence
Bessède et al. [11]	30	82 months (median)	No biochemical recurrence
Trpkov et al. [1]	9	23.8 months (mean)	No clinical or biochemical recurrence
Descazeaud et al. [9]	9	30 months (mean)	No clinical or biochemical recurrence
Köllermann et al. [13]	36	47 months for the pT0 group (median)	19.4% with biochemical recurrence
Bostwick et al. [3]	38	9.6 years (mean)	No clinical recurrence No biochemical recurrence (PSA available only for 32 of 38 patients)
Herkommer et al. [10]	13	62 months (median)	No clinical or biochemical recurrence
Köllermann et al. [22]	38	47 months (median)	18.4% with biochemical recurrence 7.9% with clinical recurrence

4. Conclusions

In summary, the absence of malignancy in the RP specimen despite previous positive biopsy is a rare and unpredictable finding, which needs special management because of possible medicolegal repercussions. It is generally associated with features of low-risk cancer and pre-operative hormonal treatment. The findings of our review strengthen the active surveillance strategy in low-risk cases instead of RP. So far, several models serving as pre-operative predictors of the pT0 stage have been proposed, but none of them have gained wide acceptance in everyday clinical practice. Although the prognosis is considered to be excellent in most of the cases, a continued close follow-up is warranted.

Author Contributions: Conceptualization, N.G., N.K., H.v.d.P.; methodology, N.K., M.K., I.L., I.K. M.C.M.; formal analysis, N.K.; writing—original draft preparation, N.K., N.G.; writing—review and editing, N.K., I.L., M.K., I.K., M.C.M., H.v.d.P., European Association of Urology (EAU) Young Academic Urologists (YAU) Robotic Urology Working Group (A. Larcher, P. Dell'Oglio, S. Goonewardene, N. Grivas, F.M. Turri, M. Covas Moschovas, R. De Groote, F. Di Maida, S. Knipper, E. Koseoglu, N Liakos, A. Martini); supervision, H.v.d.P. All authors have read and agreed to the published version of the manuscript.

Funding: This research received no external funding.

Conflicts of Interest: The authors declare no conflict of interest.

References

1. Trpkov, K.; Gao, Y.; Hay, R.; Yimaz, A. No residual cancer on radical prostatectomy after positive 10-core biopsy: Incidence biopsy findings, and DNA specimen identity analysis. *Arch. Pathol. Lab. Med.* **2006**, *130*, 811–816. [CrossRef]
2. Goldstein, N.S.; Bégin, L.R.; Grody, W.W.; Novak, J.M.; Qian, J.; Bostwick, D.G. Minimal or No Cancer in Radical Prostatectomy Specimens. *Am. J. Surg. Pathol.* **1995**, *19*, 1002–1009. [CrossRef]
3. Bostwick, D.G.; Bostwick, K.C. 'Vanishing' prostate cancer in radical prostatectomy specimens: Incidence and long-term follow-up in 38 cases. *Br. J. Urol.* **2004**, *94*, 57–58. [CrossRef] [PubMed]
4. Cao, D.; Hafez, M.; Berg, K.; Murphy, K.; Epstein, J.I. Little or no residual prostate cancer at radical prostatectomy: Vanishing cancer or switched specimen? A microsatellite analysis of specimen identity. *Am. J. Surg. Pathol.* **2005**, *29*, 467–473. [CrossRef]
5. DiGiuseppe, J.A.; Sauvageot, J.; Epstein, J.I. Increasing Incidence of Minimal Residual Cancer In Radical Prostatectomy Specimens. *Am. J. Surg. Pathol.* **1997**, *21*, 174–178. [CrossRef]
6. Truskinovsky, A.M.; Sanderson, H.; Epstein, J.I. Characterization of minute adenocarcinomas of prostate at radical prostatectomy. *Urol.* **2004**, *64*, 733–737. [CrossRef] [PubMed]
7. Bs, J.L.G.; Masterson, T.A.; Cheng, L.; Johnstone, P.A. pT0 prostate cancer after radical prostatectomy. *J. Surg. Oncol.* **2010**, *102* 331–333. [CrossRef]
8. Knipper, S.; Tilki, D.; Mazzone, E.; Mistretta, F.A.; Palumbo, C.; Pecoraro, A.; Tian, Z.; Briganti, A.; Saad, F.; Graefen, M.; et al Contemporary clinicopathological characteristics of pT0 prostate cancer at radical prostatectomy: A population-based study *Urol. Oncol. Semin. Orig. Investig.* **2019**, *37*, 696–701. [CrossRef]
9. Descazeaud, A.; Zerbib, M.; Flam, T.; Vieillefond, A.; Debré, B.; Peyromaure, M. Can pT0 Stage of Prostate Cancer be Predicted before Radical Prostatectomy? *Eur. Urol.* **2006**, *50*, 1248–1253. [CrossRef]
10. Herkommer, K.; Kuefer, R.; E Gschwend, J.; E Hautmann, R.; Volkmer, B.G. Pathological T0 prostate cancer without neoadjuvant therapy: Clinical presentation and follow-up. *Eur. Urol.* **2004**, *45*, 36–41. [CrossRef] [PubMed]
11. Bessède, T.; Soulié, M.; Mottet, N.; Rebillard, X.; Peyromaure, M.; Ravery, V.; Salomon, L. Cancerology Committee of the French Urological Association Stage pT0 After Radical Prostatectomy With Previous Positive Biopsy Sets: A Multicenter Study. *J. Urol* **2010**, *183*, 958–962. [CrossRef] [PubMed]
12. Park, J.; Jeong, I.G.; Bang, J.K.; Cho, Y.M.; Ro, J.Y.; Hong, J.H.; Ahn, H.; Kim, C.-S. Preoperative Clinical and Pathological Characteristics of pT0 Prostate Cancer in Radical Prostatectomy. *Korean J. Urol.* **2010**, *51*, 386–390. [CrossRef] [PubMed]
13. Köllermann, J.; Hopfenmüller, W.; Caprano, J.; Budde, A.; Weidenfeld, H.; Weidenfeld, M.; Helpap, B. Prognosis of stage pT0 after prolonged neoadjuvant endocrine therapy of prostate cancer: A matched-pair analysis. *Eur. Urol.* **2004**, *45*, 42–45. [CrossRef] [PubMed]
14. Bream, M.J.; Dahmoush, L.; Brown, J.A. pT0 Prostate Cancer: Predictive Clinicopathologic Features in an American Population *Curr. Urol.* **2013**, *7*, 14. [CrossRef]
15. Capitanio, U.; Briganti, A.; Suardi, N.; Gallina, A.; Salonia, A.; Freschi, M.; Rigatti, P.; Montorsi, F. When should we expect no residual tumor (pT0) once we submit incidental T1a-b prostate cancers to radical prostatectomy? *Int. J. Urol.* **2010**, *18*, 148–153 [CrossRef]
16. Moreira, D.; Gershman, B.; Rangel, L.J.; Boorjian, S.A.; Thompson, R.H.; Frank, I.; Tollefson, M.K.; Gettman, M.T.; Karnes, R.J Evaluation of pT0 prostate cancer in patients undergoing radical prostatectomy. *Br. J. Urol.* **2016**, *118*, 379–383. [CrossRef]

17. Chung, D.Y.; Goh, H.J.; Koh, D.H.; Kim, M.S.; Lee, J.S.; Jang, W.S.; Choi, Y.D. Clinical significance of multiparametric MRI and PSA density as predictors of residual tumor (pT0) following radical prostatectomy for T1a-T1b (incidental) prostate cancer. *PLoS ONE* **2018**, *13*, e0210037. [CrossRef]
18. Van der Kwast, T.H.; Têtu, B.; Candas, B.; Gomez, J.L.; Cusan, L.; Labrie, F. Prolonged neoadjuvant combined androgen blockade leads to a further reduction of prostatic tumor volume: Three versus six months of endocrine therapy. *Urology* **1999**, *53*, 523–529. [CrossRef]
19. Hellström, M.; Häggman, M.; Brändstedt, S.; De La Torre, M.; Pedersen, K.; Jarlsfeldt, I.; Wijkström, H.; Busch, C. Histopathological changes in androgen-deprived localized prostatic cancer. A study in total prostatectomy specimens. *Eur. Urol.* **1993**, *24*, 461–465. [CrossRef]
20. Smith, D.M.; Murphy, W.M. Histologic changes in prostate carcinomas treated with leuprolide (luteinizing hormone-releasing hormone effect). Distinction from poor tumor differentiation. *Cancer* **1994**, *73*, 1472–1477. [CrossRef]
21. Köllermann, J.; Feek, U.; Müller, H.; Kaulfuss, U.; Oehler, U.; Helpap, B.; Köllermann, M. Nondetected tumor (pT0) after prolonged, neoadjuvant treatment of localized prostatic carcinoma. *Eur. Urol.* **2000**, *38*, 714–720. [CrossRef] [PubMed]
22. Köllermann, J.; Caprano, J.; Budde, A.; Weidenfeld, H.; Weidenfeld, M.; Hopfenmüller, W.; Helpap, B. Follow-up of nondetectable prostate carcinoma (pT0) after prolonged PSA-monitored neoadjuvant hormonal therapy followed by radical prostatectomy. *Urology* **2003**, *62*, 476–480. [CrossRef]
23. Gurski, J.L.; Chen, Y.; Zhao, J.; Peterson, A.C.; Brand, T.C. pT0 is not benign disease: There is risk of progression in patients with no cancer in radical prostatectomy specimens. *J. Urol.* **2009**, *181*, 208. [CrossRef]

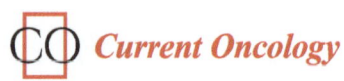

Article

Correlation of Urine Loss after Catheter Removal and Early Continence in Men Undergoing Radical Prostatectomy

Benedikt Hoeh [1,2], Felix Preisser [1,*], Mike Wenzel [1], Clara Humke [1], Clarissa Wittler [1], Jan L. Hohenhorst [2,3], Maja Volckmann-Wilde [1], Jens Köllermann [4], Thomas Steuber [3], Markus Graefen [3], Derya Tilki [3,5], Pierre I. Karakiewicz [2], Andreas Becker [1], Luis A. Kluth [1], Felix K. H. Chun [1] and Philipp Mandel [1]

1 Department of Urology, University Hospital Frankfurt, Goethe University Frankfurt am Main, 60323 Frankfurt am Main, Germany; benedikt.hoeh@gmx.de (B.H.); mike.wenzel@kgu.de (M.W.); Clara.Humke@kgu.de (C.H.); clarissa.wittler@kgu.de (C.W.); M.Volckmann@gmx.de (M.V.-W.); andreas.becker@kgu.de (A.B.); luis.kluth@kgu.de (L.A.K.); felix.chun@kgu.de (F.K.H.C.); philipp.mandel@kgu.de (P.M.)
2 Cancer Prognostics and Health Outcomes Unit, Division of Urology, University of Montréal Health Center, Montréal, QC H3T 1C5, Canada; lukas@hohenhorst.com (J.L.H.); pierrekarakiewicz@gmail.com (P.I.K.)
3 Martini-Klinik Prostate Cancer Center, University Hospital Hamburg-Eppendorf, 20246 Hamburg, Germany; steuber@uke.de (T.S.); graefen@uke.de (M.G.); dtilki@me.com (D.T.)
4 Dr. Senckenberg Institute of Pathology, University Hospital Frankfurt, 60590 Frankfurt am Main, Germany; Jens.Koellermann@kgu.de
5 Department of Urology, University Hospital Hamburg-Eppendorf, 20246 Hamburg, Germany
* Correspondence: Felix.Preisser@kgu.de; Tel.: +49-(0)69-6301-83147; Fax: +49-(0)69-6301-83140

Abstract: Background: To determine the correlation between urine loss in PAD-test after catheter removal, and early urinary continence (UC) in RP treated patients. Methods: Urine loss was measured by using a standardized, validated PAD-test within 24 h after removal of the transurethral catheter and was grouped as a loss of <1, 1–10, 11–50, and >50 g of urine, respectively. Early UC (median: 3 months) was defined as the usage of no or one safety-pad. Uni- and multivariable logistic regression models tested the correlation between PAD-test results and early UC. Covariates consisted of age, BMI, nerve-sparing approach, prostate volume, and extraprostatic extension of tumor. Results: From 01/2018 to 03/2021, 100 patients undergoing RP with data available for a PAD-test and early UC were retrospectively identified. Ultimately, 24%, 47%, 15%, and 14% of patients had a loss of urine <1 g, 1–10 g, 11–50 g, and >50 g in PAD-test, respectively. Additionally, 59% of patients reported to be continent. In multivariable logistic regression models, urine loss in PAD-test predicted early UC (OR: 0.21 vs. 0.09 vs. 0.03; for urine loss 1–10 g vs. 11–50 g vs. >50 g, Ref: <1 g; all $p < 0.05$). Conclusions: Urine loss after catheter removal strongly correlated with early continence as well as a severity in urinary incontinence.

Keywords: urinary incontinence; radical prostatectomy; pad-test; incontinence; functional outcome

Citation: Hoeh, B.; Preisser, F.; Wenzel, M.; Humke, C.; Wittler, C.; Hohenhorst, J.L.; Volckmann-Wilde, M.; Köllermann, J.; Steuber, T.; Graefen, M.; et al. Correlation of Urine Loss after Catheter Removal and Early Continence in Men Undergoing Radical Prostatectomy. *Curr. Oncol.* **2021**, *28*, 4738–4747. https://doi.org/10.3390/curroncol28060399

Received: 10 October 2021
Accepted: 13 November 2021
Published: 15 November 2021

Publisher's Note: MDPI stays neutral with regard to jurisdictional claims in published maps and institutional affiliations.

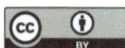

Copyright: © 2021 by the authors. Licensee MDPI, Basel, Switzerland. This article is an open access article distributed under the terms and conditions of the Creative Commons Attribution (CC BY) license (https:// creativecommons.org/licenses/by/ 4.0/).

1. Introduction

With an estimated incidence of 1.3 million cases of newly-diagnosed cases in 2018, Prostate cancer (PCa) ranks as the second most frequent cancer worldwide, accounting for approximately 15% of all cancers worldwide [1,2]. While radical prostatectomy (RP) can provide favorable cancer control in both localized and locally advanced stage disease, ensuring suitable functional outcomes represents a central issue after radical prostatectomy [3–7]. Among those, postoperative urinary incontinence has been reported to have a far-reaching negative impact on patients' quality of life, and represents a potential bothersome side-effect [4,8,9]. Recently, Ilie et al. reported a meaningful association between urinary incontinence and increased mental distress (odds ratio [OR] = 4.79) in a contemporary cohort of PCa patients treated with RP, highlighting the worrisome impact urinary incontinence can have on the quality of life in PCa patients [10]. Substantial research has been conducted to elucidate potential risk factors, such as age, body mass index (BMI), and the experience of surgeons for the postoperative urinary incontinence in patients undergoing RP with primary end-points of interest at 3 and 12 months [3,11–14]. However, current data is scarce about easily operable and reliable tools to predict early continence rates at a very timely point of convalescence.

We addressed this void by relying on a standardized, validated instrument, namely the PAD-test, to measure the urine loss within 24 h after a transurethral catheter removal. We hypothesized that urine loss (defined in the PAD-test) after catheter removal was correlated with early urinary continence rates and thus, could be used to identify patients at the highest-risk of postoperative urinary incontinence at a very early-on timepoint. We tested this hypothesis in a contemporary cohort of 100 PCa patients being treated with RP at a tertiary referral center.

2. Material and Methods

2.1. Study Population

From 01/2018 to 03/2021, 664 patients treated with RP were retrospectively identified from the prospective institutional database of the University Hospital Frankfurt. Of those, 100 patients (15.1%) were subsequently identified with data available for a PAD-test, as well as early continence follow-up assessments. Indication for RP was histologically confirmed prostate cancer. From 01/2020 ongoing, PAD-test measurements were scaled back to ensure a minimum-stay to prevent COVID-19 transmission [15]. The study was approved by the institutional review boards (ethical approval: SUG-1-2018) of the University Cancer Centre Frankfurt and the Ethical Committee at the University Hospital Frankfurt. All patients included in our study signed a written informed consent.

All surgeons, who performed RP in the current cohort, were experienced surgeons trained in high-volume prostate cancer centers. RP was routinely performed with full functional-length urethral sphincter (FFLU) and neurovascular bundle preservation (NVBP) with intraoperative frozen section technique (IFT), as previously described [16–20].

2.2. Outcome Measurements

Data regarding perioperative and early continence was ascertained by PAD-test results and the usage of pads in follow-up assessments after RP. The PAD-test was a comprehensible and validated test that measured the amount of involuntary loss of urine while performing predefined physical activities within 1 h. The PAD-test was performed within 24 h after the removal of the transurethral catheter, as previously described [17,21]. Urine loss of <1 g, 1–10 g, 11–50 g, and >50 g was defined as continent, mild incontinent, moderate incontinent, and severe incontinent, respectively (Figure 1). Early continence was defined as the use of no, or one safety-pad within 24 h, whereas a higher number of pads was considered incontinent. Early continence status was based on a voluntary self-reported standardized, established questionnaire [4]. More precisely, data regarding daily pad usage was assessed by evaluating the number of pads used, grouped as '0–one safety', '1–2', '3–5', or '>5' pads, respectively. If two follow-up assessments were available within the first six months of post-surgery ($n = 3$), the more mature assessment (closer to 6 months cut-off) was considered for further analyses.

2.3. Statistical Analyses

Descriptive statistics included frequencies and proportions for categorical variables. Medians and interquartile ranges (IQR) were reported for continuously coded variables. The chi-square test examined the statistical significance of the differences in proportions, while the Kruskal-Wallis test was used to examine differences in medians.

Uni- and multivariable logistic regression models tested the relationship between urine loss after catheter removal in PAD-tests (<1 g vs. 1–10 g vs. 11–50 g vs. >50 g) and early urinary continence (0–1 vs. ≤1 pads/24 h). Covariates consisted of age at RP (≤60 vs. 61–69 vs. ≥70 years), BMI (<25 vs. 25–30 vs. >30 kg/m^2), prostate volume

(≤40 vs. >40 mL), extraprostatic extension of tumor (pT2 vs. pT3/4), and nerve-sparing approach (no vs. yes).

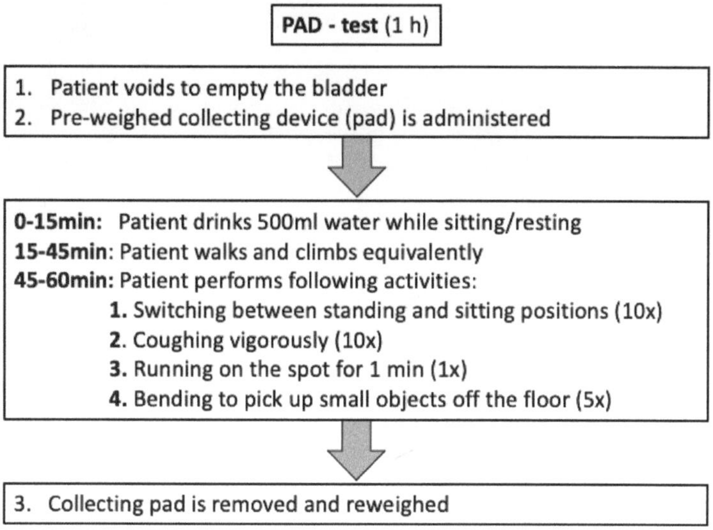

PAD - test (1 h)

1. Patient voids to empty the bladder
2. Pre-weighed collecting device (pad) is administered

0-15min: Patient drinks 500ml water while sitting/resting
15-45min: Patient walks and climbs equivalently
45-60min: Patient performs following activities:
    1. Switching between standing and sitting positions (10x)
    2. Coughing vigorously (10x)
    3. Running on the spot for 1 min (1x)
    4. Bending to pick up small objects off the floor (5x)

3. Collecting pad is removed and reweighed

Figure 1. Flowchart depicting the sequence of the PAD-test.

To test for a potential underlying selection bias, sensitivity analyses were performed between the current study cohort and patients with missing data regarding PAD-test results and early continence rates in the study period (01/2018 to 03/2021).

For all statistical analyses, R software environment for statistical computing and graphics (version 3.4.3) was used [22]. All tests were two-sided with a level of significance set at $p < 0.05$.

3. Results

3.1. Descriptive Characteristics of the Study Population

In total, 100 patients were included in the current analysis (Table 1). Of those, 74 patients (74%) underwent robotic-assisted RP, whereas 26 patients underwent (26%) open RP, respectively. The median age was 65 years (IQR: 58–59), the median PSA was 8 ng/mL (IQR: 6–12) and the median BMI was 26.1 kg/m² (IQR: 24.3–29.9). Final histopathological examination revealed in 45% an extraprostatic extension of the tumor. Nerve sparing approach (uni/bilateral) was performed in most cases (93%), and median operation time was 218 min (IQR: 189–252).

Table 1. Patient and clinicopathological characteristics of 100 patients treated with radical prostatectomy at the University Hospital Frankfurt between 01/2018 and 03/2021, with data available for both PAD-test and early continence status. All values are median (IQR) or frequencies (%).

	Study Cohort, (n = 100)
Age in years, Median (IQR)	65 (58, 69)
PSA in mg/mL, Median (IQR)	8 (6, 12)
Body Mass Index in kg/m², Median (IQR)	26.1 (24.3, 29.9)

Table 1. *Cont.*

	Study Cohort, (n = 100)
International Prostate Symptom Score, Median (IQR)	6.5 (3, 9)
Body Mass Index grouped in kg/m^2, n (%)	
≤25	33 (34%)
25–30	40 (41%)
≥30	25 (26%)
D'Amico risk classification, n (%)	
low	13 (13%)
intermediate	57 (57%)
high	30 (30%)
Surgical approach, n (%)	
robotic-assisted RP	74 (74%)
open RP	26 (26%)
Operation time in min, Median (IQR)	218 (189, 252)
Prostate volume in cm^3, Median (IQR)	40 (30, 50)
pT-stage, n (%)	
pT2a	6 (6.0%)
pT2b	1 (1.0%)
pT2c	48 (48%)
pT3a	33 (33%)
pT3b	10 (10%)
pT4	2 (2.0%)
Extraprostatic extension of tumor, n (%)	
no	55 (55%)
yes	45 (45%)
pN-stage, n (%)	
pN0	85 (85%)
pN1	4 (4.0%)
pNx	11 (11%)
cM-stage, n (%)	
M0	96 (96%)
M1	4 (4.0%)

Table 1. Cont.

	Study Cohort, (n = 100)
Gleason Grade Group RP-specimen, n (%)	
I	9 (9%)
II	53 (54%)
III	19 (19%)
IV	4 (4%)
V	13 (13%)
Nerve sparing, n (%)	
none	7 (7%)
uni/bilateral	93 (93%)
Positive surgical margin, n (%)	
R0	63 (63%)
R1	34 (34%)
Rx	3 (3%)

3.2. Perioperative and Early Continence Outcomes

PAD-test following catheter removal recorded 24%, 47%, 15%, and 14% of patients having a loss of urine <1 g (continent), 1–10 g (mild incontinent), 11–50 g (moderate incontinent), and >50 g (severe incontinent), respectively. In early follow-up assessments (median: 3 months; IQR: 2–5 months), 59% of patients were continent, defined by the usage of no or one safety-pad within 24 h. Tabulation, according to PAD-test result, exhibited 88%, 62%, 40%, and 21% urinary continence in patients with loss of urine <1 g, 1–10 g 11–50 g, and >50 g (Table 2).

Table 2. Usage of pads in early continence follow-up assessments in 100 patients treated with radical prostatectomy between 01/2018 and 10/2020 at the University Hospital Frankfurt, stratified according to urine loss in PAD-test; All values are frequencies (%).

		0–1(Safety) Pad/24 h	1–2 Pads/24 h	3–5 Pads/24 h	>5 Pads/24 h
Urine loss in g, n (%)					
<1 g	24 (24.0%)	21 (87.5%)	2 (8.3%)	1 (4.2%)	0 (0%)
1–10 g	47 (47.0%)	29 (61.7%)	12 (25.6%)	6 (12.7%)	0 (0%)
11–50 g	15 (15.0%)	6 (40.0%)	6 (40.0%)	2 (13.3%)	1 (6.7%)
>50 g	14 (14.0%)	3 (21.4%)	5 (35.7%)	2 (14.3%)	4 (28.6%)

3.3. Uni-and Multivariable Logistic Regression Models

In univariable logistic regression models, urine loss in the PAD-test was a statistically significant factor that influenced urinary continence in early assessments, and resulted in an odds ratio of 0.23 [95%-CI: 0.05–0.79; $p = 0.03$], 0.10 [95%-CI: 0.02–0.43; $p = 0.004$], and 0.04 [95%-CI: 0.01–0.20; $p < 0.001$] for 1–10 g, 11–50 g, and >50 g urine loss, respectively (Table 3). Besides age ≥ 70 years, which was associated with a lower chance of continence [OR: 0.28; 95%-CI: 0.08–0.87; $p = 0.03$], neither BMI, extraprostatic extension, prostate volume, nor nerve-sparing approach were significant risk factors in univariable analyses

After adjustment in multivariable logistic regression models, higher urine loss remained to be a factor lowering the chance for early continence (Urine loss of 1–10 g, 11–50 g, and >50 g resulted in an odds ratio of 0.21 [95%-CI: 0.04–0.79; $p = 0.03$], 0.09 [95%-CI: 0.01–0.48; $p = 0.008$], and 0.03 [95%-CI: 0.004–0.18; $p < 0.001$]). All other variables had an insignificant influence on early urinary continence in multivariable analyses.

Table 3. Uni- and multivariable logistic regression models predicting early urinary continence in 100 patients treated with radical prostatectomy between 01/2018 and 10/2020 at the University Hospital Frankfurt. Urinary continence was defined as the usage of no or one safety pad within 24 h. Extraprostatic extension was defined by pT3/pT4 in final RP-specimen stage.

	Logistic Regression Models						
	Univariable				Multivariable		
	Odds Ratio	95%-CI		p-Value	Odds Ratio	95%-CI		p-Value
PAD-test urine loss in g							
<1	Ref.				Ref.			
1–10	0.23	0.05	0.79	0.03	0.21	0.04	0.79	0.03
11–50	0.10	0.02	0.43	0.004	0.09	0.01	0.48	0.008
>50	0.04	0.01	0.20	<0.001	0.03	0.004	0.18	<0.001
Age in years							
≤60	Ref.				Ref.			
61–69	0.49	0.17	1.30	0.16	0.42	0.13	1.28	0.14
≥70	0.28	0.08	0.87	0.03	0.55	0.14	2.15	0.39
Nerve-sparing approach							
No	Ref.				Ref.			
Yes	3.96	0.81	28.67	0.11	1.52	0.23	13.51	0.68
Body Mass Index kg/m²							
<25	Ref.				Ref.			
25–30	1.55	0.60	4.02	0.36	2.04	0.66	6.56	0.22
≥30	1.06	0.37	3.05	0.91	1.06	0.29	3.86	0.93
Extraprostatic Extension							
No	Ref.				Ref.			
Yes	0.77	0.34	1.72	0.53	1.29	0.46	3.71	0.63
Prostate volume in mL							
≤40	Ref.				Ref.			
>40	1.11	0.50	2.51	0.80	0.82	0.30	2.20	0.69

3.4. Sample Selection Bias

Sensitivity analyses were performed for potential selection bias, due to differences in tumor and patient characteristics between the study cohort ($n = 100$) and patients with missing data regarding PAD-test results or early continence rates in the study period ($n = 564$). Here, no significant differences between the current study cohort and the entire cohort (all $p \geq 0.1$) were recorded.

4. Discussion

The preservation of continence after RP is a crucial aspect in the treatment of patients with PCa [1]. Several studies have demonstrated that postoperative urinary incontinence after RP can result in a substantial reduction in the patients' quality of life, and represents a potential bothersome side-effect [4,8,9]. To date, data regarding reliable measurements to predict continence rates at a very timely point of convalescence are rare. We hypothesized that urine loss (defined in a PAD-test) after catheter removal was correlated with early continence rates and thus, could be used to identify patients at the highest-risk of postoperative urinary incontinence and as such, a higher need of intensified, postoperative pelvic floor training. We relied on a contemporary cohort of 100 PCa patients being treated with RP at a tertiary referral center and made noteworthy findings.

First, PAD-test results strongly correlated with continence status in the early follow-up assessments. Patients considered to be continent according to the PAD-test results (<1 g urine loss) reported an early continence rate of 88% in follow-up assessments, whereas rates for mild incontinent (1–10 g urine loss) and moderate incontinent (11–50 g urine loss) patients were 62% and 40%. Least frequent, yet the most severe incontinence in PAD tests ($\geq$50 g urine loss) resulted in low rates of early continence (22%). This correlation can also be seen in multivariable logistic regressions for all subgroups after adjusting for further risk factors of early postoperative incontinence. A urine loss, e.g., of >50 g resulted in a strikingly decreased chance of early urinary continence (odds ratio: 0.03) compared to patients with urine loss <1 g. The current literature is scarce about the relationship between continence status after catheter removal and early continence in RP treated patients [23,24]. For example, Manfredi et al., even though ascertaining urinary continence after RP at different time points beginning with catheter removal, solely relied on the number of pads as a proxy for urinary continence throughout their study [24] Therefore, the study by Manfredi et al. could not be directly compared to the current study since pad usage represented a fairly inaccurate measurement tool, and might not represent the full bandwidth of urinary incontinence at such an early timepoint [24]. Contrary to Manfredi et al., Ates et al. relied on a more precise variable, namely the urine loss ratio (ULR), to predict early, mid-term, and long-term continence rate of PCa patients undergoing laparoscopic RP [25,26]. Urine loss ratio was defined as the weight of urine loss in the pad divided by daily micturition volume (24 h). Even though the authors were able to find a cut off 0.15 ULR, above which the level of incontinence increased in a manifold fashion, the ULR represented a labor- and time-consuming variable to harbor in everyday clinical practice, since its protocol relied on an extended collective time span of 24 h. Regarding the reduced length of stays following RP in the current era, it was questionable if such an extensive test can be implemented in routine clinical practice. By contrast, the current introduced PAD-test could be seen as a timesaving (2 vs. 24 h) measurement tool and was additionally less labor intensive. Consequently, to the best of our knowledge, the current study was the first to report a robust correlation between urine loss after catheter removal and early continence rates relying on a time-efficient, reproducible, and robust measurement tool, namely PAD-test.

Second, urine loss in the PAD-test strongly correlated with the severity of early incontinence. Instead of dichotomic ascertainment of urinary continence after catheter removal stratifying the severity of incontinence into predefined categories, made a more precise correlation possible. For example, patients with a loss of more than 50 g in PAD-test were at the highest risk (28.6%) for serious early incontinence (>5 pads/24 h), compared to patients with urine loss of 11–50 g (6.7%) or 1–10 g (0%) in a PAD-test. The same correlation trends were recorded for less profound early incontinence (3–5 pads/24 h). From a clinical point of view, current findings may be attributable to a potential malfunction of the external sphincter; either pre-existing or by an injury of the urethral sphincter during RP [18,27]. Even though full functional-length of urethral sphincter preservation was routinely performed in all patients, interindividual anatomical and tumor characteristics may have influenced the extent of preservation, and led to potential injury of the sphincter [28]. As a consequence PAD-test results did not only profoundly correlate with early continence rate, but could also be taken as a measurement tool to estimate the severity of early incontinence after RP Interestingly, preliminary data reveal clear trends that solely patients with severe urinary loss of >50 g in PAD-tests fail to regain full continence recovery in long-term follow-up (>12 months). Even though the primary focus of the current study was to investigate the correlation of PAD-test results with early continence rates, the findings added to the picture that pad-test results were of great value to estimate the severity of continence, even at a longer time of follow-up. These findings were in accordance with several previous studies, which have demonstrated a prolonged recovery time for urinary continence beyond 12 months following RP [29,30].

Finally, other variables, such as BMI, age, and prostate volume, did not meet a level of significance in the multivariable logistic regression models for early continence [31]. This could be explained by certain risk factors (e.g., age) for urinary incontinence that might simultaneously account as risk factors for PAD-test results. Theissen et al. reported that younger patients showed significantly better early continence rates relying on PAD-test results after catheter removal compared to their older counterparts [17]. Consequently, a lack of significance in the current study could be explained due to these observations.

The current study was not devoid of limitations. First and foremost, were the limitations inherent to the retrospective nature of the study and the limited sample size. Second, the population in the current study underwent open and robotic-assisted radical prostatectomy, and the differences in experience among the surgeons might be present. However, it is of note that all surgeons underwent training in high-volume prostate cancer centers. Third, since no routine bladder neck reconstruction was performed in the current study population, comparison of continence results to patients undergoing RP with bladder neck reconstruction should be interpreted accordingly [32]. Fourth and finally, a potential bias regarding the extent of postsurgical pelvic-floor training cannot be ruled out. All patients were strongly encouraged to seek professional pelvic-floor training for urinary continence recovery and were also instructed during their in-patient stay.

5. Conclusions

Urine loss after catheter removal strongly correlated with early urinary continence and could be used to estimate the severity of urinary incontinence. Therefore, PAD-test after catheter removal may identify men with a higher need of intensified, postoperative pelvic floor training. Additional studies may elucidate the correlation between PAD-test results and long-term continence rates in the future.

Author Contributions: All authors contributed substantially to the study conception and design. B.H.: Conceptualization, formal analysis, and original draft preparation; F.P.: Conceptualization, data acquisition, formal analysis, investigation, supervision, and review and editing; M.W.: Data acquisition, formal analysis, and investigation; C.H.: Conceptualization and data acquisition; C.W.: Conceptualization and data acquisition; J.L.H.: Writing and editing; M.V.-W.: Conceptualization and data acquisition; J.K.: Data acquisition; T.S.: conceptualization; M.G.: Writing—reviewing and editing; D.T.: Conceptualization, writing—reviewing and editing; P.I.K.: Conceptualization and writing—reviewing and editing; A.B.: Conceptualization and writing—reviewing and editing; L.A.K.: Conceptualization and original draft preparation; F.K.H.C.: Conceptualization, writing—reviewing and editing, and supervision; P.M.: Conceptualization, formal analysis and supervision. All authors have read and agreed to the published version of the manuscript.

Funding: The research was conducted in the absence of any commercial or financial relationships that could be construed as a potential conflict of interest.

Institutional Review Board Statement: The study was conducted according to the guidelines of the Declaration of Helsinki, and approved by the institutional review boards (Ethical approval: SUG-1-2018) of the University Cancer Centre Frankfurt and the Ethical Committee at the University Hospital Frankfurt.

Informed Consent Statement: All patients included in our study signed a written informed consent.

Data Availability Statement: The data presented in this study are available on request from the corresponding author.

Acknowledgments: B.H. was awarded a scholarship by the GIERSCH STIFTUNG.

Conflicts of Interest: The authors declare that there is no conflict of interests.

References

1. Mottet, N.; Cornford, P.; van den Bergh, R.C.N.; Briers, E.; Expert Patient Advocate (European Prostate Cancer Coalition/Europa UOMO); Santis, M.D.; Gillessen, S.; Grummet, J.; Henry, A.M.; van den Kwast, T.H.; et al. *EAU Prostate Cancer Guidelines. Edn. Presented at the EAU Annual Congress Milan 2021*; EAU Guidelines Office: Arnhem, The Netherlands, 2021; ISBN 978-94-92671-13-4
2. Bray, F.; Ferlay, J.; Soerjomataram, I.; Siegel, R.L.; Torre, L.A.; Jemal, A. Global cancer statistics 2018: GLOBOCAN estimates of incidence and mortality worldwide for 36 cancers in 185 countries. *A Cancer J. Clin.* **2018**, *68*, 394–424. [CrossRef]
3. Haese, A.; Knipper, S.; Isbarn, H.; Heinzer, H.; Tilki, D.; Salomon, G.; Michl, U.; Steuber, T.; Budäus, L.; Maurer, T.; et al. A comparative study of robot-assisted and open radical prostatectomy in 10 790 men treated by highly trained surgeons for both procedures. *BJU Int.* **2019**, *123*, 1031–1040. [CrossRef]
4. Pompe, R.S.; Tian, Z.; Preisser, F.; Tennstedt, P.; Beyer, B.; Michl, U.; Graefen, M.; Huland, H.; Karakiewicz, P.I.; Tilki, D. Short- and Long-term Functional Outcomes and Quality of Life after Radical Prostatectomy: Patient-reported Outcomes from a Tertiary High-volume Center. *Eur. Urol. Focus* **2017**, *3*, 615–620. [CrossRef] [PubMed]
5. Hamdy, F.C.; Donovan, J.L.; Lane, J.A.; Mason, M.; Metcalfe, C.; Holding, P.; Davis, M.; Peters, T.J.; Turner, E.L.; Martin, R.M.; et al 10-Year Outcomes after Monitoring, Surgery, or Radiotherapy for Localized Prostate Cancer. *N. Engl. J. Med.* **2016**, *13*, 1415–1424 [CrossRef]
6. Wilt, T.J.; Brawer, M.K.; Jones, K.M.; Barry, M.J.; Aronson, W.J.; Fox, S.; Gingrich, J.R.; Wei, J.T.; Gilhooly, P.; Grob, B.M.; et al. Radical Prostatectomy versus Observation for Localized Prostate Cancer. *N. Engl. J. Med.* **2012**, *367*, 203–213. [CrossRef]
7. Hoeh, B.; Preisser, F.; Wenzel, M.; Humke, C.; Wittler, C.; Köllermann, J.; Bodelle, B.; Bernatz, S.; Steuber, T.; Tilki, D.; et al Feasibility and outcome of radical prostatectomy following inductive neoadjuvant therapy in patients with suspicion of rectal infiltration. *Urol. Oncol. Semin. Orig. Investig.* **2021**. [CrossRef] [PubMed]
8. Whiting, P.F.; Moore, T.H.; Jameson, C.M.; Davies, P.; Rowlands, M.-A.; Burke, M.; Beynon, R.; Savovic, J.; Donovan, J.L. Symptomatic and quality-of-life outcomes after treatment for clinically localised prostate cancer: A systematic review. *BJU Int* **2016**, *118*, 193–204. [CrossRef]
9. Borges, R.C.; Tobias-Machado, M.; Gabriotti, E.N.; Dos Santos Figueiredo, F.W.; Bezerra, C.A.; Glina, S. Post-radical prostatectomy urinary incontinence: Is there any discrepancy between medical reports and patients' perceptions? *BMC Urol.* **2019**, *19*, 32 [CrossRef] [PubMed]
10. Ilie, G.; White, J.; Mason, R.; Rendon, R.; Bailly, G.; Lawen, J.; Bowes, D.; Patil, N.; Wilke, D.; Macdonald, C.; et al. Current Mental Distress Among Men with a History of Radical Prostatectomy and Related Adverse Correlates. *Am. J. Men's Health* **2020**, *14* [CrossRef] [PubMed]
11. Mandel, P.; Graefen, M.; Michl, U.; Huland, H.; Tilki, D. The effect of age on functional outcomes after radical prostatectomy *Urol. Oncol. Semin. Orig. Investig.* **2015**, *33*, 203.e11–203.e18. [CrossRef]
12. Mandel, P.; Kretschmer, A.; Chandrasekar, T.; Nguyen, H.; Buchner, A.; Stief, C.G.; Tilki, D. The effect of BMI on clinicopathologic and functional outcomes after open radical prostatectomy. *Urol. Oncol. Semin. Orig. Investig.* **2014**, *32*, 297–302. [CrossRef] [PubMed]
13. Holm, H.V.; Fosså, S.D.; Hedlund, H.; Schultz, A.; Dahl, A.A. How Should Continence and Incontinence after Radical Prostatectomy be Evaluated? A Prospective Study of Patient Ratings and Changes with Time. *J. Urol.* **2014**, *192*, 1155–1161. [CrossRef] [PubMed]
14. Ficarra, V.; Novara, G.; Rosen, R.C.; Artibani, W.; Carroll, P.R.; Costello, A.; Menon, M.; Montorsi, F.; Patel, V.R.; Stolzenburg, J.-U. et al. Systematic Review and Meta-analysis of Studies Reporting Urinary Continence Recovery After Robot-assisted Radical Prostatectomy. *Eur. Urol.* **2012**, *62*, 405–417. [CrossRef] [PubMed]
15. Moschovas, M.C.; Sighinolfi, M.C.; Rocco, B.; Bhat, S.; Onol, F.; Rogers, T.; Patel, V. Balancing the Effects of COVID-19 Against Potential Progression and Mortality in High-risk Prostate Cancer. *Eur. Urol.* **2020**, *78*, e14–e15. [CrossRef] [PubMed]
16. Preisser, F.; Theissen, L.; Wild, P.; Bartelt, K.; Kluth, L.; Köllermann, J.; Graefen, M.; Steuber, T.; Huland, H.; Tilki, D.; et al Implementation of Intraoperative Frozen Section During Radical Prostatectomy: Short-term Results from a German Tertiary-care Center. *Eur. Urol. Focus* **2021**, *7*, 95–101. [CrossRef]
17. Theissen, L.; Preisser, F.; Wenzel, M.; Humke, C.; Roos, F.C.; Kluth, L.A.; Becker, A.; Banek, S.; Bodelle, B.; Köllermann, J.; et al Very Early Continence After Radical Prostatectomy and Its Influencing Factors. *Front. Surg.* **2019**, *6*, 60. [CrossRef]
18. Schlomm, T.; Heinzer, H.; Steuber, T.; Salomon, G.; Engel, O.; Michl, U.; Haese, A.; Graefen, M.; Huland, H. Full Functional-Length Urethral Sphincter Preservation During Radical Prostatectomy. *Eur. Urol.* **2011**, *60*, 320–329. [CrossRef]
19. Beyer, B.; Schlomm, T.; Tennstedt, P.; Boehm, K.; Adam, M.; Schiffmann, J.; Sauter, G.; Wittmer, C.; Steuber, T.; Graefen, M.; et al A Feasible and Time-efficient Adaptation of NeuroSAFE for da Vinci Robot-assisted Radical Prostatectomy. *Eur. Urol.* **2013** *66*, 138–144. [CrossRef]
20. Spinelli, M.G.; Cozzi, G.; Grasso, A.; Talso, M.; Varisco, D.; El Rahman, D.A.; Acquati, P.; Albo, G.; Rocco, B.; Maggioni, A.; et al Ralp & Rocco Stitch: Original Technique. *Urol. J.* **2011**, *78*, 35–38. [CrossRef]
21. Hahn, I.; Fall, M. Objective quantification of stress urinary incontinence: A short, reproducible, provocative pad-test. *Neurourol Urodyn.* **1991**, *10*, 475–481. [CrossRef]

22. RCT. R: A Language and Environment for Statistical Computing. 2017. Available online: https://wwwr-projectorg2017 (accessed on 10 October 2021).
23. Harke, N.N.; Wagner, C.; Liakos, N.; Urbanova, K.; Addali, M.; Hadaschik, B.A.; Witt, J.H. Superior early and long-term continence following early micturition on day 2 after robot-assisted radical prostatectomy: A randomized prospective trial. *World J. Urol.* **2020**, *39*, 771–777. [CrossRef]
24. Manfredi, M.; Checcucci, E.; Fiori, C.; Garrou, D.; Aimar, R.; Amparore, D.; De Luca, S.; Bombaci, S.; Stura, I.; Migliaretti, G.; et al. Total anatomical reconstruction during robot-assisted radical prostatectomy: Focus on urinary continence recovery and related complications after 1000 procedures. *BJU Int.* **2019**, *124*, 477–486. [CrossRef]
25. Ates, M.; Teber, D.; Gozen, A.S.; Tefekli, A.; Hruza, M.; Sugiono, M.; Erdogan, S.; Rassweiler, J. A New Postoperative Predictor of Time to Urinary Continence after Laparoscopic Radical Prostatectomy: The Urine Loss Ratio. *Eur. Urol.* **2007**, *52*, 178–185. [CrossRef]
26. Tienza, A.; Akin, Y.; Rassweiler, J.; Gözen, A.S. A match-pair analysis of continence in intermediate and high-risk prostate cancer patients after robot-assisted radical prostatectomy: The role of urine loss ratio and predictive analysis. *Prostate Int.* **2017**, *6*, 94–98. [CrossRef] [PubMed]
27. Kim, M.; Park, M.; Pak, S.; Choi, S.-K.; Shim, M.; Song, C.; Ahn, H. Integrity of the Urethral Sphincter Complex, Nerve-sparing, and Long-term Continence Status after Robotic-assisted Radical Prostatectomy. *Eur. Urol. Focus* **2018**, *5*, 823–830. [CrossRef] [PubMed]
28. Wenzel, M.; Preisser, F.; Mueller, M.; Theissen, L.H.; Welte, M.N.; Hoeh, B.; Humke, C.; Bernatz, S.; Bodelle, B.; Würnschimmel, C.; et al. Effect of prostatic apex shape (Lee types) and urethral sphincter length in preoperative MRI on very early continence rates after radical prostatectomy. *Int. Urol. Nephrol.* **2021**, *53*, 1297–1303. [CrossRef] [PubMed]
29. Mandel, P.; Preisser, F.; Graefen, M.; Steuber, T.; Salomon, G.; Haese, A.; Michl, U.; Huland, H.; Tilki, D. High Chance of Late Recovery of Urinary and Erectile Function Beyond 12 Months After Radical Prostatectomy. *Eur. Urol.* **2016**, *71*, 848–850. [CrossRef]
30. Lee, J.K.; Assel, M.; Thong, A.E.; Sjoberg, D.D.; Mulhall, J.P.; Sandhu, J.; Vickers, A.J.; Ehdaie, B. Unexpected Long-term Improvements in Urinary and Erectile Function in a Large Cohort of Men with Self-reported Outcomes Following Radical Prostatectomy. *Eur. Urol.* **2015**, *68*, 899–905. [CrossRef]
31. Heesakkers, J.; Farag, F.; Bauer, R.M.; Sandhu, J.; De Ridder, D.; Stenzl, A. Pathophysiology and Contributing Factors in Postprostatectomy Incontinence: A Review. *Eur. Urol.* **2016**, *71*, 936–944. [CrossRef]
32. Massanova, M.; Bada, M.; Crocetto, F.; Barone, B.; Arcaniolo, D.; Silvestri, T.; De Concilio, B.; Zeccolini, G.; Mazzon, G.; Celia, A. Bowel suture technique for bladder neck reconstruction during RALP and its impact on early continence recovery. *Minerva Urol. E Nefrol.* **2020**, *72*, 640–641. [CrossRef]

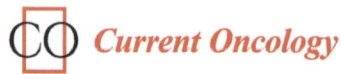

Article

Prospective Randomized Phase II Study of Stereotactic Body Radiotherapy (SBRT) vs. Conventional Fractionated Radiotherapy (CFRT) for Chinese Patients with Early-Stage Localized Prostate Cancer †

Darren M. C. Poon [1,2,*], Daisy Lam [1], Kenneth C. W. Wong [1], Cheuk-Man Chu [3], Michael Cheung [1], Frankie Mo [1], Joyce Suen [1], Chi-Fai Ng [4] and Anthony T. C. Chan [1]

[1] Department of Clinical Oncology, State Key Laboratory of Translational Oncology, Sir YK Pao Centre for Cancer, Hong Kong Cancer Institute and Prince of Wales Hospital, The Chinese University of Hong Kong, Hong Kong, China; lcm306@ha.org.hk (D.L.); wcw979@ha.org.hk (K.C.W.W.); clm314@ha.org.hk (M.C.); frankie@clo.cuhk.edu.hk (F.M.); j_suen@clo.cuhk.edu.hk (J.S.); anthonytcchan@cuhk.edu.hk (A.T.C.C.)
[2] Comprehensive Oncology Centre, Hong Kong Sanatorium & Hospital, Hong Kong, China
[3] Department of Imaging and Interventional Radiology, Prince of Wales Hospital, The Chinese University of Hong Kong, Hong Kong, China; charmantchu@gmail.com or cmchu@doctorcare.hk
[4] Department of Surgery, Prince of Wales Hospital, The Chinese University of Hong Kong, Hong Kong, China; ngcf@surgery.cuhk.edu.hk
* Correspondence: mc_poon@clo.cuhk.edu.hk; Tel.: +852-3505-3380
† Presentations: Presented in part at the 2019 Asian Congress of European Society of Medical Oncology, Singapore, 23–25 November 2018, and at the 2019 American Society of Clinical Oncology Genitourinary Symposium, San Francisco, CA, USA, 14–16 February 2019.

Abstract: Background: Stereotactic body radiotherapy (SBRT) has potential radiobiologic and economic advantages over conventional fractionated radiotherapy (CFRT) in localized prostate cancer (PC). This study aimed to compare the effects of these two distinct fractionations on patient-reported quality of life (PRQOL) and tolerability. Methods: In this prospective phase II study, patients with low and intermediate-risk localized PC were randomly assigned in a 1:1 ratio to the SBRT (36.25 Gy/5 fractions/2 weeks) or CFRT (76 Gy/38 fractions/7.5 weeks) treatment groups. The primary endpoint of variation in PRQOL at 1 year was assessed by changes in the Expanded Prostate Cancer Index Composite (EPIC) questionnaire scores and analysed by z-tests and t-tests. Results: Sixty-four eligible Chinese men were treated (SBRT, n = 31; CFRT, n = 33) with a median follow-up of 2.3 years. At 1 year, 40.0%/46.9% of SBRT/CFRT patients had a >5-point decrease in bowel score ($p = 0.08/0.28$) respectively, and 53.3%/46.9% had a >2-point decrease in urinary score ($p = 0.21/0.07$). There were no significant differences in EPIC score changes between the arms at 3, 6, 9 and 12 months, but SBRT was associated with significantly fewer grade ≥ 1 acute and 1-year late gastrointestinal toxicities (acute: 35% vs. 87%, $p < 0.0001$; 1-year late: 64% vs. 84%, $p = 0.03$), and grade ≥ 2 acute genitourinary toxicities (3% vs. 24%, $p = 0.04$) compared with CFRT. Conclusion: SBRT offered similar PRQOL and less toxicity compared with CFRT in Chinese men with localized PC.

Keywords: dose fractionation (radiation); patient reported outcomes; prostate cancer; quality of life; radiation tolerance; stereotactic body radiotherapy

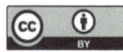

1. Introduction

External beam radiotherapy (EBRT) is an effective curative treatment option for localized prostate cancer (PC) [1]. Conventional fractionated radiotherapy (CFRT), with daily dose fractionation of 1.8–2 Gy over 8 to 9 weeks, has been commonly administered worldwide [2]. However, such a protracted total treatment time, together with the mounting incidence of PC, poses burdens for the healthcare system [3]. Epidemiological studies have estimated that, optimally, 60% of PC patients require radiotherapy (RT) at some point in their illness [4,5]. In a recent U.S. modeling study, for low-risk PC patients, RT is the most expensive initial treatment option, and results in the highest 10-year cumulative cost [6]. However, even in high-income countries, disparities in access to standard-of-care RT exist because of socio-geographical factors [7].

The unique radiobiologic characteristics of PC open new possibilities for shortening the overall radiation treatment time. In theory, a low alpha/beta ratio entails a more pronounced linear-quadratic dose response, with greater killing per unit dose at higher doses [8], i.e., an increased fraction sensitivity. The low alpha/beta ratio (range: 0.9–2.2) of PC, which has been reported across low-, intermediate- and high-risk patient groups [9,10], suggests that the therapeutic ratio could potentially be enhanced by hypofractionation. Clinical trials published in the past several years showed non-inferiority of moderately hypofractionated RT (MHRT; fraction size 2.4–3.4 Gy over 4 to 6 weeks) for biochemical disease-free survival, and similar toxicity compared with CFRT [11–14]. MHRT is now the recommended EBRT option [15].

With the emergence of high-precision RT techniques such as image guidance systems, further shortening of overall treatment times with stereotactic body RT (SBRT; 5–6 fractions of extremely high-dose radiation, $\geq$500 cGy per fraction over 2 to 3 weeks) is hypothetically feasible. Ample prospective, single-arm trials have demonstrated promising efficacy and favorable toxicity of SBRT that is largely comparable to CFRT. In the pooled analysis of multi-institutional prospective phase II studies, SBRT showed 5-year biochemical relapse-free survival (bRFS) rates of 93%, 95%, 84% and 81% for all, low-, intermediate- and high-risk patients, respectively [16]. In a recent meta-analysis including 6116 patients among 38 prospective studies, the overall 5- and 7-year bRFS rates were 95.3% and 93.7%, whereas the estimated late grade $\geq$ 3 genitourinary (GU) and gastrointestinal (GI) toxicity rates were 2.0% and 1.1%, respectively [17]. In another meta-analysis of 7 phase III trials in men with localized PC (n = 6795), the 5-year cumulative incidence of late grade $\geq$ 2 GU toxicity was comparable between ultrahypofractionated RT, hypofractionated RT and CFRT, at 18%, 20.4% and 19.4%, respectively (p = 0.92; random effects model) [18].

Two phase III trials of SBRT and CFRT were ongoing at the time of our study: PACE (NCT01584258) for low- or intermediate-risk PC patients (8% and 92%, respectively) and HYPO-RT-PC (ISRCTN45905321) in PC patients with intermediate and high risks (89% and 11%). The latest published results of HYPRO-RT-PC confirmed highly similar failure-free survival at 5 years (84% in both arms, hazard ratio = 1.002, log-rank p = 0.99) [19]. There was a small increase in early side-effects such as urinary toxicities in the SBRT group, but toxicity was otherwise similar at up to 5-year follow-up. For PACE-B, while efficacy results are not yet mature, short-term toxicity findings were similar between-arms: radiation therapy oncology group (RTOG) grade $\geq$ 2 GI toxicities were reported in 10% (SBRT) vs. 12% (CFRT; p = 0.38) and grade $\geq$ 2 GU toxicities in 23% vs. 27% of patients (p = 0.16), respectively [20].

While further efficacy and long-term safety results are needed, the growing body of evidence supports potential radiobiologic and economic benefits of SBRT for PC. Our present phase II study was designed to provide evidence in the form of a prospective, randomized trial evaluation and head-to-head comparison of the patient-reported quality of life (PRQOL) and treatment-related toxicities with SBRT vs. CFRT in low- and intermediate-risk localized PC.

2. Results

2.1. Demographic Characteristics

Between January 2015 and May 2017, 68 patients were enrolled (Figure 1); four patients were ineligible. The baseline characteristics of 64 patients who received the protocol treatment with follow-up were well-balanced and are listed in Table 1. The median age was 69.5 years and the median pre-treatment prostate-specific antigen (PSA) was 8.1 ng/mL. In general, 93% had a Zubrod performance score of 0. National Comprehensive Cancer Network (NCCN) low- and intermediate-risk patients were equally represented in both arms.

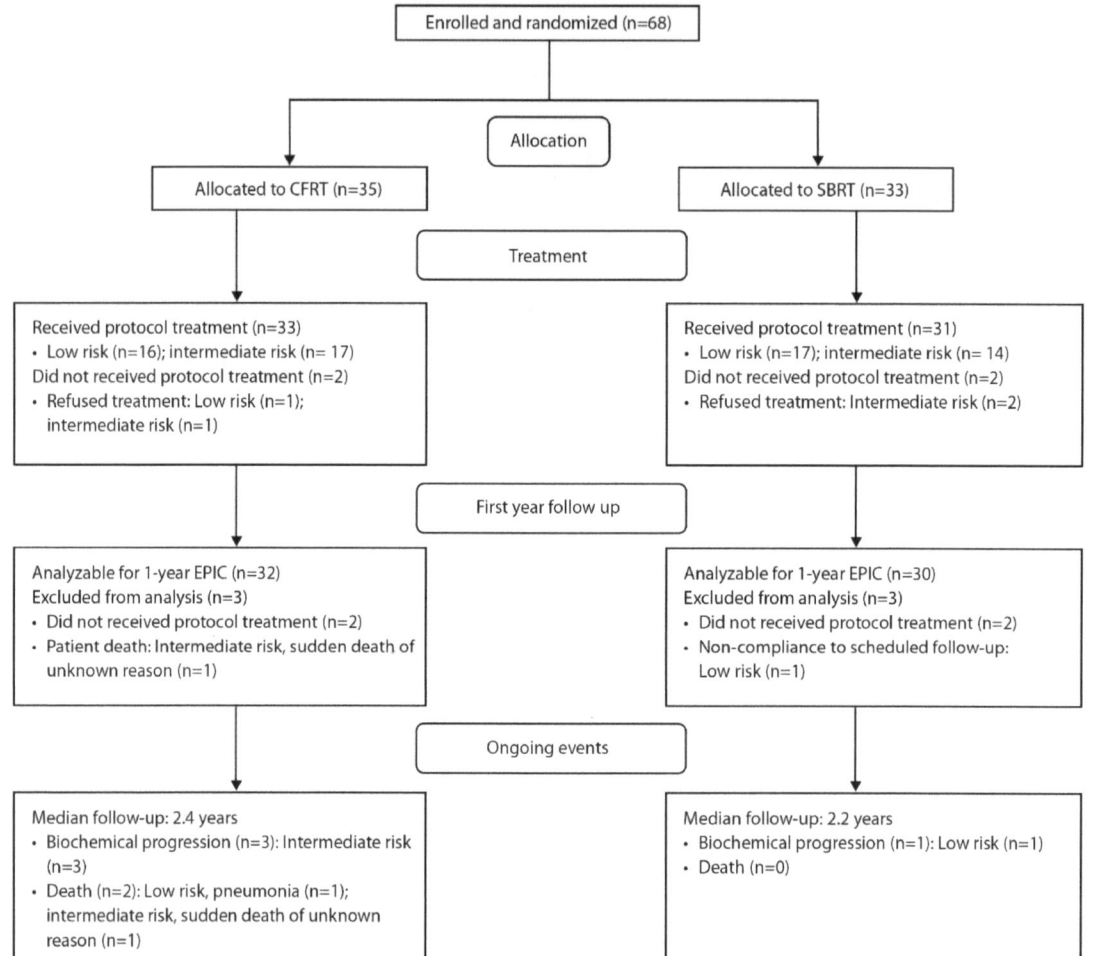

Figure 1. CONSORT diagram showing enrollment, random assignment and follow-up of the study participants. Abbreviations: SBRT, stereotactic body radiotherapy; CFRT, conventional fractionated radiotherapy; EPIC, Expanded Prostate Cancer Index Composite questionnaire.

Table 1. Patient baseline characteristics.

Patient Characteristics	SBRT (n = 31)	CFRT (n = 33)
Age		
Mean (SD)	69.4 (6.0)	69.0 (6.8)
Median (range)	68 (53–78)	70 (55–81)
Zubrod Performance		
0	30 (96%)	30 (90%)
1	1 (3%)	3 (10%)
Clinical T Stage		
1a	1 (3%)	0
1c	16 (51%)	15 (45%)
2a	7 (22%)	10 (30%)
2b	5 (16%)	3 (9%)
2c	2 (6%)	5 (15%)
Gleason Score		
5	3 (9%)	0
6	16 (51%)	22 (66%)
7	12 (38%)	11 (33%)
PSA		
Mean (SD)	9.2 (5.0)	8.6 (5.4)
Median (Q1–Q3)	8.8 (6.0–11.8)	7.6 (5.8–10.3)
NCCN Risk Group		
Low	16 (51%)	16 (48%)
Intermediate	15 (48%)	17 (51%)

Abbreviations: SD, standard deviation; PSA, prostate-specific antigen; Q1–Q3, first to third quartile; NCCN, National Comprehensive Cancer Network risk classification; SBRT, stereotactic body radiotherapy; CFRT, conventional fractionated radiotherapy.

2.2. Treatments Received

Of 64 eligible patients, 31 received SBRT and 33 received CFRT. Neoadjuvant androgen-deprivation therapy (ADT) was given in 10 patients (SBRT: 4; CFRT: 6). A total of 6 months of ADT with luteinizing hormone-releasing hormone agonists were prescribed 3 months prior to RT. Median follow-up from the beginning of RT was 2.2 (range: 1.7–2.7) and 2.4 (range: 1.8–2.9) years for the SBRT and CFRT arms, respectively. All 64 patients were analyzed, with no protocol violations, and none was lost to follow-up.

2.3. PRQOL

The Expanded Prostate Cancer Index Composite (EPIC) questionnaire completion compliance rate was 100% (64/64) before treatment and 96.9% (62/64) at 1 year. Given the median follow-up of 2.2–2.4 years, the 2-year or later EPIC results will not be presented here. There were no significant differences in change of score between the arms with respect to the urinary and bowel, as well as the sexual and hormonal, EPIC domains at 3, 6, 9 and 12 months (Figure 2). At 1 year, 12 (40.0%) SBRT and 15 (46.9%) CFRT patients had a >5-point reduction in EPIC bowel score compared with baseline (SBRT, $p = 0.28$; CFRT, $p = 0.08$). Regarding the EPIC urinary domain, 16 (53.3%) SBRT and 15 (46.9%) CFRT patients had a >2-point score reduction at 1 year compared with baseline (SBRT, $p = 0.07$; CFRT, $p = 0.21$; Table 2). In the SBRT arm, compared with pre-treatment assessment, 9 patients (30%) had a >11-point reduction in 1-year EPIC sexual score compared with baseline ($p = 0.28$) and 13 patients (43%) had a >3-point reduction in 1-year EPIC hormonal score compared with baseline ($p = 0.27$). In the CFRT arm, eight patients (25%) experienced a >11-point reduction in EPIC sexual score at 1 year ($p = 0.12$) and eight patients (25%) had a >3-point reduction in 1-year EPIC hormonal score ($p = 0.06$).

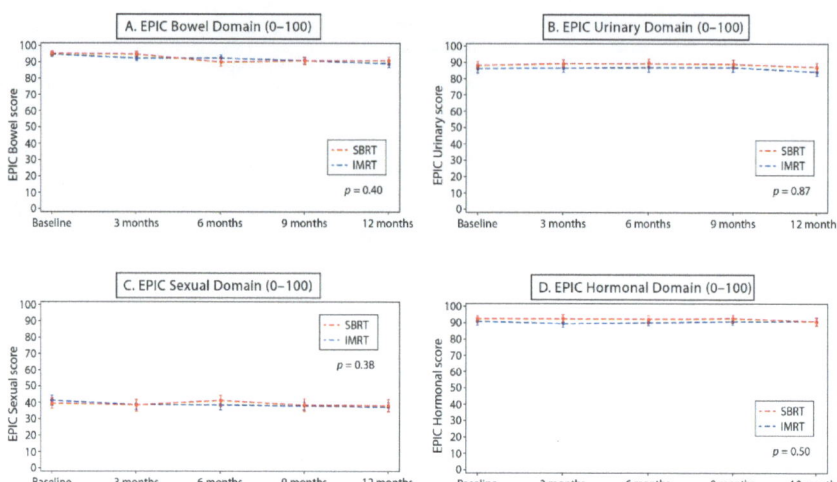

Figure 2. Mean (95% confidence interval) Expanded Prostate Cancer Index Composite questionnaire (EPIC) score over time for stereotactic body radiotherapy (SBRT) and conventional fractionated radiotherapy (CFRT): (**A**) bowel domain; (**B**) urinary domain; (**C**) sexual domain; and (**D**) hormonal domain. Abbreviations: EPIC, Expanded Prostate Cancer Index Composite questionnaire; SBRT stereotactic body radiotherapy; CFRT, conventional fractionated radiotherapy.

Table 2. Patient-reported quality of life: Expanded Prostate Cancer Index Composite questionnaire (EPIC) score change at 1 year from baseline.

Domain	SBRT	p-Value	CFRT	p-Value
Bowel				
Patients, no.	30		32	
Mean (SD)	−4.2 (12.5)	0.40 **	−5.8 (9.9)	
Median	0.0		−1.8	
>5-point reduction, no (%) [†]	12 (40%)	0.28 *	15 (46.9%)	0.08 *
Urinary				
Patients, no.	30		32	
Mean (SD)	−1.3 (12.9)	0.87 **	−2.3 (12.7)	
Median	−2.1		0.0	
>2-point reduction, no (%) [‡]	16 (53.3%)	0.07 *	15 (46.9%)	0.21 *
Sexual				
Patients, no.	30		32	
Mean (SD)	−1.9 (15.3)	0.38 **	−3.8 (18.3)	
Median	0.3		−1.8	
>11-point reduction, no (%) [§]	9 (30%)	0.28 *	8 (25%)	0.12 *
Hormonal				
Patients, no.	30		32	
Mean (SD)	−1.3 (13.8)	0.50 **	0.2 (13.6)	
Median	0.0		0.0	
>3-point reduction, no (%) [¶]	13 (43%)	0.27 *	8 (25%)	0.06 *

Abbreviations: EPIC, Expanded Prostate Cancer Index Composite questionnaire; SD, standard deviation; SBRT stereotactic body radiotherapy; CFRT, conventional fractionated radiotherapy. * p-value from one-sided, one sample z-test (before vs. after). ** p-value for the comparison between SBRT and CFRT. [†] Rate $\leq 35\%$, acceptable rate $\geq 60\%$, unacceptable (see Statistical Analysis section in Methods on details of the acceptability/unacceptability thresholds). [‡] Rate $\leq 40\%$, acceptable; rate $\geq 65\%$, unacceptable. [§] Rate $\leq 35\%$, acceptable; rate $\geq 60\%$ unacceptable. [¶] Rate $\leq 38\%$, acceptable; rate $\geq 63\%$, unacceptable.

2.4. Acute and Late Toxicities

There were no grade ≥ 3 acute toxicities reported in either arm. SBRT patients experienced significantly fewer ≥ grade 1 acute GI toxicities (cumulative number: 35% vs. 87%, $p < 0.0001$) and grade ≥ 2 acute GU toxicities (cumulative number: 3% vs. 24%, $p = 0.0426$) compared with CFRT patients. At the 1-year follow-up, two grade 3 GU late toxicities, one in each arm (SBRT: non-infective cystitis [3%]; CFRT: urinary incontinence [3%]), were reported. SBRT patients experienced significantly fewer grade ≥1 late GI toxicities (cumulative number: 64% vs. 84%, $p = 0.033$) and a similar rate of grade ≥ 1 late GU toxicities (cumulative number: 93% vs. 100%, $p = 0.2307$) than CFRT patients (Table 3).

Table 3. Acute and 1-year late gastrointestinal (GI) and genitourinary (GU) adverse events according to treatment assignment.

Adverse Event (Maximum Grade)	SBRT ($n = 31$)	CFRT ($n = 33$)	p-Value
Acute GI Toxicity			
None reported	20 (64%)	4 (12%)	
1	9 (29%)	22 (66%)	
2	2 (6%)	7 (21%)	$p < 0.0001$ [†]
≥3	0	0	
≥1 (Total)	11 (35%)	29 (87%)	
Acute GU Toxicity			
None reported	3 (9%)	0	
1	26 (83%)	25 (75%)	
2	1 (3%)	8 (24%)	$p = 0.0426$ [‡]
≥3	0	0	
≥1 (Total)	27 (87%)	33 (100%)	
1-Year Late GI Toxicity			
None reported	11 (35%)	5 (15%)	
1	16 (51%)	22 (66%)	
2	4 (12%)	6 (18%)	$p = 0.033$ [†]
≥3	0	0	
≥1 (Total)	20 (64%)	28 (84%)	
1-Year Late GU Toxicity			
None reported	2 (6%)	0	
1	23 (74%)	25 (75%)	
2	5 (16%)	7 (21%)	$p = 0.2307$ [†]
≥3	1 (3%)	1 (3%)	
≥1 (Total)	29 (93%)	33 (100%)	

Abbreviations: Gastrointestinal (GI) toxicity, toxicities including abdominal pain, bloating, constipation, diarrhea, fecal incontinence, hemorrhoids, proctitis, rectal hemorrhage, and rectal pain; genitourinary (GU) toxicity, toxicities including non-infective cystitis, hematuria, urinary frequency, urgency, retention, incontinence, and urinary tract pain; SBRT, stereotactic body radiotherapy; CFRT, conventional fractionated radiotherapy. [†] p for comparison of treatment group of grade ≥ 1 vs. grade < 1; [‡] p for comparison of treatment group of grade ≥ 2 vs. grade < 2.

2.5. Disease Control

At 1 year, two patients in the CFRT group had died of diseases unrelated to their PC (community-acquired pneumonia and sudden death of unknown reason). The overall survival rates at 1 year for the whole cohort, SBRT and CFRT patients were 98.4%, 100% and 97%, respectively ($p = 0.08$). Biochemical progressions (Phoenix criteria, PSA nadir + 2 ng/mL [21]) occurred in two CFRT patients, resulting in 98.4%, 100% and 97% biochemical failure-free survival at 1 year for all patients, SBRT and CFRT groups, respectively ($p = 0.08$).

3. Discussion

In this phase II study of SBRT vs. CFRT in low- and intermediate-risk localized PC, SBRT resulted in a similar PRQOL in terms of the proportion of patients with significant reductions in EPIC bowel and urinary scores at 1 year from baseline, and seemingly favorable physician-scored acute and late toxicities compared with CFRT. Our results suggest that SBRT is a safe, tolerable alternative to CFRT for patients with early-stage localized PC.

MHRT, based on non-inferiority to CFRT in several randomized landmark studies, is currently the recommended EBRT option for localized PC [15], but was not recognized as such when our study was conceived. In comparison to CFRT, SBRT offers similar benefits to MHRT in terms of patient convenience and resource utilization, with much shorter travel and treatment times, and potentially higher cost-effectiveness [22].

Even more important in establishing the role of SBRT in managing localized PC is its safety and tolerability. Whereas HYPO-RT-PC observed higher levels of self-reported acute urinary and bowel symptoms in patients receiving SBRT vs. CFRT, PACE-B did not (or even found slightly less acute toxicity in the SBRT arm). This might have been due to (i) the inclusion of high-risk patients in HYPO-RT-PC and low-risk patients in PACE-B, (ii) an SBRT dosage difference (HYPO-RT-PC: 42.7 Gy/7 fractions [frs]/2.5 weeks vs. PACE-B 36.25 Gy/5 frs/1–2 weeks) and/or (iii) the majority (70%) of controls in PACE-B receiving MHRT (62 Gy/20 frs/4 weeks). The present study found lower levels of GI and GU toxicity in patients receiving SBRT vs. CFRT, with more pronounced differences that could be attributable to an underpowered sample size.

Our results corroborate previous reports with regard to the favorable physician-scored toxicity of SBRT in localized PC, with <5% acute and late grade $\geq$ 3 GI and GU complications [17]. Aside from similar 1-year late GU toxicities between the two arms, fewer grade $\geq$ 1 acute/1-year late GI and grade $\geq$ 2 GU toxicities were reported with SBRT in our study. Interestingly, there was disagreement between patient-reported outcomes (PROs) and physician-scored toxicities, with seemingly favorable side effects with SBRT but similar PROs between the two treatment arms. This highlights the well-known challenges in assessing treatment-related outcomes, particularly PROs, in open-label cancer trials [23–25]. By integrating both PROs and physician-scored toxicities collectively, our study demonstrated that SBRT is not inferior to CFRT in treating localized PC.

Relatively few studies assessed the tolerability and efficacy of SBRT in intermediate risk compared with low-risk PC. Half of our study involved intermediate-risk patients demonstrating that SBRT is feasible and comparable to CFRT in this subgroup. Nonetheless, because we included the seminal vesicles (SVs) for irradiation (Supplementary Methods), the risk of possible adverse consequences with SBRT in the intermediate-risk group patients may be higher. The recent RTOG-0938 study [26], which evaluated two regimens of ultra hypofractionation (36.25 Gy/5 frs/2 weeks and 51.6 Gy/12 frs/2 weeks) for low-risk PC without incorporation of SVs in the high-dose zone, reported a seemingly lower proportion of EPIC score decline in patients randomized to the SBRT arm (36.25 Gy/5 frs/2 weeks) than ours. Specifically, only 29.8% of their SBRT patients had a >5-point reduction in EPIC bowel score from baseline at 1 year, compared with 40.0% of our SBRT patients. Similarly, 45.7% of their patients and 53.3% of our patients had a >2-point reduction in 1-year EPIC urinary score from baseline. Although a cross-trial comparison would be inappropriate statistically, the numerical difference in the proportion of patients with EPIC score decline between the two studies may be partly attributed to the SV irradiation in the intermediate risk group. However, the degree of EPIC deterioration was similar between SBRT and CFRT in this study, suggesting that such an influence is more likely related to the larger irradiation volume than the dose-fractionation in intermediate-risk disease.

This study has several limitations. First, this trial only compared SBRT to CFRT, and not the currently recommended MHRT. However, since various studies have established the non-inferiority of MHRT to CFRT, we expect that the results of a SBRT vs. MHRT comparison will be similar. Second, the limited data on long-term PROs and efficacy can be attributed to the relatively short follow-up. While follow-up of our cohorts will continue, previous retrospective series and pooled-analysis demonstrated comparable long-term efficacy and tolerability to other definitive treatments, suggesting that our preliminary results will likely be sustained [16,17,27]. Third, endorectal balloons (ERBs) were used only in the SBRT arm, thus their potential benefits, e.g., reducing intra-fractional prostatic motion and displacing the posterior part of the rectum out of the high-dose zone, could have contributed to the better tolerability in the SBRT arm. However, such benefits could have been outweighed by the considerable detrimental dosimetric effect of ERBs on the rectum via the displacement of the anterior rectal wall into the ultra-high-dose zone with SBRT, which was shown in a prior dosimetric study [28]. Furthermore, 7–8 weeks of daily ERB application in the CFRT arm would have been impractical and disturbing for the patients.

4. Materials and Methods

4.1. Trial Design

This was a single-institution, unblinded randomized phase II study with 1:1 random assignment to SBRT (36.25 Gy in 5 frs over 2 weeks) or CFRT (76 Gy in 38 frs over 7.5 weeks). Participants were randomly assigned by the minimization method to either SBRT or CFRT, and stratified by the risk of localized PC using the NCCN risk classification (low vs. intermediate). The study was approved by the institutional review board (CUHK/NTEC CREC Ref. No. 2013.483-T) and registered at ClinicalTrials.gov (NCT02339701).

4.2. Study Patients

Men aged $\geq$ 18 years with a histologic diagnosis of prostate adenocarcinoma and NCCN low- or intermediate-risk (T1-2, Gleason score $\leq$ 7 and PSA < 20 ng/mL) localized disease were eligible for the study. Additional criteria were Zubrod performance status < 2, no nodal or distant metastasis, and no prior bilateral orchiectomy, chemotherapy, RT, cryosurgery, or definitive surgery for PC. Patients with another invasive cancer, other than localized basal or squamous cell skin carcinoma, were ineligible. Only patients who were willing and able to complete the EPIC questionnaire and signed and understood the informed consent were enrolled.

4.3. Treatments

The prescription doses to planning target volume (PTV)-1/PTV-2 in the SBRT and CFRT arms were 36.25 Gy/32.5 Gy in five frs and 76 Gy/70 Gy in 38 frs, respectively. The patients were treated with volumetric modulated arc therapy (VMAT) using a Varian TrueBeam 2.0 linear accelerator with Millennium 120 MLC (Supplementary Methods). Dose constraints to normal tissues (bladder, rectum, penile bulb) were as listed in the protocol (in Supplementary Materials). Neoadjuvant androgen-deprivation therapy (ADT) was optional, given at physician's discretion for intermediate-risk PC patients.

4.4. Patient Assessments

At baseline, patient history, physical examination, toxicity and performance status were assessed. Pre-treatment assessment also included PSA measurement and the EPIC questionnaire [29]. The serine protease PSA is almost produced exclusively by prostate epithelial cells, and it is thought that prostate tumor growth leads to leakage of PSA into the blood [30]. Early-stage PC tumors secrete PSA, which is useful as a biomarker for monitoring response to therapy, and predicting pathologic stages over time [30].

In this study, the traditional Chinese version of EPIC was used (see Clinical Trial Protocol in Supplementary Materials), which was translated and culturally adapted from the original English version in a validation study [31]. Both versions of the instrument are now available on the University of Michigan Department of Urology website (https://medicine.umich.edu/dept/urology/research/epic, accessed on 17 December 2021).

Patients were evaluated weekly during RT for performance status and toxicities. An acute adverse event was defined as the first occurrence of worst severity of the adverse event from the beginning of RT until ≤30 days after the completion of RT. Both acute and late adverse events were evaluated with the Common Terminology Criteria for Adverse Events (version 4.0). Assessments were performed and the EPIC questionnaire collected every 3 months for the first 2 years, every 6 months for the next 3 years and annually thereafter.

4.5. Study Endpoints

The primary endpoint of this study was to evaluate and compare the PRQOL by the proportion of patients with >5-point and >2-point reductions in the EPIC bowel and urinary domains, respectively, at 1 year compared with baseline, between the two treatment arms. Additional endpoints included the sexual and hormonal EPIC scores, acute and late toxicities, bRFS, and overall survival.

4.6. Statistical Analysis

As in the RTOG 0415 and RTOG 0938 studies, the proportion of patients with a change in EPIC bowel domain score (baseline to 1-year) worse than 5 points and a change in urinary domain score worse than 2 points were considered to be clinically meaningful endpoints for the tolerability and safety of radical prostate RT [12,26]. These thresholds were selected from an analysis of EPIC scores in 108 patients who received standard RT treatment in RTOG 0415, based on the universal notion that half of a standard deviation constitutes a threshold of discrimination for changes in health-related QOL for chronic diseases [26,32]. EPIC change scores were compared between treatment arms using a t-test, p-values < 0.05 were considered statistically significant. All analyses were conducted using Statistical Analysis Software (SAS for Windows, version 9.3).

5. Conclusions

SBRT had similar PRQOL and less toxicity than CFRT in this phase II study of Chinese men with localized PC. In corroboration with the latest phase III results, our results support SBRT as a safe and tolerable treatment option in low- and intermediate-risk PC.

Supplementary Materials: The following are available online at https://www.mdpi.com/article/10.3390/curroncol29010003/s1, Supplementary Methods and Clinical Trial Protocol.

Author Contributions: Conception and design: D.M.C.P., F.M.; provision of study materials or patients: D.L., K.C.W.W., C.-M.C., M.C. and C.-F.N.; collection and assembly of data: D.M.C.P. and F.M.; data analysis and interpretation: D.M.C.P. and F.M.; manuscript writing: all authors; final approval of manuscript: all authors. All authors have read and agreed to the published version of the manuscript.

Funding: This study did not receive any specific grants from funding agencies in the public, commercial, or not-for-profit sectors.

Institutional Review Board Statement: The study was conducted according to the guidelines of the Declaration of Helsinki, and approved by the Joint Chinese University of Hong Kong—New Territories East Cluster Clinical Research Ethics Committee (Ref. No. 2013.483-T; date of approval: 20 November 2013) and registered at ClinicalTrials.gov (NCT02339701).

Informed Consent Statement: Informed consent was obtained from all subjects involved in the study.

Data Availability Statement: Request to obtain the study data may be addressed to the corresponding author. The data are not publicly available due to ethical (privacy) and legal considerations.

Conflicts of Interest: The authors declare that they have no conflict of interest.

References

1. Hamdy, F.C.; Donovan, J.L.; Lane, J.A.; Mason, M.; Metcalfe, C.; Holding, P.; Davis, M.; Peters, T.J.; Turner, E.L.; Martin, R.M.; et al. 10-Year Outcomes after Monitoring, Surgery, or Radiotherapy for Localized Prostate Cancer. *N. Engl. J. Med.* **2016**, *375*, 1415–1424. [CrossRef]
2. Swisher-McClure, S.; Mitra, N.; Woo, K.; Smaldone, M.; Uzzo, R.; Bekelman, J.E. Increasing use of dose-escalated external beam radiation therapy for men with nonmetastatic prostate cancer. *Int. J. Radiat. Oncol. Biol. Phys.* **2014**, *89*, 103–112. [CrossRef] [PubMed]
3. Nguyen, P.L.; Gu, X.; Lipsitz, S.R.; Choueiri, T.K.; Choi, W.W.; Lei, Y.; Hoffman, K.E.; Hu, J.C. Cost implications of the rapid adoption of newer technologies for treating prostate cancer. *J. Clin. Oncol.* **2011**, *29*, 1517–1524. [CrossRef]
4. Barton, M.B.; Jacob, S.; Shafiq, J.; Wong, K.; Thompson, S.R.; Hanna, T.P.; Delaney, G.P. Estimating the demand for radiotherapy from the evidence: A review of changes from 2003 to 2012. *Radiother Oncol.* **2014**, *112*, 140–144. [CrossRef]
5. Delaney, G.; Jacob, S.; Barton, M. Estimating the optimal external-beam radiotherapy utilization rate for genitourinary malignancies. *Cancer* **2005**, *103*, 462–473. [CrossRef]
6. Gustavsen, G.; Gullet, L.; Cole, D.; Lewine, N.; Bishoff, J.T. Economic burden of illness associated with localized prostate cancer in the United States. *Future Oncol.* **2020**, *16*, 4265–4277. [CrossRef] [PubMed]
7. Yan, M.; Gouveia, A.G.; Cury, F.L.; Moideen, N.; Bratti, V.F.; Patrocinio, H.; Berlin, A.; Mendez, L.C.; Moraes, F.Y. Practical considerations for prostate hypofractionation in the developing world. *Nat. Rev. Urol.* **2021**, *18*, 669–685. [CrossRef]
8. McMahon, S.J. The linear quadratic model: Usage, interpretation and challenges. *Phys. Med. Biol.* **2018**, *64*, 01TR. [CrossRef]
9. Miralbell, R.; Roberts, S.A.; Zubizarreta, E.; Hendry, J.H. Dose-fractionation sensitivity of prostate cancer deduced from radiotherapy outcomes of 5, 969 patients in seven international institutional datasets: Alpha/beta = 1.4 (0.9 − 2.2) Gy. *Int. J. Radiat. Oncol. Biol. Phys.* **2012**, *82*, e17–e24. [CrossRef] [PubMed]
10. Vogelius, I.R.; Bentzen, S.M. Meta-analysis of the alpha/beta ratio for prostate cancer in the presence of an overall time factor: Bad news, good news, or no news? *Int. J. Radiat. Oncol. Biol. Phys.* **2013**, *85*, 89–94. [CrossRef] [PubMed]
11. Dearnaley, D.; Syndikus, I.; Mossop, H.; Khoo, V.; Birtle, A.; Bloomfield, D.; Graham, J.; Kirkbride, P.; Logue, J.; Malik, Z.; et al. Conventional versus hypofractionated high-dose intensity-modulated radiotherapy for prostate cancer: 5-year outcomes of the randomised, non-inferiority, phase 3 CHHiP trial. *Lancet Oncol.* **2016**, *17*, 1047–1060. [CrossRef]
12. Lee, W.R.; Dignam, J.J.; Amin, M.B.; Bruner, D.W.; Low, D.; Swanson, G.P.; Shah, A.B.; D'Souza, D.P.; Michalski, J.M.; Dayes, I.S.; et al. Randomized Phase III Noninferiority Study Comparing Two Radiotherapy Fractionation Schedules in Patients With Low-Risk Prostate Cancer. *J. Clin. Oncol.* **2016**, *34*, 2325–2332. [CrossRef] [PubMed]
13. Catton, C.N.; Lukka, H.; Gu, C.S.; Martin, J.M.; Supiot, S.; Chung, P.W.M.; Bauman, G.S.; Bahary, J.P.; Ahmed, S.; Cheung, P.; et al. Randomized Trial of a Hypofractionated Radiation Regimen for the Treatment of Localized Prostate Cancer. *J. Clin. Oncol.* **2017**, *35*, 1884–1890. [CrossRef] [PubMed]
14. Arcangeli, G.; Saracino, B.; Arcangeli, S.; Gomellini, S.; Petrongari, M.G.; Sanguineti, G.; Strigari, L. Moderate Hypofractionation in High-Risk, Organ-Confined Prostate Cancer: Final Results of a Phase III Randomized Trial. *J. Clin. Oncol.* **2017**, *35*, 1891–1897. [CrossRef] [PubMed]
15. Morgan, S.C.; Hoffman, K.; Loblaw, D.A.; Buyyounouski, M.K.; Patton, C.; Barocas, D.; Bentzen, S.; Chang, M.; Efstathiou, J.; Greany, P.; et al. Hypofractionated Radiation Therapy for Localized Prostate Cancer: An ASTRO, ASCO, and AUA Evidence-Based Guideline. *J. Clin. Oncol.* **2018**, *36*, JCO1801097. [CrossRef]
16. King, C.R.; Freeman, D.; Kaplan, I.; Fuller, D.; Bolzicco, G.; Collins, S.; Meier, R.; Wang, J.; Kupelian, P.; Steinberg, M.; et al. Stereotactic body radiotherapy for localized prostate cancer: Pooled analysis from a multi-institutional consortium of prospective phase II trials. *Radiother Oncol.* **2013**, *109*, 217–221. [CrossRef] [PubMed]
17. Jackson, W.C.; Silva, J.; Hartman, H.E.; Dess, R.T.; Kishan, A.U.; Beeler, W.H.; Gharzai, L.A.; Jaworski, E.M.; Mehra, R.; Hearn, J.W.D.; et al. Stereotactic Body Radiation Therapy for Localized Prostate Cancer: A Systematic Review and Meta-Analysis of Over 6000 Patients Treated On Prospective Studies. *Int. J. Radiat. Oncol. Biol. Phys.* **2019**, *104*, 778–789. [CrossRef]
18. Lehrer, E.J.; Kishan, A.U.; Yu, J.B.; Trifiletti, D.M.; Showalter, T.N.; Ellis, R.; Zaorsky, N.G. Ultrahypofractionated versus hypofractionated and conventionally fractionated radiation therapy for localized prostate cancer: A systematic review and meta-analysis of phase III randomized trials. *Radiother Oncol.* **2020**, *148*, 235–242. [CrossRef] [PubMed]
19. Widmark, A.; Gunnlaugsson, A.; Beckman, L.; Thellenberg-Karlsson, C.; Hoyer, M.; Lagerlund, M.; Kindblom, J.; Ginman, C.; Johansson, B.; Bjornlinger, K.; et al. Ultra-hypofractionated versus conventionally fractionated radiotherapy for prostate cancer: 5-year outcomes of the HYPO-RT-PC randomised, non-inferiority, phase 3 trial. *Lancet* **2019**, *394*, 385–395. [CrossRef]
20. Brand, D.H.; Tree, A.C.; Ostler, P.; van der Voet, H.; Loblaw, D.A.; Chu, W.; Ford, D.; Tolan, S.; Jain, S.; Martin, A.; et al. Intensity-modulated fractionated radiotherapy versus stereotactic body radiotherapy for prostate cancer (PACE-B): Acute toxicity findings from an international, randomised, open-label, phase 3, non-inferiority trial. *Lancet Oncol.* **2019**, *20*, 1531–1543. [CrossRef]
21. Roach, M., 3rd; Hanks, G.; Thames, H., Jr.; Schellhammer, P.; Shipley, W.U.; Sokol, G.H.; Sandler, H. Defining biochemical failure following radiotherapy with or without hormonal therapy in men with clinically localized prostate cancer: Recommendations of the RTOG-ASTRO Phoenix Consensus Conference. *Int. J. Radiat. Oncol. Biol. Phys.* **2006**, *65*, 965–974. [CrossRef]
22. Hodges, J.C.; Lotan, Y.; Boike, T.P.; Benton, R.; Barrier, A.; Timmerman, R.D. Cost-effectiveness analysis of stereotactic body radiation therapy versus intensity-modulated radiation therapy: An emerging initial radiation treatment option for organ-confined prostate cancer. *J. Oncol. Pract.* **2012**, *8* (Suppl. 3), e31s–e37s. [CrossRef] [PubMed]

23. Rammant, E.; Ost, P.; Swimberghe, M.; Vanderstraeten, B.; Lumen, N.; Decaestecker, K.; Bultijnck, R.; De Meerleer, G.; Sarrazyn, C.; Colman, R.; et al. Patient- versus physician-reported outcomes in prostate cancer patients receiving hypofractionated radiotherapy within a randomized controlled trial. *Strahlenther Onkol.* **2019**, *195*, 393–401. [CrossRef]
24. Atkinson, T.M.; Wagner, J.S.; Basch, E. Trustworthiness of Patient-Reported Outcomes in Unblinded Cancer Clinical Trials. *JAMA Oncol.* **2017**, *3*, 738–739. [CrossRef]
25. Roydhouse, J.K.; Fiero, M.H.; Kluetz, P.G. Investigating Potential Bias in Patient-Reported Outcomes in Open-label Cancer Trials. *JAMA Oncol.* **2019**, *5*, 457–458. [CrossRef]
26. Lukka, H.R.; Pugh, S.L.; Bruner, D.W.; Bahary, J.P.; Lawton, C.A.F.; Efstathiou, J.A.; Kudchadker, R.J.; Ponsky, L.E.; Seaward, S.A.; Dayes, I.S.; et al. Patient Reported Outcomes in NRG Oncology RTOG 0938, Evaluating Two Ultrahypofractionated Regimens for Prostate Cancer. *Int. J. Radiat. Oncol. Biol. Phys.* **2018**, *102*, 287–295. [CrossRef] [PubMed]
27. King, C.R.; Collins, S.; Fuller, D.; Wang, P.C.; Kupelian, P.; Steinberg, M.; Katz, A. Health-related quality of life after stereotactic body radiation therapy for localized prostate cancer: Results from a multi-institutional consortium of prospective trials. *Int. J Radiat. Oncol. Biol. Phys.* **2013**, *87*, 939–945. [CrossRef] [PubMed]
28. Wong, A.T.; Schreiber, D.; Agarwal, M.; Polubarov, A.; Schwartz, D. Impact of the use of an endorectal balloon on rectal dosimetry during stereotactic body radiation therapy for localized prostate cancer. *Pract. Radiat. Oncol.* **2016**, *6*, 262–267. [CrossRef]
29. Wei, J.T.; Dunn, R.L.; Sandler, H.M.; McLaughlin, P.W.; Montie, J.E.; Litwin, M.S.; Nyquist, L.; Sanda, M.G. Comprehensive comparison of health-related quality of life after contemporary therapies for localized prostate cancer. *J. Clin. Oncol.* **2002**, *20*, 557–566. [CrossRef] [PubMed]
30. Payne, H.; Cornford, P. Prostate-specific antigen: An evolving role in diagnosis, monitoring, and treatment evaluation in prostate cancer. *Urol. Oncol.* **2011**, *29*, 593–601. [CrossRef] [PubMed]
31. Lee, T.K.; Poon, D.M.C.; Ng, A.C.F.; Ho, T.; Singh-Carlson, S.; Joffres, M.; Oshan, G.; Kohli, J.; Kwan, W. Cultural adaptation and validation of the Chinese version of the expanded prostate cancer index composite. *Asia Pac. J. Clin. Oncol.* **2018**, *14* (Suppl. 1), 10–15. [CrossRef] [PubMed]
32. Norman, G.R.; Sloan, J.A.; Wyrwich, K.W. Interpretation of changes in health-related quality of life: The remarkable universality of half a standard deviation. *Med. Care* **2003**, *41*, 582–592. [CrossRef] [PubMed]

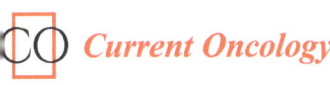

Article

Acute Toxicity and Quality of Life in a Post-Prostatectomy Ablative Radiation Therapy (POPART) Multicentric Trial

Raffaella Lucchini [1,2], Ciro Franzese [3,4,*], Suela Vukcaj [5], Giorgio Purrello [1,2], Denis Panizza [1,6], Valeria Faccenda [6,7], Stefano Andreoli [8], Gian Luca Poli [8], Davide Baldaccini [4], Lorenzo Lo Faro [3,4], Stefano Tomatis [4], Luigi Franco Cazzaniga [5], Marta Scorsetti [3,4] and Stefano Arcangeli [1,2]

1. School of Medicine and Surgery, University of Milan Bicocca, 20126 Milan, Italy
2. Department of Radiation Oncology, ASST Monza, 20900 Monza, Italy
3. Department of Biomedical Sciences, Humanitas University, Via Rita Levi Montalcini 4Pieve Emanuele, 20090 Milan, Italy
4. Department of Radiotherapy and Radiosurgery, Humanitas Clinical and Research Center—IRCCS, Rozzano, 20089 Milan, Italy
5. Department of Radiation Oncology, ASST Papa Giovanni XXIII, 24127 Bergamo, Italy
6. Department of Medical Physics, ASST Monza, 20900 Monza, Italy
7. Department of Physics, University of Milan, 20122 Milan, Italy
8. Department of Medical Physics, ASST Papa Giovanni XXIII, 24127 Bergamo, Italy
* Correspondence: ciro.franzese@hunimed.eu

Abstract: Background: The aim of this study was to investigate the feasibility of ultrahypofractionated radiotherapy to the prostate bed in patients with biochemical and/or clinical relapse following radical prostatectomy who were enrolled in the prospective, observational, multicentric POPART trial (NCT04831970). Methods: Patients with post-radical prostatectomy PSA levels of ≥ 0.1–2.0 ng/mL and/or local relapse at PSMA PET/CT or multiparametric MRI were treated with Linac-based SBRT on the prostate bed up to a total dose of 32.5 Gy in five fractions every other day (EQD2$_{1.5}$ = 74.2 Gy). Maximum acute toxicity was assessed using the Common Terminology Criteria for Adverse Events version 5 scale. International Consultation on Incontinence Questionnaire—Short Form (ICIQ-SF) and Prostate Cancer Index Composite for Clinical Practice (EPIC-CP) scores were assessed at baseline and during the follow-up. Results: From April 2021 to June 2022, thirty men with a median age of 72 years (range 55–82) were enrolled in three centers. The median PSA level before RT was 0.30 ng/mL (range 0.18–1.89 ng/mL). At 3 months post-treatment, no GI or ≥ 2 GU side effects were reported; three patients (10%) experienced Grade 1 GU toxicity. No changes in ICIQ-SF or in the urinary domains of EPIC-CP were observed, while a transient worsening was registered in the bowel domain. At the same time point, all but two patients, who progressed distantly, were found to be biochemically controlled with a median post-treatment PSA level of 0.07 ng/mL (range 0–0.48 ng/mL). Conclusions: Our preliminary findings show that SBRT can be safely extended to the postoperative setting, without an increase in short-term toxicity or a significant decline in QoL. Long-term results are needed to confirm this strategy.

Keywords: prostate cancer; postoperative setting; SBRT

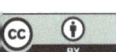

1. Introduction

Regardless of the two settings (adjuvant or salvage), external-beam radiation therapy (RT) for prostate cancer is usually a protracted course, since a total dose of 64 Gy to 72 Gy is needed to be effective [1,2]. In addition, a randomized trial [3] has recently proven the benefit of extending salvage RT to the pelvic lymph nodes in combination with short-term androgen deprivation therapy (ADT) in patients with a detectable or rising prostate-specific antigen (PSA) level after prostatectomy. All these strategies share a typical rate of 1.8 Gy to 2.0 Gy per treatment, taking up to 39 fractions over the course of 8 weeks to be completed, which is extremely time-consuming and barely convenient for both patients and the healthcare system.

Since the end of the 1990s, dose–response analyses of patients with prostate cancer treated with both external-beam RT and brachytherapy have led to the assumption that the α/β ratio of prostate cancer is lower than that for most other tumors and approaches a value characteristic of late-responding tissues. Values between 1.2 and 3.9 Gy have been proposed [4–6]. Therefore, delivering the same equivalent dose at 2 Gy per fraction (EQD2) to the prostate using a larger than conventional (2 Gy) fraction size would not affect late side effects and would result in a sparing effect on early responding normal tissues. Hypofractionation would thus reduce early side effects (if overall treatment time is left constant) or could be used to shorten overall treatment time owing to the increased therapeutic index. This strategy is expected to be at least isoeffective in terms of tumor control but with the associated advantages of cost, logistics and patient convenience. However, while non-inferiority trials [7–10] have confirmed these premises and validated moderate hypofractionation as an established treatment modality in the radical setting, such an approach has traditionally been hampered in the postoperative setting, likely due to the concerns that high radiation doses in the anastomosis (where most recurrences occur) may lead to tissue injury. To date, few studies [11,12] have explored the use of hypofractionation for salvage RT in patients with biochemical recurrence after prostatectomy, showing excellent outcomes in terms of both efficacy and toxicity. However, differences in follow-up radiation techniques and treatment schedules prevent any definitive conclusion. Data are even more scarce for Stereotactic Body Radiation Therapy (SBRT), which is on the shortest end of the hypofractionation spectrum, with only a phase II trial reporting on the Quality of-Life Outcomes and Toxicity Profile of 100 patients who received post-prostatectomy SBRT doses of 30–34 Gy in five fractions to the prostate bed, either with MRI-guided RT or standard computed tomography-guided RT [13].

In this study, we aimed to report on the short-term physician-scored genitourinary (GU) and gastrointestinal (GI) toxicities and the Quality of Life (QoL) of a cohort of patients enrolled in a post-prostatectomy SBRT multicentric trial.

2. Methods

2.1. Study Design

The POPART trial was a multicentric, prospective, observational trial (NCT04831970) aimed at evaluating the feasibility of postoperative SBRT for prostate cancer in terms of toxicity and QoL. The study was approved by the Ethical Committees of the participating centers. All participants provided written informed consent prior to trial enrollment in agreement with the Declaration of Helsinki [14].

2.2. Eligibility

Patients eligible for this study must have had adenocarcinoma of the prostate treated with radical prostatectomy (any type of radical prostatectomy was permitted, including retropubic, perineal, laparoscopic or robotically assisted; there was no time limit for the date of radical prostatectomy). Additional factors were required as inclusion criteria, such as a post-radical prostatectomy PSA level between 0.1 and 2.0 ng/mL; adverse pathologic features (pathologic T3/T4 disease with or without positive surgical margins) and/or a rising prostate-specific antigen (PSA) level > 0.1 ng/mL on at least two consecutive measurements; and no distant metastases on [^{18}F]-PSMA positron emission tomography (PET) within 60 days prior to registration. ADT was allowed, and its prescription was left at the physician's discretion.

2.3. Treatment Planning and Radiation Delivery

The patients were immobilized in the supine position using the FeetFix (CIVCO Medical Solutions, Coralville, IA, USA) system anchored to the couch for ankle fixation with their arms placed over their chest. To assess anatomical reproducibility and organ motion mitigation, before simulation and each treatment, the patients were administered a micro-enema and asked to fill their bladder by drinking 500 mL of still water.

The clinical target volume (CTV) was delineated according to the Groupe Francophone de Radiothérapie Urologique (GFRU) Guideline [15]. The planning target volume (PTV) included CTV with a 5 mm isotropic 3D margin, except for at the rectum interface, where the margin was kept at 3 mm. Volumetric Modulated Arc Therapy (VMAT) treatment consisted of two 6 MV or 10 MV flattening filter free (FFF) full arcs optimized to ensure that the 95% isodose covered at least 95% of the PTV. SBRT was scheduled in 5 fractions every other day for a total dose of either 31 Gy or 32.5 Gy, according to the adjuvant or salvage intent. The corresponding EQD2 considering an α/β ratio of 1.5 Gy was 68.2 Gy and 74.3 Gy, respectively. Mandatory dose–volume constraints were defined for both target coverage and the avoidance of normal adjacent tissues, including the rectum, rectum wall, bladder, bladder wall and penile bulb, as shown in Table 1. Accurate patient setup was obtained using kilovoltage cone-beam CT (CBCT) before each session to check the anatomical reproducibility.

Table 1. Treatment Planning Dose–Volume Constraints for Post-prostatectomy SBRT.

PTV D95%	D95% ≥ 95%	≥30.875 Gy
PTV Maximum	Dmax < 107%	<34.800 Gy
Rectal Wall Maximum	Dmax < 107%	<34.800 Gy
Rectal Wall D (1 cc) (Dose to 1 cc)	<100% of Prescribed Dose	<32.500 Gy
Rectal wall D50% (Dose to 50% Volume)		<22.500 Gy
Bladder Wall Maximum	Dmax < 107%	<34.800 Gy
Bladder Wall D (10 cc) (Dose to 10 cc)	<100% of Prescribed Dose	<32.500 Gy
Bladder Wall D25% (Dose to 25% Volume)	<100% of Prescribed Dose	<32.500 Gy
Bladder Wall D50% (Dose to 50% Volume)		<24.000 Gy
Small/Large Bowel Maximum		<20.000/25.000 Gy
Penile Bulb	<100% of Prescribed Dose	3 cc 24.000 Gy
Femur Maximum		<30.000 Gy

2.4. Toxicity and Quality of Life Assessment

Toxicity, as defined by the National Cancer Institute Common Terminology Criteria for Adverse Events v.5.0, was assessed at baseline, at the end of treatment and every 3 months thereafter. The ICIQ-SF and the Expanded Prostate Cancer Index Composite for Clinical Practice (EPIC-CP) bowel and urinary QoL [16,17] scores were collected once prior to treatment and thereafter at the aforementioned time points via questionnaires. Paired t-test and the Wilcoxon signed-rank test were used to compare pretreatment and post-treatment EPIC-CP domain scores. The incidence of acute treatment-related GU and GI toxicities, patient QoL and PSA outcomes were computed from the start of the treatment to the last follow-up.

3. Results

3.1. Population Characteristics

From April 2021 to 30 June 2022, patients (median age, 72 years; range, 55–82) were enrolled in the multicentric POPART trial and completed the study treatment. Their baseline demographic and clinical characteristics, as well as treatment parameters, are shown in Table 2. The majority (74%) had a biochemical relapse only, while eight patients (26%) also had a local relapse. The median PSA level before RT was 0.30 ng/mL (range 0.18–1.89 ng/mL). Four patients (13%) received ADT. At baseline, the median ICIQ-SF score was 1 (range 0–8). The median PTV was 72 cc (range 14.8–250.2 cc).

Table 2. Patients, Disease and Treatment Characteristics.

Age	
Median	72 [range 55–82]
PSA pre-prostatectomy (ng/mL)	
Median	6.04 [range 3.30–17.25]
Gleason score	
6 (3 + 3)	4 (13%)
7 (3 + 4)	12 (40%)
7 (4 + 3)	11 (37%)
8 (4 + 4)	2 (6.5%)
9 (4 + 5)	1 (3.5%)
ISUP Grade Group	
1	4 (13%)
2	12 (40%)
3	11 (37%)
4	2 (6.5%)
5	1 (3.5%)
Pathological T stage	
pT2	19 (64%)
pT3a	8 (26%)
pT3b	3 (10%)
Positive Margins	
R1	11 (37%)
R1 and positive apex	8 (26%)
Time from prostatectomy (months)	
Median	54.5 [range 7–155]
Clinical relapse	
Yes	8 (26%)
No	22 (74%)
PSA pre-SBRT (ng/mL)	
Median	0.30 [range 0.18–1.89]
ADT	
Yes	4 (13%)
No	26 (87%)
CTV (cc)	
Median	29.39 [range 4.40–149.00]
PTV (cc)	
Median	72 [range 14.8–250.2]

3.2. Treatment Outcome

All patients completed the treatment according to the protocol's schedule. After SBRT completion, only one instance of Grade 2 acute GI toxicity was documented; no ≥ Grade 2 acute GU toxicity was observed, and three patients experienced Grade 1 GU side effects. At the three-month follow-up, no GI or ≥Grade 2 GU side effects were reported; Grade 1 GU toxicity was detected in three patients (10%) (Table 3). Three months after SBRT, all but two patients, who progressed in new distant sites, were found to be biochemically controlled with a median post-treatment PSA level of 0.07 ng/mL (range 0–0.48 ng/mL).

Table 3. Maximum acute toxicity during radiation or within 3 months after RT.

	0	1	2	≥3
GI	29 (97%)	—	1 (3%)	—
GU	27 (90%)	3 (10%)	—	—

3.3. Quality of Life

The ICIQ-SF assessed at baseline and 3 months after treatment remained unchanged with a median score of 1 (range 1–8). In agreement with the results of the ICIQ-SF, there was no significant decline in the median EPIC-CP scores in the urinary domains at the end of the treatment and 3 months after. Conversely, in the bowel domain, a transient worsening was observed at the end of SBRT with a median value of 1.8 ($\pm$0.2) from the baseline of 0.7 ($\pm$0.1), but this returned to the pre-treatment level at a later time point, with a median score of 0.8 ($\pm$0.1) at 3 months (Table 4).

Table 4. Patients reported HRQOL using EPIC-CP.

	Mean $\pm$ SD Score		
	Baseline	End of Treatment	3 Months
Urinary incontinence	1.6 $\pm$ 0.1	1.8 $\pm$ 0.1	1.6 $\pm$ 0.1
Urinary irritation/obstruction	1.2 $\pm$ 0.1	1.8 $\pm$ 0.2	1.6 $\pm$ 0.1
Bowel symptoms	0.7 $\pm$ 0.1	1.8 $\pm$ 0.2	0.8 $\pm$ 0.1
Sexual dysfunctions	5.3 $\pm$ 0.2	5.3 $\pm$ 0.2	5.8 $\pm$ 0.2
Hormonal symptoms	1.1 $\pm$ 0.1	1.3 $\pm$ 0.1	1.6 $\pm$ 0.1

4. Discussion

It has been established that, in the salvage setting, for each additional Gy, there is an approximately 2.5% improvement in 5 y biochemical relapse-free survival (bRFS) [18]. However, two phase III dose-escalation studies using conventional schedules showed only increased rates of GI side effects without providing any benefits to the patients [1,2]. Due to the low α/β ratio of prostate cancer, hypofractionation might represent a window of opportunity aimed at maintaining the same local control (isoeffective) while potentially decreasing the risk of treatment-related toxicities, as already proven in the primary setting [7–10]. Historically, in the postoperative setting, the use of hypofractionation has for a long time been discouraged because microscopic relapse in the prostate bed can only be inferred because of some concerns that high radiation doses absorbed by tissues, which have been already injured by surgery, could have resulted in an increased risk of developing major toxicities. Indeed, some evidence became available from a number of retrospective studies of salvage moderately hypofractionated RT with small sample sizes and different endpoints. Their results were summarized in a systematic review [11], involving more than 1200 patients, which showed that an EQD2 dose > 70 Gy was associated with better bRFS (namely, 83%, 85.4% and 100% in three studies) and a 5-year $\geq$ Grade 2 toxicity ranging between 7.3% and 18.1%. Another metanalysis [12] on five retrospective studies of moderate hypofractionation in the salvage setting in 369 patients reported encouraging results of 3-year bRFS of 73% and late $\geq$ Grade 2 GU and GI toxicities of 6% and 3%, respectively. However, differences in the number of patients, fractionation schedules and the duration of follow-up raise some uncertainties and lower the quality of the evidence. More robust data came from a phase II single trial [19] reporting on 61 patients treated with a salvage hypofractionated regimen of 15 fractions of 3.4 Gy each: with a median follow-up of 16 months, only two cases of acute (primary endpoint) and late > Grade 3 GU events were documented, along with bRFS rates of 95.1%. When approaching extreme hypofractionation, the latest evidence was provided by the largest prospective study of post-prostatectomy SBRT [13] reporting on 100 participants treated with a median prostate bed dose of 32 Gy in five fractions: at a median follow-up of 29.5 months, acute and late Grade 2 GU toxicities were both 9%, while acute and late Grade 2 GI toxicities were 5% and 0%, respectively. Interestingly, those treated with MRI-guided RT (MRgRT) showed a 30% reduction in any grade acute GI toxicity and improved bowel QoL.

Our prospective study is among the few reporting on early toxicity and QoL assessment following postoperative SBRT. Besides the Scimitar trial [13], only a metanalysis [20] is available on extreme hypofractionation in the salvage setting, including 11 retrospective series, which showed acceptable rates of acute and late GU and GI toxicity; however, in all but two, the radiation target was a macroscopic recurrence and not the prostate bed. When our study was conceived, we designed two slightly different SBRT regimens according to the adjuvant or salvage setting. As a matter of fact, all patients received salvage SBRT for biochemical recurrence, and none were treated on the basis of negative prognostic findings at pathologic specimen examination with PSA controlled. This attitude likely acknowledged the results from the Artistic metanalysis [21], which suggested that early salvage RT is the preferable treatment policy, as it can spare many patients from the overtreatment of upfront RT and its associated adverse events. Likewise, ADT was left to the physician's discretion because, at that time, there was no compelling evidence that it added clear benefit in the salvage setting. Recently, a randomized trial [3] for the first time showed that the combination of short-term ADT with salvage RT extended to treat the pelvic lymph nodes led to significant reductions in progression in patients with a detectable or rising PSA after prostatectomy. This benefit however came at the cost of a significant increase in the risk of late $\geq$ Grade 2 blood or bone marrow events (p = 0.0060), attributable to the addition of pelvic nodal RT. In view of the detrimental prognosis of such hematologic toxicity, namely leukopenia, associated with extended-field RT [22,23], hypofractionation to the prostate bed may only result in providing a protective effect against leukotoxicity [24], thus increasing its therapeutic gain.

In our series, the rates of clinically relevant acute and subacute side effects and QoL were almost negligible and nearly equivalent to those reported in the retrospective series employing moderate hypofractionation, mostly with IMRT [11,12,25–27]. These results also compare favorably to the acute $\geq$ Grade 2 GU toxicity of 0–8% and the $\geq$Grade 2 GI toxicity of 33–58% observed in patients receiving similar doses on two prior phase I SBRT trials [28,29] and with two phase II trials using either moderate hypofractionation [19] or extreme hypofractionation [13]. Notably, in the latter study, the authors attributed the improvements in GI toxicity and QoL to the narrower PTV margins obtained with MRgRT (3 mm) compared to the 5 mm used with standard computed tomography-guided RT (CTgRT). In our study, treating the prostate bed with a similar schedule on a Linac platform and using an anisotropic expansion for PTV of 5 mm in each direction, except for at the rectum interface (3 mm), resulted in a single instance of acute Grade 2 GI toxicity. Although the real-time tracking of the anterior rectal wall was not an option, as for MRgRT, the PTV margin's drop to 3 mm posteriorly was still considered safe due to the short beam-on time enabled by the flattering filter free (FFF) modality, as well as the intrafraction motion mitigation protocol obtained by a strict bowel and bladder set-up, which ensured target stabilization and anatomical reproducibility. Furthermore, the use of [^{18}F]-PSMA PET before treatment excluded distant metastases, even at low PSA levels, thus aiding patient selection and accordingly improving oncologic outcomes, as already elucidated in the Empire 1 phase II/III trial [30], where patients whose treatment was guided by another form of advanced imaging (^{18}F-Fluciclovine PET/CT) exhibited a remarkable benefit in 5-year bRFS.

5. Conclusions

Despite the follow-up being too short to consider our SBRT schedule safe in the long term, we believe that our findings are encouraging, at least at early time points, and that they highlight that highly focused radiation in a few fractions to the prostate bed with robust conformality and modulation, abrupt dose fall off and image guidance can be safely extended to the postoperative setting, thus broadening the attractiveness of extreme hypofractionation and enhancing its already unmatched cost-effectiveness profile.

Author Contributions: R.L. is the leading author and participated in the data collection, data analysis, manuscript drafting, table/figure creation, and manuscript revision. C.F. and S.V. contributed equally to this work and participated in the data analysis, manuscript drafting, table/figure creation, and manuscript revision. D.P. and V.F. organized and performed the analysis of the dataset. G.P., S.A. (Stefano Andreoli), G.L.P., D.B. and L.L.F. participated in the data collection and data analysis. S.T. is a senior author who aided in the data analysis and manuscript revision. L.F.C. and M.S. aided in the study design. S.A. (Stefano Arcangeli) is the principal investigator and developed the concept of the study and the design, aided in data collection, and drafted and revised the manuscript. All authors have read and agreed to the published version of the manuscript.

Funding: This research received no external funding.

Institutional Review Board Statement: This study was conducted according to the guidelines of the Declaration of Helsinki and approved by Ethics Committee of Comitato Etico Brianza, Humanitas Cancer Center and ASST-PG23 (3435, 19 March 2021).

Informed Consent Statement: Informed consent was obtained from all subjects involved in the study.

Data Availability Statement: The datasets supporting the conclusions of this article are included within the article.

Conflicts of Interest: The authors declare no conflict of interests.

References

1. Ghadjar, P.; Hayoz, S.; Bernhard, J.; Zwahlen, D.R.; Hölscher, T.; Gut, P.; Polat, B.; Hildebrandt, G.; Müller, A.-C.; Plasswilm, L.; et al. Dose-intensified Versus Conventional-dose Salvage Radiotherapy for Biochemically Recurrent Prostate Cancer After Prostatectomy: The SAKK 09/10 Randomized Phase 3 Trial. *Eur. Urol.* **2021**, *80*, 306–315. [CrossRef]
2. Qi, X.; Li, H.-Z.; Gao, X.-S.; Qin, S.-B.; Zhang, M.; Li, X.-M.; Ma, M.-W.; Bai, Y.; Li, X.-Y.; Wang, D. Toxicity and Biochemical Outcomes of Dose-Intensified Postoperative Radiation Therapy for Prostate Cancer: Results of a Randomized Phase III Trial. *Int. J. Radiat. Oncol. Biol. Phys.* **2020**, *106*, 282–290. [CrossRef] [PubMed]
3. Pollack, A.; Karrison, T.G.; Balogh, A.G.; Gomella, L.G.; Low, D.A.; Bruner, D.W.; Wefel, J.S.; Martin, A.-G.; Michalski, J.M.; Angyalfi, S.J.; et al. The addition of androgen deprivation therapy and pelvic lymph node treatment to prostate bed salvage radiotherapy (NRG Oncology/RTOG 0534 SPPORT): An international, multicentre, randomised phase 3 trial. *Lancet* **2022**, *399*, 1886–1901. [CrossRef]
4. Proust-Lima, C.; Taylor, J.M.; Sécher, S.; Sandler, H.; Kestin, L.; Pickles, T.; Bae, K.; Allison, R.; Williams, S. Confirmation of a Low α/β Ratio for Prostate Cancer Treated by External Beam Radiation Therapy Alone Using a Post-Treatment Repeated-Measures Model for PSA Dynamics. *Int. J. Radiat. Oncol. Biol. Phys.* **2011**, *79*, 195–201. [CrossRef] [PubMed]
5. Miralbell, R.; Roberts, S.A.; Zubizarreta, E.; Hendry, J.H. Dose-Fractionation Sensitivity of Prostate Cancer Deduced From Radiotherapy Outcomes of 5,969 Patients in Seven International Institutional Datasets: $\alpha/\beta = 1.4$ (0.9–2.2) Gy. *Int. J. Radiat. Oncol Biol Phys.* **2012**, *82*, e17–e24. [CrossRef] [PubMed]
6. Dasu, A.; Toma-Dasu, I. Prostate alpha/beta revisited—An analysis of clinical results from 14 168 patients. *Acta Oncol.* **2012**, *51*, 963–974. [CrossRef]
7. Hoffman, K.E.; Voong, K.R.; Levy, L.B.; Allen, P.K.; Choi, S.; Schlembach, P.J.; Lee, A.K.; McGuire, S.E.; Nguyen, Q.; Pugh, T.J.; et al. Randomized trial of hypofraction- ated dose-escalated intensity modulated radiation therapy versus conventionally fractionated intensity modulated radiation therapy for localized prostate cancer. *Int. J. Radiat. Oncol. Biol. Phys.* **2016**, *96*, S32. [CrossRef]
8. Dearnaley, D.; Syndikus, I.; Sumo, G.; Bidmead, M.; Bloomfield, D.; Clark, C.; Gao, A.; Hassan, S.; Horwich, A.; Huddart, R.; et al. Conventional versus hypofractionated high-dose intensity-modulated radiotherapy for prostate cancer: 5-year out-comes of the randomised, non-inferiority, phase 3 CHHiP trial. *Lancet Oncol.* **2016**, *17*, 1047–1060. [CrossRef]
9. Catton, C.N.; Lukka, H.; Gu, C.-S.; Martin, J.M.; Supiot, S.; Chung, P.W.M.; Bauman, G.S.; Bahary, J.-P.; Ahmed, S.; Cheung, P.; et al. Randomized trial of a hypofractionated radiation regimen for the treatment of localized prostate cancer. *J. Clin. Oncol.* **2017**, *35*, 1884–1890. [CrossRef]
10. Lee, W.R.; Dignam, J.J.; Amin, M.B.; Bruner, D.W.; Low, D.; Swanson, G.P.; Shah, A.B.; D'Souza, D.P.; Michalski, J.M.; Dayes, I.S.; et al. Randomized phase III noninferiority study comparing two radiotherapy fractionation schedules in patients with low-risk prostate cancer. *J. Clin. Oncol.* **2016**, *34*, 2325–2332. [CrossRef]
11. Siepe, G.; Buwenge, M.; Nguyen, N.P.; Macchia, G.; Deodato, F.; Cilla, S.; Mattiucci, G.C.; Capocaccia, I.; Cammelli, S.; Guido, A.; et al. Postoperative Hypofractionated Radiation Therapy in Prostate Carcinoma: A Systematic Review. *Anticancer Res.* **2018**, *38*, 1221–1230. [CrossRef] [PubMed]
12. Viani, G.A.; Gouveia, A.G.; Leite, E.T.T.; Moraes, F.Y. Moderate hypofractionation for salvage radiotherapy (HYPO-SRT) in patients with biochemical recurrence after prostatectomy: A cohort study with meta-analysis. *Radiother. Oncol.* **2022**, *171*, 7–13. [CrossRef] [PubMed]

13. Ma, T.M.; Ballas, L.K.; Wilhalme, H.; Sachdeva, A.; Chong, N.; Sharma, S.; Yang, T.; Basehart, V.; Reiter, R.E.; Saigal, C.; et al Quality-of-Life Outcomes and Toxicity Profile Among Patients with Localized Prostate Cancer After Radical Prostatectomy Treated with Stereotactic Body Radiation: The SCIMITAR Multi-Center Phase 2 Trial. *Int. J. Radiat. Oncol. Biol. Phys.* **2022**, in press [CrossRef] [PubMed]
14. World Medical Association. World Medical Association Declaration of Helsinki: Ethical principles for medical research involving human subjects. *JAMA* **2013**, *310*, 2191–2194. [CrossRef]
15. Robin, S.; Jolicoeur, M.; Palumbo, S.; Zilli, T.; Crehange, G.; De Hertogh, O.; Derashodian, T.; Sargos, P.; Salembier, C.; Supiot, S.; et al. Prostate Bed Delineation Guidelines for Postoperative Radiation Therapy: On Behalf of the Francophone Group of Urological Radiation Therapy. *Int. J. Radiat. Oncol. Biol. Phys.* **2020**, *109*, 1243–1253. [CrossRef]
16. Wagner, A.A.; Cheng, P.J.; Carneiro, A.; Dovirak, O.; Khosla, A.; Taylor, K.N.; Crociani, C.M.; McAnally, K.C.; Percy, A.; Dewey, L.E.; et al. Clinical Use of Expanded Prostate Cancer Index Composite for Clinical Practice to Assess Patient Reported Prostate Cancer Quality of Life Following Robot-Assisted Radical Prostatectomy. *J. Urol.* **2016**, *197*, 109–114. [CrossRef]
17. Parzen, J.S.; Quinn, T.J.; Thompson, A.B.; Chang, P.; Collins, S.P.; Suy, S.; Michalski, J.M.; Mantz, C.A.; Seymour, Z.; Hamstra, D.A Evaluating the correlation between early and late quality-of-life declines using the Expanded Prostate Cancer Index Composite for Clinical Practice (EPIC-CP) after definitive stereotactic body radiotherapy, intensity-modulated radiotherapy, or brachytherapy for prostate cancer. *J. Clin. Oncol.* **2021**, *39*, 214. [CrossRef]
18. King, C.R. The dose–response of salvage radiotherapy following radical prostatectomy: A systematic review and meta-analysis *Radiother. Oncol.* **2016**, *121*, 199–203. [CrossRef]
19. Leite, E.T.T.; Ramos, C.C.A.; Ribeiro, V.A.B.; Salvajoli, B.P.; Nahas, W.C.; Salvajoli, J.V.; Moraes, F.Y. Hypofractionated Radiation Therapy to the Prostate Bed With Intensity-Modulated Radiation Therapy (IMRT): A Phase 2 Trial. *Int. J. Radiat. Oncol. Biol. Phys.* **2020**, *109*, 1263–1270. [CrossRef]
20. Schröder, C.; Tang, H.; Windisch, P.; Zwahlen, D.R.; Buchali, A.; Vu, E.; Bostel, T.; Sprave, T.; Zilli, T.; Murthy, V.; et al. Stereotactic Radiotherapy after Radical Prostatectomy in Patients with Prostate Cancer in the Adjuvant or Salvage Setting: A Systematic Review. *Cancers* **2022**, *14*, 696. [CrossRef]
21. Vale, C.L.; Fisher, D.; Kneebone, A.; Parker, C.; Pearse, M.; Richaud, P.; Sargos, P.; Sydes, M.R.; Brawley, C.; Brihoum, M.; et al Adjuvant or early salvage radiotherapy for the treatment of localised and locally advanced prostate cancer: A prospectively planned systematic review and meta-analysis of aggregate data. *Lancet* **2020**, *396*, 1422–1431. [CrossRef] [PubMed]
22. Cozzarini, C.; Chiorda, B.N.; Sini, C.; Fiorino, C.; Briganti, A.; Montorsi, F.; Di Muzio, N. Hematologic Toxicity in Patients Treated With Postprostatectomy Whole-Pelvis Irradiation With Different Intensity Modulated Radiation Therapy Techniques Is Not Negligible and Is Prolonged: Preliminary Results of a Longitudinal, Observational Study. *Int. J. Radiat. Oncol. Biol. Phys.* **2016**, *95*, 690–695. [CrossRef] [PubMed]
23. Iorio, G.C.; Spieler, B.O.; Ricardi, U.; Pra, A.D. The Impact of Pelvic Nodal Radiotherapy on Hematologic Toxicity: A Systematic Review with Focus on Leukopenia, Lymphopenia and Future Perspectives in Prostate Cancer Treatment. *Crit. Rev. Oncol. Hematol.* **2021**, *168*, 103497. [CrossRef] [PubMed]
24. Sanguineti, G.; Giannarelli, D.; Petrongari, M.G.; Arcangeli, S.; SanGiovanni, A.; Saracino, B.; Farneti, A.; Faiella, A.; Conte, M. Arcangeli, G. Leukotoxicity after moderately Hypofractionated radiotherapy versus conventionally fractionated dose escalated radiotherapy for localized prostate Cancer: A secondary analysis from a randomized study. *Radiat. Oncol.* **2019**, *14*, 23. [CrossRef]
25. Tramacere, F.; Arcangeli, S.; Pignatelli, A.; Bracci, S.; Vinella, M.; Portaluri, M. Postoperative Hypofractionated Radiotherapy for Prostate Cancer. *Anticancer Res.* **2018**, *38*, 2951–2956. [CrossRef] [PubMed]
26. Ferrera, G.; D'Alessandro, S.; Cuccia, F.; Serretta, V.; Trapani, G.; Savoca, G.; Mortellaro, G.; Casto, A.L. Post-operative hypofractionated radiotherapy for prostate cancer: A mono-institutional analysis of toxicity and clinical outcomes. *J. Cancer Res. Clin. Oncol.* **2021**, *148*, 89–95. [CrossRef]
27. Mahase, S.; Nagar, H. Hypofractionated Postoperative Radiotherapy for Prostate Cancer: Is the Field Ready Yet? *Eur. Urol. Open Sci.* **2020**, *22*, 9–16. [CrossRef]
28. Ballas, L.K.; Luo, C.; Chung, E.; Kishan, A.U.; Shuryak, I.; Quinn, D.I.; Dorff, T.; Jhimlee, S.; Chiu, R.; Abreu, A.; et al. Phase 1 Trial of SBRT to the Prostate Fossa After Prostatectomy. *Int. J. Radiat. Oncol. Biol. Phys.* **2018**, *104*, 50–60. [CrossRef]
29. Sampath, S.; Frankel, P.; del Vecchio, B.; Ruel, N.; Yuh, B.; Liu, A.; Tsai, T.; Wong, J. Stereotactic Body Radiation Therapy to the Prostate Bed: Results of a Phase 1 Dose-Escalation Trial. *Int. J. Radiat. Oncol. Biol. Phys.* **2019**, *106*, 537–545. [CrossRef]
30. Jani, A.B.; Schreibmann, E.; Goyal, S.; Halkar, R.; Hershatter, B.; Rossi, P.J.; Shelton, J.W.; Patel, P.R.; Xu, K.M.; Goodman, M.; et al 18F-fluciclovine-PET/CT imaging versus conventional imaging alone to guide postprostatectomy salvage radiotherapy for prostate cancer (EMPIRE-1): A single centre, open-label, phase 2/3 randomised controlled trial. *Lancet* **2021**, *397*, 1895–1904. [CrossRef]

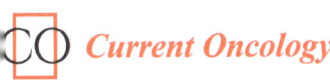

Article

Is an Endorectal Balloon Beneficial for Rectal Sparing after Spacer Implantation in Prostate Cancer Patients Treated with Hypofractionated Intensity-Modulated Proton Beam Therapy? A Dosimetric and Radiobiological Comparison Study

Dalia Ahmad Khalil [1], Jörg Wulff [2], Danny Jazmati [1,*], Dirk Geismar [2], Christian Bäumer [1], Paul-Heinz Kramer [2], Theresa Steinmeier [1], Stefanie Schulze Schleithoff [2], Stephan Tschirdewahn [3], Boris Hadaschik [3] and Beate Timmermann [1,2,4]

[1] Department of Particle Therapy, University Hospital Essen, West German Proton Therapy Centre Essen (WPE), West German Cancer Center (WTZ), 45147 Essen, Germany
[2] Faculty of Physics, TU Dortmund University, 44227 Dortmund, Germany
[3] Department of Urology, University Hospital Essen, University of Duisburg-Essen, 45147 Essen, Germany
[4] German Cancer Consortium (DKTK), 45147 Essen, Germany
* Correspondence: danny.jazmati@uk-essen.de

Abstract: Background: The aim of this study is to examine the dosimetric influence of endorectal balloons (ERB) on rectal sparing in prostate cancer patients with implanted hydrogel rectum spacers treated with dose-escalated or hypofractionated intensity-modulated proton beam therapy (IMPT). Methods: Ten patients with localized prostate cancer included in the ProRegPros study and treated at our center were investigated. All patients underwent placement of hydrogel rectum spacers before planning. Two planning CTs (with and without 120 cm^3 fluid-filled ERB) were applied for each patient. Dose prescription was set according to the h strategy, with 72 Gray (Gy)/2.4 Gy/5× weekly to prostate + 1 cm of the seminal vesicle, and 60 Gy/2 Gy/5× weekly to prostate + 2 cm of the seminal vesicle. Planning with two laterally opposed IMPT beams was performed in both CTs. Rectal dosimetry values including dose-volume statistics and normal tissue complication probability (NTCP) were compared for both plans (non-ERB plans vs. ERB plans). Results: For ERB plans compared with non-ERB, the reductions were 8.51 ± 5.25 Gy (RBE) (p = 0.000) and 15.76 ± 11.11 Gy (p = 0.001) for the mean and the median rectal doses, respectively. No significant reductions in rectal volumes were found after high dose levels. The use of ERB resulted in significant reduction in rectal volume after receiving 50 Gy (RBE), 40 Gy (RBE), 30 Gy (RBE), 20 Gy (RBE), and 10 Gy (RBE) with p values of 0.034, 0.008, 0.003, 0.001, and 0.001, respectively. No differences between ERB and non-ERB plans for the anterior rectum were observed. ERB reduced posterior rectal volumes in patients who received 30 Gy (RBE), 20 Gy (RBE), or 10 Gy (RBE), with p values of 0.019, 0.003, and 0.001, respectively. According to the NTCP models, no significant reductions were observed in mean or median rectal toxicity (late rectal bleeding $\geq$ 2, necrosis or stenosis, and late rectal toxicity $\geq$ 3) when using the ERB. Conclusion: ERB reduced rectal volumes exposed to intermediate or low dose levels. However, no significant reduction in rectal volume was observed in patients receiving high or intermediate doses. There was no benefit and also no disadvantage associated with the use of ERB for late rectal toxicity, according to available NTCP models.

Keywords: endorectal balloon; proton therapy; intensity-modulated therapy; prostate cancer; dose-escalated radiation therapy; hypofractionated radiation therapy

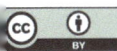

1. Introduction

Despite advances in radiotherapy (RT) techniques, rectal morbidity related to prostate radiation treatment cannot be entirely avoided and carries implications for quality of life

(QOL). Escalation of radiation dosage for prostate cancer patients has evolved over the past decade with the development of modern three-dimensional conformal radiotherapy (3D-CRT) and the more advanced intensity-modulated radiotherapy (IMRT) together with image-guided radiotherapy (IGRT). Several randomized studies have demonstrated that dose escalation offers improved local control and biochemical control rates compared with conventional doses [1–6]. However, the relative biological effectiveness (RBE) achieved by escalating the total dose delivered to the prostate by 8–10 Gray (Gy) has been shown to significantly increase the risk of rectal toxicity by about 10% [2,7–9]. The results of several trials have been published relating rectal dose-volume characteristics to radiotherapy induced rectal toxicity [10–14]. Based on these reports, the efforts of radiation oncologists in the past decade have been directed not only towards utilizing modern radiotherapy techniques for patients with prostate cancer, but also to incorporating mechanical tools to increase the separation between prostate and rectum, such as implantation of rectum-prostate spacers and/or the use of endorectal balloons (ERBs).

Significant reduction of intra-fractional prostate motion during radiotherapy achieved by using ERB was shown in a systematic review of 21 articles [15]. The dosimetric effect of ERB in reducing rectal radiation exposure during 3D-CRT, IMRT, or stereotactic body radiation therapy for prostate cancer has been demonstrated in several studies [16–23]. However, there have been few trials in the field of proton therapy that have investigated the role of ERB [24–28].

The pencil beam scanning (PBS) technique is highly sensitive to organ motion [29], therefore ERB has more frequently been used in our institution to stabilize the position and shape of the rectum and hence fix the position of the prostate during treatment. It is unclear whether the benefit of ERB is retained when decreasing the dose exposure in the rectum. Our goal was to explore the dosimetric impact of ERB on rectal dosage and normal tissue complication probability (NTCP) values in prostate cancer patients with implanted rectum spacers who were treated with dose-escalated or hypofractionated IMPT.

2. Materials and Methods

Since August 2015, a prospective single-center register evaluating proton therapy for patients with localized prostate cancer (ProRegPros) has been carried out at the West German Proton Therapy Centre Essen (WPE). Two computed tomography (CT) scans respectively before and after the insertion of the ERB, were obtained for each of 10 consecutive patients undergoing prostate cancer treatment. All patients had been diagnosed with T1–T4, N0, M0, and PSA $\leq$ 50 ng/mL. All patients were treated with dose escalated or moderate hypofractionated IMPT with 72 Gy (RBE) in 30 fractions. All the patients had been diagnosed with intermediate- to high-risk prostate symptoms (T1–T4, N0, M0, PSA $\leq$ 50 ng/mL, Gleason score 7a–9) and had no indication of lymph node irradiation. Patients were in good general health with no life-limiting conditions, and each had a life expectancy of more than five years.

All patients selected for analysis underwent hydrogel rectal spacer insertion and fiducial marker implantation one week before planned CT application.

Written informed consent was obtained from all patients for their inclusion in the register. The register was approved by the ethical committee of the University of Duisburg Essen.

2.1. CT-MRI Simulation

All patients drank 350 mL water on an empty bladder 30 min prior to simulation. Patients were immobilized in a supine position using a thermoplastic pelvic cast. The first planning CT was acquired in 1 mm slices for each patient. Then, the thermoplastic pelvic cast was removed and the ERB catheter was inserted with the patient in a knees-raised position, then the catheter was filled with 120 cm^3 of fluid. The patient was positioned and immobilized again using the laser alignment and immobilization mask markings placed during the first CT, and the second CT was acquired in 1 mm slices. A T1/T2-weighted MRI scan was performed for each patient.

2.2. Target Volumes and OARs Delineation

Within our in-house standard framework, taking into account national and international recommendations and guidelines, we determined target volume and dose. Planning and contouring for each patient were performed using the same methods. For each patient in every CT, the prostate, seminal vesicles, clinical target volumes (CTV,) and organs at risk (OARs) were contoured using a combination of CT and magnetic resonance imaging (MRI) for accurate prostate delineation. Two CTVs were defined; low risk CTV1 (prostate + 5 mm peri-prostatic tissue + 2 cm of the seminal vesicles), and high risk CTV2 (prostate + 1 cm of the seminal vesicles). Margins of 5 mm in every direction were added to the CTV to create the corresponding planning target volumes (PTVs), except at the seminal vesicle region where a 7 mm margin was applied [29]. Dose prescription was 60 Gy (RBE) in 2 Gy to PTV1 and 72 Gy (RBE) in 2.4 Gy to PTV2, in 30 fractions using simultaneous integrated boost (SIB). The rectum was contoured as a solid organ extending from just above the anal verge to the sigmoid flexure. Extra contours were generated for the anterior and posterior rectum.

2.3. SIB-IMPT Planning Process

Dose calculation and optimization of IMPT plans were performed using a pencil beam algorithm with the RayStation treatment planning system version 6 (RaySearch Laboratories, Stockholm, Sweden). For all patients, fixed geometry plans were generated in both CTs using two laterally opposed IMPT beams with the same optimization goals. A margin of 3.5% proton beam range + 2 mm was included in the PTV in the beam direction to account for field-specific range uncertainty. For greater consistency, all contours were generated by the same senior radiation oncologist who also created all the treatment plans. For all dose concepts, a generic relative biological effectiveness (RBE) factor of 1.1 (relative to that of Co-60) was assumed.

2.4. DVH Analysis and Rectal NTCP Calculation

The dose-volume histogram (DVH) of the rectum was assessed and the following parameters were calculated:
- For the whole rectum: RV (rectal volume in cc), Dmax, Dmean, Dmedian, and RVxGy = percentage of rectal volume received X dose in Gy (RV72Gy, RV70Gy, RV65Gy, RV60Gy, RV55Gy, RV50Gy, RV40Gy, RV30Gy, RV20Gy, and RV10Gy).
- For the anterior rectum: Dmax and Ant-RVxGy = percentage of anterior rectal volume received x dose in Gy.
- For the posterior rectum: Dmax and Post-RVxGy = percentage of posterior rectal volume received x dose in Gy.

NTCPs are able to predict the toxicity of radiation therapy to organs at risk. These biological models can be used to predict the risk of various complications.

For the rectal NTCP calculation, the following biological models available in RayStation were employed:
- Layman Kutcher Burman (LKB) model for late rectal bleeding ≥ 2 with D50 = 81.8 Gy, $\gamma = 3$, $m = 0.22$, $n = 0.29$, and $\alpha/\beta = 3$ [30].
- Poisson-LQ model for necrosis or stenosis with D50 = 80 Gy, $\gamma = 2.2$, $S = 1$, and $\alpha/\beta = 3$ [27].
- LKB model for late effects grade ≥ 3 with D50 = 80 Gy, $m = 0.15$, $n = 0.06$, and $\alpha/\beta = 3.9$ [31].

We compared the rectal DVH parameters and rectal NTCP values of the non-rectal balloon plans (non-ERB group) with those of the rectal balloon plans (ERB group). The differences in DVH and NTCP indices were calculated (Δ = mean value of non-ERB plans − mean value of ERB plans). Statistical analysis was conducted using the IBM SPSS Statistics program V22. The Mann–Whitney U test was applied to compare means between the non-ERB and ERB plans.

3. Results

3.1. DVH Analysis

The 120 cm^3 fluid-filled ERBs significantly increased rectal volume in ERB patients compared to non-ERB patients. Analysis of the DVH of the whole rectum confirmed that the ERB plans could attain lower values of Dmax, D1, Dmean, and Dmedian in comparison with non-ERB plans. However, the differences in Dmax and D1 were not statistically significant. There was a minimal statistically insignificant reduction in RV72Gy in favor of non-ERB plans compared with ERB. Otherwise, the ERB plans were able to lower the rectal volumes exposed to different radiation doses compared with the non-ERB plans with an insignificant reduction in RV70Gy, RV65Gy, RV60Gy, and RV55Gy and a significant reduction in RV50Gy, RV40Gy, RV30Gy, RV20Gy, and RV10Gy (Table 1, Figure 1).

Table 1. DVH analysis for the whole rectum comparing between the non-ERB plans and ERB plans.

	Study Group	Mean	SD	Range	Diff (Δ)[d] Mean	Diff (Δ)[d] SD	p Value
RV[a]	non-ERB	90.79	42.34	42.08–183.51	137.35	32.58	0.000
	ERB	228.14	31.65	179.79–267.54			
D_{max}[b]	non-ERB	73.62	0.77	72.6–74.8	0.64	0.85	0.103
	ERB	72.98	0.55	72.6–74.4			
D_{mean}[b]	non-ERB	31.42	4.98	24.20–42.29	8.51	5.25	0.000
	ERB	22.91	3.0	18.79–27.53			
D_{median}[b]	non-ERB	26.34	9.66	13.06–45.25	15.76	11.11	0.001
	ERB	10.57	5.89	4.39–21.52			
D1[b]	non-ERB	72.49	0.53	71.59–73.29	0.11	0.52	0.363
	ERB	72.38	0.16	72.21–72.78			
RV72Gy[c]	non-ERB	3.42	1.73	0.34–5.60	−0.38	2.24	0.734
	ERB	3.80	1.07	1.96–5.30			
RV70Gy[c]	non-ERB	7.90	3.4	2.12–13.29	0.58	4.42	0.597
	ERB	7.32	2.03	3.89–9.84			
RV65Gy[c]	non-ERB	13.98	4.3	5.93–21.28	1.66	5.45	0.257
	ERB	12.31	2.54	7.66–15.98			
RV60Gy[c]	non-ERB	18.74	4.85	9.63–27.32	1.10	6.99	0.345
	ERB	17.64	5.62	11.17–31.51			
RV55Gy[c]	non-ERB	23.37	6.37	13.11–37.72	4.02	8.15	0.082
	ERB	19.35	3.15	14.85–23.96			
RV50Gy[c]	non-ERB	26.87	5.59	16.49–37.51	4.58	7.37	0.034
	ERB	22.29	3.43	17.52–27.51			
RV40Gy[c]	non-ERB	34.50	6.19	23.45–46.37	6.82	8.02	0.008
	ERB	27.68	3.74	22.36–33.83			
RV30Gy[c]	non-ERB	42.67	6.60	32.64–54.68	9.57	8.23	0.003
	ERB	33.10	4.4	27.05–40.37			
RV20Gy[c]	non-ERB	52.33	7.75	42.85–65.88	12.87	8.75	0.001
	ERB	39.46	5.09	32.58–47.58			
RV10Gy[c]	non-ERB	64.57	8.55	54.38–81.85	15.78	8.91	0.001
	ERB	48.77	6.13	40.99–57.68			

[a] Rectal volume in cm^3; [b] Dose in Gy; [c] RVXGy = Percentage of rectal volume received x dose; [d] Δ difference between the non-ERB plans and the ERB plans (mean value non-ERB plans - mean value ERB plans).

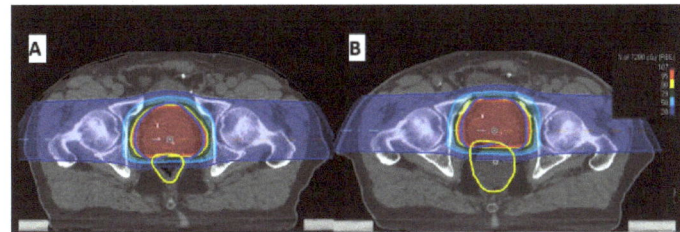

Figure 1. Example of IMPT dose distribution for cT2N0M0 Prostate cancer patient. (**A**) non-ERB plan. (**B**) ERB plan.

In the results of the analysis carried out for the anterior rectum, we found that ERB reduced the values of Dmax, D1, RV72Gy, RV70Gy, RV65Gy, RV60Gy, RV55G, RV50G, RV40G, RV30Gy, RV20Gy, and RV10Gy, but no statistically significant differences were attained (Table 2).

Table 2. DVH analysis for the anterior rectum comparing between the non-ERB plans and ERB plans.

	Study Group	Mean	SD	Range	Diff (Δ) [c]		p Value
					Mean	SD	
Ant-D$_{max}$ [a]	non-ERB	73.62	0.77	72.6–74.8	0.64	0.85	0.103
	ERB	72.98	0.545	72.6–74.4			
Ant-D1 [a]	non-ERB	72.77	0.72	71.31–73.73	0.21	0.69	0.326
	ERB	72.56	0.23	72.30–73.01			
Ant-RV72Gy [b]	non-ERB	5.99	3.17	0.66–12.32	−1.14	3.71	0.290
	ERB	7.13	2.1	3.78–10.29			
Ant-RV70Gy [b]	non-ERB	14.44	5.36	4.98–21.80	−0.95	6.49	0.705
	ERB	15.39	3.98	8.28–20.98			
Ant-RV65Gy [b]	non-ERB	22.84	5.75	11.39–31.05	−1.22	8.41	0.940
	ERB	24.05	5.7	14.79–31.02			
Ant-RV60Gy [b]	non-ERB	31.74	7.51	18.49–41.66	0.93	9.11	0.545
	ERB	30.81	6.61	21.55–39.18			
Ant-RV55Gy [b]	non-ERB	38.66	8.32	25.13–48.53	1.19	10.52	0.734
	ERB	37.47	7.16	28.65–48.53			
Ant-RV50Gy [b]	non-ERB	47.34	7.41	31.36–56.39	3.88	11.14	0.226
	ERB	43.46	7.29	34.42–54.28			
Ant-RV40Gy [b]	non-ERB	59.11	7.64	42.45–68.87	6.6	11.88	0.174
	ERB	52.51	8.60	42.48–65.22			
Ant-RV30Gy [b]	non-ERB	69.25	7.9	52.49–78.39	7.65	12.21	0.059
	ERB	61.60	9.05	50.20–76.17			
Ant-RV20Gy [b]	non-ERB	78.84	9.65	61.83–89.52	8.31	12.81	0.059
	ERB	70.53	9.03	58.28–84.13			
Ant-RV10Gy [b]	non-ERB	85.2	9.44	71.7–96.11	4.17	11.75	0.174
	ERB	81.03	7.9	68.21–91.01			

[a] Dose in Gy; [b] RVXGy =Percentage of ant-rectal volume received X dose; [c] Δ difference between the non-ERB plans and the ERB plans (mean value non-ERB plans - mean value ERB plans).

For the posterior rectum, the Dmax and D1 were reduced in ERB plans in comparison with non-ERB plans, without statistical significance. There were no statistically significant differences between the two groups in terms of RV72Gy, RV70G, RV65Gy, RV60Gy, RV55Gy, or RV40Gy (Figure 2). Statistically significant differences were found between the two groups for rectal volumes after receiving 30 Gy, 20 Gy, and 10 Gy (Table 3).

Table 3. DVH analysis for the posterior rectum comparing between the non-ERB plans and ERB plans

	Study Group	Mean	SD	Range	Diff (Δ) [c] Mean	Diff (Δ) [c] SD	p Value
D_{max} [a]	non-ERB	60.24	9.16	47.60–72.60	3.83	12.41	0.406
	ERB	56.41	10.54	42.80–70.60			
D1 [a]	non-ERB	37.36	11.82	23.66–57.94	11.11	13.93	0.059
	ERB	72.56	0.23	72.3–73.01			
Post-RV72Gy [b]	non-ERB	0.11	0.35	0–1.14	0.11	0.36	0.317
	ERB	0	0	0			
Post-RV70Gy [b]	non-ERB	0.51	1.6	0–5.06	0.51	1.6	0.503
	ERB	0	0	0–0.02			
Post-RV65Gy [b]	non-ERB	1.08	3.31	0–10.49	1.06	3.29	0.829
	ERB	0.03	0.07	0–0.22			
Post-RV60Gy [b]	non-ERB	1.67	4.5	0–14.4	1.56	4.44	0.518
	ERB	0.11	0.23	0–0.71			
Post-RV55Gy [b]	non-ERB	2.38	5.47	0–17.67	2.14	5.39	0.435
	ERB	0.24	0.46	0–1.45			
Post-RV50Gy [b]	non-ERB	3.01	6.39	0–20.57	2.55	6.25	0.286
	ERB	0.451	0.70	0–2.25			
Post-RV40Gy [b]	non-ERB	4.98	8.05	0.2–27.09	3.83	7.79	0.069
	ERB	1.148	1.309	0.06–4.03			
Post-RV30Gy [b]	non-ERB	11.59	10.90	0.88–36.46	8.86	9.92	0.019
	ERB	2.7	2.26	0.33–6.68			
Post-RV20Gy [b]	non-ERB	21.92	14.84	3.8–349.00	15.76	12.94	0.003
	ERB	6.165	3.711	1.59–10.87			
Post-RV10Gy [b]	non-ERB	39.54	17.17	14.87–71.37	25.66	14.21	0.001
	ERB	13.88	6.695	3.97–22.05			

[a] Dose in Gy; [b] RVXGy =Percentage of post-rectal volume receiving X dose; [c] Δ difference between the non-ERB plans and the ERB plans (mean value non-ERB plans - mean value ERB plans).

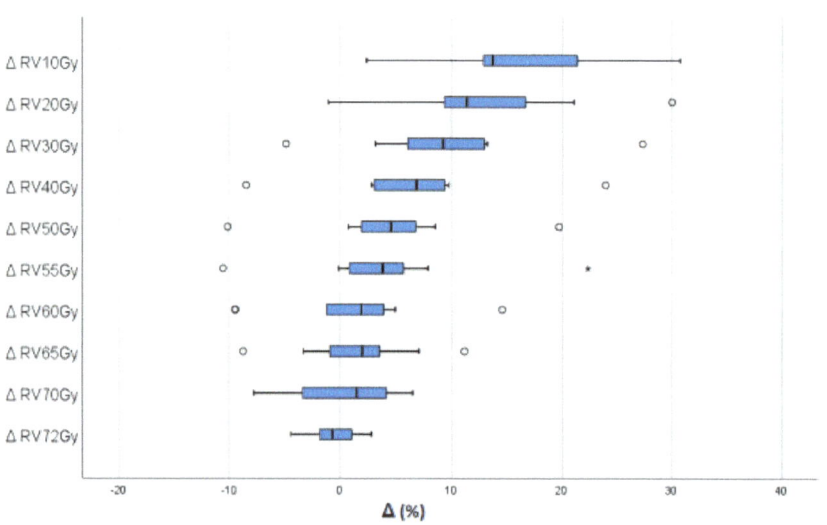

Figure 2. Box plot illustrates the difference (Δ) in percentage of rectal volume received x dose between the non-ERB plans and ERB plans (mean value non-ERB plans- mean value ERB plans).

3.2. NTCP Results

No statistically significant differences between the two study groups were determined for the risk of NTCP with late rectal toxicities. Comparisons of NTCP results for late rectal bleeding ≥ 2, necrosis or stenosis, and late rectal toxicity ≥ 3 are presented in Table 4 and Figure 3.

Table 4. NTCP results for the whole rectum comparing between the non-ERB plans and ERB plans.

NTCP [a]	Study Group	Mean	SD	Range	Diff (Δ) [b] Mean	Diff (Δ) [b] SD	p Value
Late rectal bleeding ≥ 2	non-ERB	2.6	0.97	2–5	−0.5	1.18	0.150
	ERB	3.1	1.1	1–5			
Necrosis/stenosis	non-ERB	5.5	1.78	1–7	−0.1	2.02	0.728
	ERB	5.6	2.22	1–8			
Late rectal toxicity ≥ 3	non-ERB	13.1	1.37	11–15	−0.2	3.82	0.593
	ERB	13.3	3.02	7–17			

[a] NTCP results in %; [b] Δ difference between the non-ERB plans and the ERB plans (mean value non-ERB plans - mean value ERB plans).

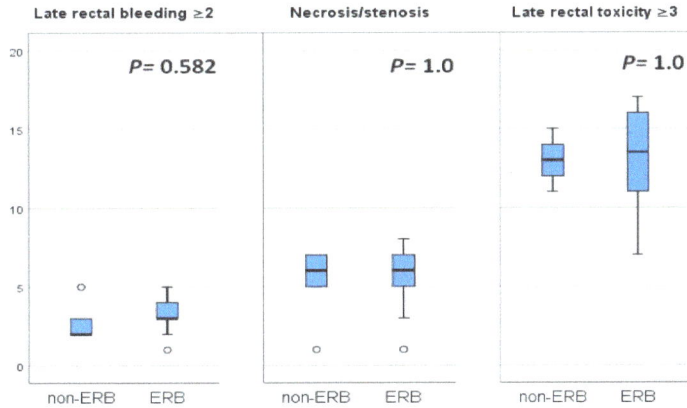

Figure 3. Blox plot comparing median and full range of variation of the rectal NTCP rates for late rectal bleeding ≥2, necrosis/stenosis, and late toxicity ≥3 for non ERB plans vs. ERB plans.

4. Discussion

Few trials have been conducted into the use of proton therapy for prostate patients in order to investigate the effectiveness of ERB utilization to achieve rectal sparing [24], reduction of the interfraction prostate motion [26], or removal of rectal gas [25]. Our aim was to investigate whether insertion of 120 cm^3 fluid-filled ERB could spare rectal space and hence reduce rectal NTCPs in patients who had undergone prior placement of hydrogel rectal spacers and received treatment with dose-escalated or hypofractionated IMPT to the prostate and the seminal vesicle.

In this study, ERB increased the rectal volume by 137.35 ± 32.58 cm^3. The reduction in mean radiation dose received by the whole rectum in the ERB plans compared to non-ERB plans was 8.51 ± 5.25 Gy (RBE) ($p = 0.000$), and for Dmedian the reduction was 15.76 ± 11.11 Gy (RBE) ($p = 0.001$). Regarding the maximum dose delivered to the rectum, we recorded a 0.64 Gy (RBE) difference in Dmax, a 0.11 Gy (RBE) difference in D1 of the rectum, and a 0.21 Gy difference in D1 of the anterior rectum in favor of the ERB plans, but with no statistical significance. We found that ERB could reduce Dmax in the posterior rectum, but with no statistical significance. Furthermore, D1 was reduced in ERB plans by 11.11 ± 13.93 Gy (RBE) with a marginal statistical significance ($p = 0.059$). Our results are similar to those reported by Elsayed et al., who applied 3D-CRT with 59.4 Gy (RBE) + 10 Gy (RBE) high dose-rate (HDR) brachytherapy to 12 patients. The authors found that for teletherapy applied with a PTV including prostate + 9 mm safety margins, the application of a 60 cm^3 air-filled ERB led to a decrease in Dmax of the anterior rectal wall and the rectum as a complete organ, but with no statistical significance. However, owing to the dose distribution obtained from the 3D-CRT, the authors demonstrated a reduction in the Dmax of the posterior rectal wall of 18.6 Gy (RBE) (47.1 Gy for non-ERB vs. 28.5 Gy for ERB), which was found to be significant ($p = 0.01$) [32].

Regarding rectal volumes receiving different dose levels, we found no statistically significant differences of rectal volumes at high or intermediate dose levels. Furthermore through separate analysis of the anterior rectum, we found that the ERB plans led to no significant differences in comparison with non-ERB plans in any of the DVH parameters examined. In the case of intermediate and low dosage levels, the differences in rectal volume between non-ERB and ERB plans were found to be 4.58, 6.82, 9.57, 12.87, and 15.78% for RV50Gy (RBE), RV40Gy (RBE), RV30Gy (RBE), RV20Gy (RBE), and RV10Gy (RBE), respectively, which were statistically significant. Further analysis of the posterior rectum confirmed that the ERB reduced Post-RV30Gy (RBE) by 8.89 ± 9.92% ($p = 0.019$) Post-RV20Gy by 15.76 ± 12.94% ($p = 0.003$), and the Post-RV10Gy by 25.66 ± 14.21% ($p = 0.001$).

Our results are in agreement with those reported by Hille et al., who used 3D-CRT and applied 72 Gy with conventional fractionation. The authors found that after inclusion of the prostate, the entire, and the proximal seminal vesicles as CTV, a 60 cm^3 air-filled ERB led to a significant decrease of the rectal wall receiving 40 Gy and 50 Gy, while no significant decrease of the rectal wall receiving 60 Gy, 65 Gy, or 70 Gy could be found [33]

Other trials applying 3D-CRT demonstrated that insertion of ERB could lower rectal volumes exposed to high doses. In an early study in 2002, Wachter et al. used 3D-CRT with 66 Gy for prostate cancer, and tested the role of a 40 cm^3 air-filled ERB on the rectal dose. The authors found that for PTV prostate-only plans, the proportion of the rectum volume receiving doses larger than 90% could be reduced from 24% without ERB to 20% with ERB. However, for PTV prostate + seminal vesicle plans, the volume increased from 41% without ERB to 48% with ERB, due to posterior displacement of the seminal vesicle resulting from application of the ERB [34]. Van Lin et al. conducted a study testing 40, 80 and 100 cm^3 air-filled ERB vs. non-ERB plans, using three-dimensional conformal radiation therapy (DCRT) and IMRT delivered to two different PTVs with and without seminal vesicle involvement. They found that in cases of 3D-CRT the application of an ERB resulted in a statistically significant reduction of the mean rectal wall dose, which was the case for rectal wall volume irradiated to a dose level of 70 Gy or more and for that irradiated to a dose level of 50 Gy or more. However, in case of IMRT, the authors reported no statistically significant reduction in the rectal wall dose parameters for any of the ERBs [16]. In contrast the results obtained by Van Lin et al., Patel et al. conducted a planning study to detect the beneficial effect of 60 cm^3 air-filled ERB on rectal dosimetry. They generated radiotherapy plans for five patients, delivering 76 Gy either with 3DCRT or IMRT to target volumes with and without inclusion of the seminal vesicle, and proved that inflation of the ERB in all cases and even in the context of IMRT resulted in significant decreases in the absolute volume of rectal wall receiving greater than 60, 65, or 70 Gy [23].

Vargas et al. published the only trial to have investigated the role of ERB in rectal sparing for patients treated with proton therapy. They analyzed 20 proton plans for 15 patients who received doses of 78–82 Gy, and found that ERB decreased the volume of the rectum radiated by doses from 10 to 65 Gy ($p \leq 0.05$), while no benefit was observed for doses $\geq$ 70 Gy [24]. No hydrogel prostate rectum spacers were used in their trial.

Based on NTCP calculations, we found that the probability of late rectal toxicity was not reduced by the application of ERB. The mean NTCP for late rectal bleeding $\geq$ grade 2 was 2.6 ± 0.97% for non-ERB plans vs. 3.1± 1.1% for ERB ($p = 0.15$). For necrosis or stenosis it was 5.5 ± 1.78% for non-ERB vs. 5.6 ± 2.22% for ERB ($p = 0.72$); for late rectal toxicity ≥ 3 it was 13.1 ± 1.37% for non-ERB vs. 13.3 ± 3.02% for ERB (p = 0.593). Our results are similar to those reported by Van Lin et al., who used the LKB model with Emami parameters (n = 0.12, m = 0.15, and D50 = 80 Gy) for calculation of late rectal NTCP. In their trial, no statistically significant reduction in NTCP could be demonstrated for the combination of IMRT with ERBs (40, 80, and 100 cm^3 air-filled). However, according to their analysis, ERB could improve the results of 3D-CRT plans, with a statistically significant reduction in rectal NTCP for 100 cm^3 air-filled ERB compared to non-ERB (15% vs. 24%, respectively, p < 0.0001) [16].

It has been proven that the exposure of rectal volume to intermediate and high radiation doses is associated with developing late rectal toxicities. Storey et al. reported a significant correlation between the percentage of the rectum irradiated to 70 Gy or greater and the likelihood of developing late rectal complications in patients treated with up to 78 Gy [35]. Kupelian et al. tested a short-course IMRT (70 Gy with 2.5 Gy per fraction) and demonstrated that only the volume of rectum receiving 70 Gy (with a cutoff of 15 cc) was a significant predictor of rectal bleeding [11]. Huang et al. also observed a significant effect on volume at rectal doses of 60, 70, 75.6, and 78 Gy and concluded that the risk of developing rectal complications increased exponentially as larger volumes were irradiated [36]. Zapatero et al. reported that rectal Dmean and the percentage of the rectum receiving >60 Gy were correlated with grade 2 rectal bleeding or worse [37]. Meanwhile, other investigators have demonstrated the likelihood of rectal toxicity for rectal volumes receiving an intermediate dose. Tucker and colleagues found that the incidence of grade 2 or worse late rectal bleeding increased within 2 years when ≥80% of the rectal wall was exposed to doses > 32 Gy [38]. Jackson et al. reported that rectal bleeding was significantly correlated with volumes exposed to 46 Gy in prostate cancer patients who received 70.2 or 75.6 Gy [39].

The strength of the current study is limited by the small number of patients involved. Nevertheless, since the data include internal controls, the dataset is particularly homogeneous and thus highly relevant.

5. Conclusions

Our study suggests that ERB could reduce rectal volumes exposed to intermediate or low doses of radiation treatment in prostate cancer patients with implanted rectum spacers during their treatment with hypofractionated or dose-escalated IMPT. We could not find any benefit associated with ERB in terms of reducing rectal volumes receiving high to intermediate dose levels. Supported by previous trials, these results can explain the lack of benefit obtained from ERB in reducing NTCP values for late rectal toxicity in those patients. We conclude that the application of ERB adds little benefit for patients treated with IMPT, due to high capability of this technique to conform the dose to the target, which in turn reduces the volume of the rectum exposed to high doses. Furthermore, reduction of the rectum volume receiving a high dose can be achieved using spacer implantation. However, the potential effect of ERB in reducing volumetric changes in the rectum cannot be neglected, and nor can variabilities in rectal positioning during treatment, especially in patients undergoing proton therapy due to the high sensitivity of PBS dose distribution to inter- and intrafractional motion. This issue is currently under investigation at our center, and results will be reported soon. Therefore, at our center we are currently continuing to use the endorectal balloon to reduce motion.

Author Contributions: D.A.K., D.J., T.S. and J.W. wrote parts of the manuscript. B.T., D.G., D.A.K. and J.W. designed the study. B.H., C.B., P.-H.K., S.T., S.S.S. and D.G. contributed significantly to the discussion on the interpretation of the results. All authors have read and agreed to the published version of the manuscript.

Funding: This research received no external funding.

Institutional Review Board Statement: The study was conducted in accordance with the Declaration of Helsinki, and approved by the Institutional Review Board University of Duisburg Essen (CT-MRI Simulation DRKS00005363l).

Informed Consent Statement: Informed consent was obtained from all subjects involved in the study.

Data Availability Statement: All data and materials can be accessed via DAK, in compliance with data protection guidelines.

Conflicts of Interest: The authors declare no conflict of interest.

References

1. Michalski, J.M.; Moughan, J.; Purdy, J.; Bosch, W.; Bruner, D.W.; Bahary, J.P.; Lau, H.; Duclos, M.; Parliament, M.; Morton, G.; et al. Effect of Standard vs Dose-Escalated Radiation Therapy for Patients With Intermediate-Risk Prostate Cancer: The NRG Oncology RTOG 0126 Randomized Clinical Trial. *JAMA Oncol.* **2018**, *4*, e180039. [CrossRef]
2. Kuban, D.A.; Tucker, S.L.; Dong, L.; Starkschall, G.; Huang, E.H.; Cheung, M.R.; Lee, A.K.; Pollack, A. Long-term results of the M. D. Anderson randomized dose-escalation trial for prostate cancer. *Int. J. Radiat. Oncol. Biol. Phys.* **2008**, *70*, 67–74. [CrossRef]
3. Zietman, A.L.; Bae, K.; Slater, J.D.; Shipley, W.U.; Efstathiou, J.A.; Coen, J.J.; Bush, D.A.; Lunt, M.; Spiegel, D.Y.; Skowronski, R.; et al. Randomized Trial Comparing Conventional-Dose With High-Dose Conformal Radiation Therapy in Early-Stage Adenocarcinoma of the Prostate: Long-Term Results From Proton Radiation Oncology Group/American College of Radiology 95-09. *J. Clin. Oncol.* **2010**, *28*, 1106–1111. [CrossRef]
4. Heemsbergen, W.D.; Al-Mamgani, A.; Slot, A.; Dielwart, M.F.; Lebesque, J.V. Long-term results of the Dutch randomized prostate cancer trial: Impact of dose-escalation on local, biochemical, clinical failure, and survival. *Radiother. Oncol.* **2014**, *110*, 104–109. [CrossRef]
5. Beckendorf, V.; Guerif, S.; Le Prisé, E.; Cosset, J.-M.; Bougnoux, A.; Chauvet, B.; Salem, N.; Chapet, O.; Bourdain, S.; Bachaud, J.-M.; et al. 70 Gy Versus 80 Gy in Localized Prostate Cancer: 5-Year Results of GETUG 06 Randomized Trial. *Int. J. Radiat. Oncol. Biol. Phys.* **2011**, *80*, 1056–1063. [CrossRef]
6. Dearnaley, D.P.; Jovic, G.; Syndikus, I.; Khoo, V.; Cowan, R.A.; Graham, J.D.; Aird, E.G.; Bottomley, D.; Huddart, R.A.; Jose, C.C.; et al. Escalated-dose versus control-dose conformal radiotherapy for prostate cancer: Long-term results from the MRC RT01 randomised controlled trial. *Lancet Oncol.* **2014**, *15*, 464–473. [CrossRef]
7. Peeters, S.T.; Heemsbergen, W.D.; Koper, P.C.; Van Putten, W.L.; Slot, A.; Dielwart, M.F.; Bonfrer, J.M.; Incrocci, L.; Lebesque, J.V. Dose-Response in Radiotherapy for Localized Prostate Cancer: Results of the Dutch Multicenter Randomized Phase III Trial Comparing 68 Gy of Radiotherapy With 78 Gy. *J. Clin. Oncol.* **2006**, *24*, 1990–1996. [CrossRef]
8. Dearnaley, D.P.; Sydes, M.R.; Graham, J.D.; Aird, E.G.; Bottomley, D.; Cowan, R.A.; Huddart, R.A.; Jose, C.C.; Matthews, J.H.; Millar, J.; et al. Escalated-dose versus standard-dose conformal radiotherapy in prostate cancer: First results from the MRC RT01 randomised controlled trial. *Lancet Oncol.* **2007**, *8*, 475–487. [CrossRef]
9. Delobel, J.-B.; Gnep, K.; Ospina, J.D.; Beckendorf, V.; Chira, C.; Zhu, J.; Bossi, A.; Messai, T.; Acosta, O.; Castelli, J.; et al. Nomogram to predict rectal toxicity following prostate cancer radiotherapy. *PLoS ONE* **2017**, *12*, e0179845. [CrossRef]
10. Vargas, C.; Martinez, A.; Kestin, L.L.; Yan, D.; Grills, I.; Brabbins, D.S.; Lockman, D.M.; Liang, J.; Gustafson, G.S.; Chen, P.Y.; et al. Dose-volume analysis of predictors for chronic rectal toxicity after treatment of prostate cancer with adaptive image-guided radiotherapy. *Int. J. Radiat. Oncol. Biol. Phys.* **2005**, *62*, 1297–1308. [CrossRef]
11. Kupelian, P.A.; Reddy, C.A.; Carlson, T.P.; Willoughby, T.R. Dose/volume relationship of late rectal bleeding after external beam radiotherapy for localized prostate cancer: Absolute or relative rectal volume? *Cancer J.* **2002**, *8*, 62–66. [CrossRef]
12. Marzi, S.; Arcangeli, G.; Saracino, B.; Petrongari, M.G.; Bruzzaniti, V.; Iaccarino, G.; Landoni, V.; Soriani, A.; Benassi, M. Relationships Between Rectal Wall Dose–Volume Constraints and Radiobiologic Indices of Toxicity for Patients With Prostate Cancer. *Int. J. Radiat. Oncol.* **2007**, *68*, 41–49. [CrossRef]
13. Ishikawa, H.; Tsuji, H.; Kamada, T.; Hirasawa, N.; Yanagi, T.; Mizoe, J.-E.; Akakura, K.; Suzuki, H.; Shimazaki, J.; Tsujii, H. Risk factors of late rectal bleeding after carbon ion therapy for prostate cancer. *Int. J. Radiat. Oncol. Biol. Phys.* **2006**, *66*, 1084–1091. [CrossRef] [PubMed]
14. Wachter, S.; Gerstner, N.; Goldner, G.; Pötzi, R.; Wambersie, A.; Pötter, R. Rectal sequelae after conformal radiotherapy of prostate cancer: Dose-volume histograms as predictive factors. *Radiother. Oncol.* **2001**, *59*, 65–70. [CrossRef] [PubMed]
15. Afkhami Ardekani, M.; Ghaffari, H.; Navaser, M.; Zoljalali Moghaddam, S.H.; Refahi, S. Effectiveness of rectal displacement devices in managing prostate motion: A systematic review. *Strahlenther. Onkol.* **2021**, *197*, 97–115. [CrossRef] [PubMed]
16. van Lin, E.N.; Hoffmann, A.L.; van Kollenburg, P.; Leer, J.W.; Visser, A.G. Rectal wall sparing effect of three different endorectal balloons in 3D conformal and IMRT prostate radiotherapy. *Int. J. Radiat. Oncol. Biol. Phys.* **2005**, *63*, 565–576. [CrossRef]
17. Wong, A.T.; Schreiber, D.; Agarwal, M.; Polubarov, A.; Schwartz, D. Impact of the use of an endorectal balloon on rectal dosimetry during stereotactic body radiation therapy for localized prostate cancer. *Pract. Radiat. Oncol.* **2016**, *6*, 262–267. [CrossRef] [PubMed]
18. Teh, B.S.; Lewis, G.D.; Mai, W.; Pino, R.; Ishiyama, H.; Butler, E.B. Long-term outcome of a moderately hypofractionated intensity-modulated radiotherapy approach using an endorectal balloon for patients with localized prostate cancer. *Cancer Commun.* **2018**, *38*, 1–9. [CrossRef]

19. Wortel, R.C.; Oomen-de Hoop, E.; Heemsbergen, W.D.; Pos, F.J.; Incrocci, L. Moderate Hypofractionation in Intermediate- and High-Risk, Localized Prostate Cancer: Health-Related Quality of Life From the Randomized, Phase 3 HYPRO Trial. *Int. J. Radiat. Oncol. Biol. Phys.* **2018**, *103*, 823–833. [CrossRef]
20. Deville, C.; Both, S.; Bui, V.; Hwang, W.-T.; Tan, K.-S.; Schaer, M.; Tochner, Z.; Vapiwala, N. Acute gastrointestinal and genitourinary toxicity of image-guided intensity modulated radiation therapy for prostate cancer using a daily water-filled endorectal balloon. *Radiat. Oncol.* **2012**, *7*, 76. [CrossRef]
21. Vlachaki, M.T.; Teslow, T.N.; Ahmad, S. Impact of Endorectal Balloon in the Dosimetry of Prostate and Surrounding Tissues in Prostate Cancer Patients Treated with IMRT. *Med. Dosim.* **2007**, *32*, 281–286. [CrossRef] [PubMed]
22. Smeenk, R.J.; van Lin, E.N.; van Kollenburg, P.; Kunze-Busch, M.; Kaanders, J.H. Anal wall sparing effect of an endorectal balloon in 3D conformal and intensity-modulated prostate radiotherapy. *Radiother. Oncol.* **2009**, *93*, 131–136. [CrossRef]
23. Patel, R.R.; Orton, N.; Tomé, W.A.; Chappell, R.; Ritter, M.A. Rectal dose sparing with a balloon catheter and ultrasound localization in conformal radiation therapy for prostate cancer. *Radiother. Oncol.* **2003**, *67*, 285–294. [CrossRef] [PubMed]
24. Vargas, C.; Mahajan, C.; Fryer, A.; Indelicato, D.; Henderson, R.H.; McKenzie, C.; Horne, D.; Chellini, A.; Lawlor, P.; Li, Z.; et al. Rectal Dose–Volume Differences Using Proton Radiotherapy and a Rectal Balloon or Water Alone for the Treatment of Prostate Cancer. *Int. J. Radiat. Oncol. Biol. Phys.* **2007**, *69*, 1110–1116. [CrossRef] [PubMed]
25. Wootton, L.S.; Kudchadker, R.J.; Beddar, A.S.; Lee, A.K. Effectiveness of a novel gas-release endorectal balloon in the removal of rectal gas for prostate proton radiation therapy. *J. Appl. Clin. Med. Phys.* **2012**, *13*, 190–197. [CrossRef]
26. Hedrick, S.G.; Fagundes, M.; Robison, B.; Blakey, M.; Renegar, J.; Artz, M.; Schreuder, N. A comparison between hydrogel spacer and endorectal balloon: An analysis of intrafraction prostate motion during proton therapy. *J. Appl. Clin. Med. Phys.* **2017**, *18*, 106–112. [CrossRef]
27. Agren Cronqvist, A.K.; Kallman, P.; Turesson, I.; Brahme, A. Volume and heterogeneity dependence of the dose-response relationship for head and neck tumours. *Acta Oncol.* **1995**, *34*, 851–860. [CrossRef]
28. Vanneste, B.G.L.; van Wijk, Y.; Lutgens, L.C.; Van Limbergen, E.J.; van Lin, E.N.; van de Beek, K.; Lambin, P.; Hoffmann, A.L. Dynamics of rectal balloon implant shrinkage in prostate VMAT: Influence on anorectal dose and late rectal complication risk. *Strahlenther. Onkol.* **2018**, *194*, 31–40. [CrossRef]
29. Qamhiyeh, S.; Geismar, D.; Pöttgen, C.; Stuschke, M.; Farr, J. The effects of motion on the dose distribution of proton radiotherapy for prostate cancer. *J. Appl. Clin. Med. Phys.* **2012**, *13*, 3–11. [CrossRef]
30. Rancati, T.; Fiorino, C.; Gagliardi, G.; Cattaneo, G.M.; Sanguineti, G.; Borca, V.C.; Cozzarini, C.; Fellin, G.; Foppiano, F.; Girelli, G.; et al. Fitting late rectal bleeding data using different NTCP models: Results from an Italian multi-centric study (AIROPROS0101). *Radiother. Oncol.* **2004**, *73*, 21–32. [CrossRef]
31. Dale, E.; Hellebust, T.P.; Skjønsberg, A.; Høgberg, T.; Olsen, D.R. Modeling normal tissue complication probability from repetitive computed tomography scans during fractionated high-dose-rate brachytherapy and external beam radiotherapy of the uterine cervix. *Int. J. Radiat. Oncol. Biol. Phys.* **2000**, *47*, 963–971. [CrossRef]
32. Elsayed, H.; Bolling, T.; Moustakis, C.; Müller, S.-B.; Schüller, P.; Ernst, I.; Willich, N.; Könemann, S. Organ Movements and Dose Exposures in Teletherapy of Prostate Cancer using a Rectal Balloon. *Strahlenther. Onkol.* **2007**, *183*, 617–624. [CrossRef]
33. Hille, A.; Schmidberger, H.; Töws, N.; Weiss, E.; Vorwerk, H.; Hess, C.F. The Impact of Varying Volumes in Rectal Balloons on Rectal Dose Sparing in Conformal Radiation Therapy of Prostate Cancer. A prospective three-dimensional analysis. *Strahlenther. Onkol.* **2005**, *181*, 709–716. [CrossRef]
34. Wachter, S.; Gerstner, N.; Dorner, D.; Goldner, G.; Colotto, A.; Wambersie, A.; Pötter, R. The influence of a rectal balloon tube as internal immobilization device on variations of volumes and dose-volume histograms during treatment course of conformal radiotherapy for prostate cancer. *Int. J. Radiat. Oncol. Biol. Phys.* **2002**, *52*, 91–100. [CrossRef]
35. Storey, M.R.; Pollack, A.; Zagars, G.; Smith, L.; Antolak, J.; Rosen, I. Complications from radiotherapy dose escalation in prostate cancer: Preliminary results of a randomized trial. *Int. J. Radiat. Oncol. Biol. Phys.* **2000**, *48*, 635–642. [CrossRef]
36. Huang, E.H.; Pollack, A.; Levy, L.; Starkschall, G.; Dong, L.; Rosen, I.; Kuban, D.A. Late rectal toxicity: Dose-volume effects of conformal radiotherapy for prostate cancer. *Int. J. Radiat. Oncol. Biol. Phys.* **2002**, *54*, 1314–1321. [CrossRef]
37. Zapatero, A.; García-Vicente, F.; Modolell, I.; Alcántara, P.; Floriano, A.; Cruz-Conde, A.; Torres, J.J.; Pérez-Torrubia, A. Impact of mean rectal dose on late rectal bleeding after conformal radiotherapy for prostate cancer: Dose–volume effect. *Int. J. Radiat. Oncol. Biol. Phys.* **2004**, *59*, 1343–1351. [CrossRef]
38. Tucker, S.L.; Dong, L.; Cheung, R.; Johnson, J.; Mohan, R.; Huang, E.H.; Liu, H.H.; Thames, H.D.; Kuban, D. Comparison of rectal dose–wall histogram versus dose–volume histogram for modeling the incidence of late rectal bleeding after radiotherapy. *Int. J. Radiat. Oncol. Biol. Phys.* **2004**, *60*, 1589–1601. [CrossRef]
39. Jackson, A.; Skwarchuk, M.W.; Zelefsky, M.J.; Cowen, D.M.; Venkatraman, E.S.; Levegrun, S.; Burman, C.M.; Kutcher, G.J.; Fuks, Z.; Liebel, S.A.; et al. Late rectal bleeding after conformal radiotherapy of prostate cancer. II. Volume effects and dose-volume histograms. *Int. J. Radiat. Oncol. Biol. Phys.* **2001**, *49*, 685–698. [CrossRef]

Disclaimer/Publisher's Note: The statements, opinions and data contained in all publications are solely those of the individual author(s) and contributor(s) and not of MDPI and/or the editor(s). MDPI and/or the editor(s) disclaim responsibility for any injury to people or property resulting from any ideas, methods, instructions or products referred to in the content.

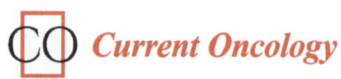

Systematic Review

Salvage Radical Prostatectomy for Radio-Recurrent Prostate Cancer: An Updated Systematic Review of Oncologic, Histopathologic and Functional Outcomes and Predictors of Good Response

Bernhard Grubmüller [1], Victoria Jahrreiss [1], Stephan Brönimann [1], Fahad Quhal [1,2], Keiichiro Mori [1,3], Axel Heidenreich [4], Alberto Briganti [5], Derya Tilki [6] and Shahrokh F. Shariat [1,7,8,9,10,11,12,*]

1. Department of Urology, Medical University of Vienna, 1090 Vienna, Austria; berhard.grubmueller@meduniwien.ac.at (B.G.); Victoria.jahrreiss@meduniwien.ac.at (V.J.); stephan.Broenimann@meduniwien.ac.at (S.B.); fahad.quhal@meduniwien.ac.at (F.Q.); Keiichiro.mori@meduniwien.ac.at (K.M.)
2. Department of Urology, King Fahad Specialist Hospital, Dammam 32253, Saudi Arabia
3. Department of Urology, The Jikei University School of Medicine, Tokyo 105-8461, Japan
4. Department of Urology, University Hospital Cologne, 50923 Cologne, Germany; axel.heidenreich@uk-koeln.de
5. Department of Urology and Division of Experimental Oncology, URI, Urological Research Institute, IRCCS San Raffaele Scientific Institute, 20132 Milan, Italy; briganti.alberto@hsr.it
6. Department of Urology, University Hospital-Hamburg Eppendorf, 20251 Hamburg, Germany; dtilki@me.com
7. Karl Landsteiner Institute of Urology and Andrology, 3100 St. Pölten, Austria
8. Department of Urology, University of Texas Southwestern, Dallas, TX 75390, USA
9. Department of Urology and Division of Medical Oncology, Weill Medical College of Cornell University, New York, NY 10065, USA
10. Department of Urology, Second Faculty of Medicine, Charles University, 150 06 Prague, Czech Republic
11. Institute for Urology and Reproductive Health, I.M. Sechenov First Moscow State Medical University, 119992 Moscow, Russia
12. Division of Urology, Department of Special Surgery, Jordan University Hospital, The University of Jordan, Amman 11942, Jordan
* Correspondence: shahrokh.shariat@meduniwien.ac.at; Tel.: +43-1-40400-26150; Fax: +43-1-40400-32230

Abstract: A valid treatment option for recurrence after definite radiotherapy (RT) for localized prostate cancer (PC) is salvage radical prostatectomy (SRP). However, data on SRP are scarce, possibly resulting in an underutilization. A systematic review was performed using MEDLINE (Pubmed), Embase, and Web of Science databases including studies published between January 1980 and April 2020. Overall, 23 English language articles including a total number of 2323 patients were selected according to PRISMA criteria. The overall median follow-up was 37.5 months (IQR 35.5–52.5). Biochemical-recurrence (BCR)-free probability ranged from 34% to 83% at five years, respectively, and from 31% to 37% at 10 years. Cancer specific survival (CSS) and overall survival (OS) ranged from 88.7% to 98% and 64% to 95% at five years and from 72% to 83% and 65% to 72% at 10 years, respectively. Positive surgical margins ranged from 14% to 45.8% and pathologic organ-confined disease was reported from 20% to 57%. The rate of pathologic > T2-disease ranged from 37% to 80% and pN1 disease differed between 0% to 78.4%. Pre-SRP PSA, pre-SRP Gleason Score (GS), pathologic stage after SRP, and pathologic lymph node involvement seemed to be the strongest prognostic factors for good outcomes. SRP provides accurate histopathological and functional outcomes, as well as durable cancer control. Careful patient counseling in a shared decision-making process is recommended.

Keywords: prostate cancer; salvage radical prostatectomy; primary radiotherapy; recurrence

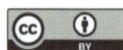

1. Introduction

Radiation therapy (RT) is a standard and widely used primary treatment strategy with the intention to cure non-metastatic prostate cancer (PC) [1]. Despite adequate delivery, up to 40% of patients eventually suffer from biochemical recurrence (BCR) [2–4]. Despite several studies having shown acceptable oncologic and functional results for salvage radical prostatectomy (SRP) of radio-recurrent PC [5–7], most of these patients are still treated with systemic palliative androgen deprivation therapy (ADT) [1,2], with all its downsides, including the very high failure rate and systemic side effects [8–10]. A systematic review of the literature published in 2012 by Chade et al. [11] reported on the steadily improving outcomes of SRP resulting from surgical expertise and improved patient selection. Thanks to novel surgical techniques such as the robot-assisted approach [12] and the earlier detection of locoregional recurrent disease with novel superior imaging modalities in the BCR setting (i.e., PSMA-PET) [13], outcomes of salvage local surgical interventions promise to further improve [14]. Most guidelines recommend performing SRP in case of BCR after primary RT (1) in centers with great experience, (2) after confirmatory biopsy of the local relapse, (3) without clinical evidence of metastatic disease [1,15]. The aim of SRP is to cure with local therapy, to delay time to clinical progression and death, to prevent local symptoms, and/or to achieve a local cytoreduction that would allow a better response to subsequent therapies. Additionally, systemic treatment-related toxicity can in some cases be delayed or avoided completely.

Despite progress in this field, exact data on ideal patient selection and predictors of response for SRP is still scarce but urgently needed to help guide clinical decision making for individual patients. Several confounding studies have addressed the oncologic, histopathological, and functional outcomes of SRP over a long period of time. For this reason, we aimed to conduct an updated systematic review of the literature concerning histopathologic and oncologic outcomes for SRP with the aim of identifying predictors of response.

Considering the interventional aim of this meta-analysis, oncologic outcomes (BCR-rate, overall survival (OS), cancer-specific survival (CSS), histopathological outcomes (T stage, N stage, and positive surgical margins (PSM)), as well as functional outcomes (erectile function (EF), urinary continence) have been assessed.

The secondary aim was to compare histopathological outcomes after SRP, the usage of minimally invasive surgery (laparoscopic/robotic) and time to SRP in studies published before and after 2010. Another secondary aim was to compare outcomes of open versus laparoscopic/robotic SRP. Therefore, analyses were conducted among (1) studies published 1988–2009 and 2010–2020, and (2) open vs. laparoscopic/robotic cases.

2. Methods

2.1. Search Strategy

Databases which are considered the most relevant for our topic will be searched. For this reason, this review is based on systematic searches in the MEDLINE (Pubmed), Embase, and Web of Science databases according to the Preferred Reporting Items for Systematic Reviews and Meta-analysis (PRISMA) guidelines [16]. These electronic databases were searched in April 2020 to identify reports on oncologic, histopathologic, and functional outcomes of SRP for radio-recurrent PC.

Initially, medical subject headings (MeSH) were used followed by free-text terms using the following controlled vocabulary for the further search strategy: "radical AND salvage therapy" OR "salvage AND therapy" OR "salvage therapy" OR "salvage AND prostatectomy" OR "salvage AND prostatectomy AND prostate cancer". The temporal limit was set to January 1980 and only articles in English were considered for review.

2.2. Study Selection

A flow diagram adhering the PRISMA guidelines for reporting of systematic reviews was used in reporting of the selection process and the results (Figure 1).

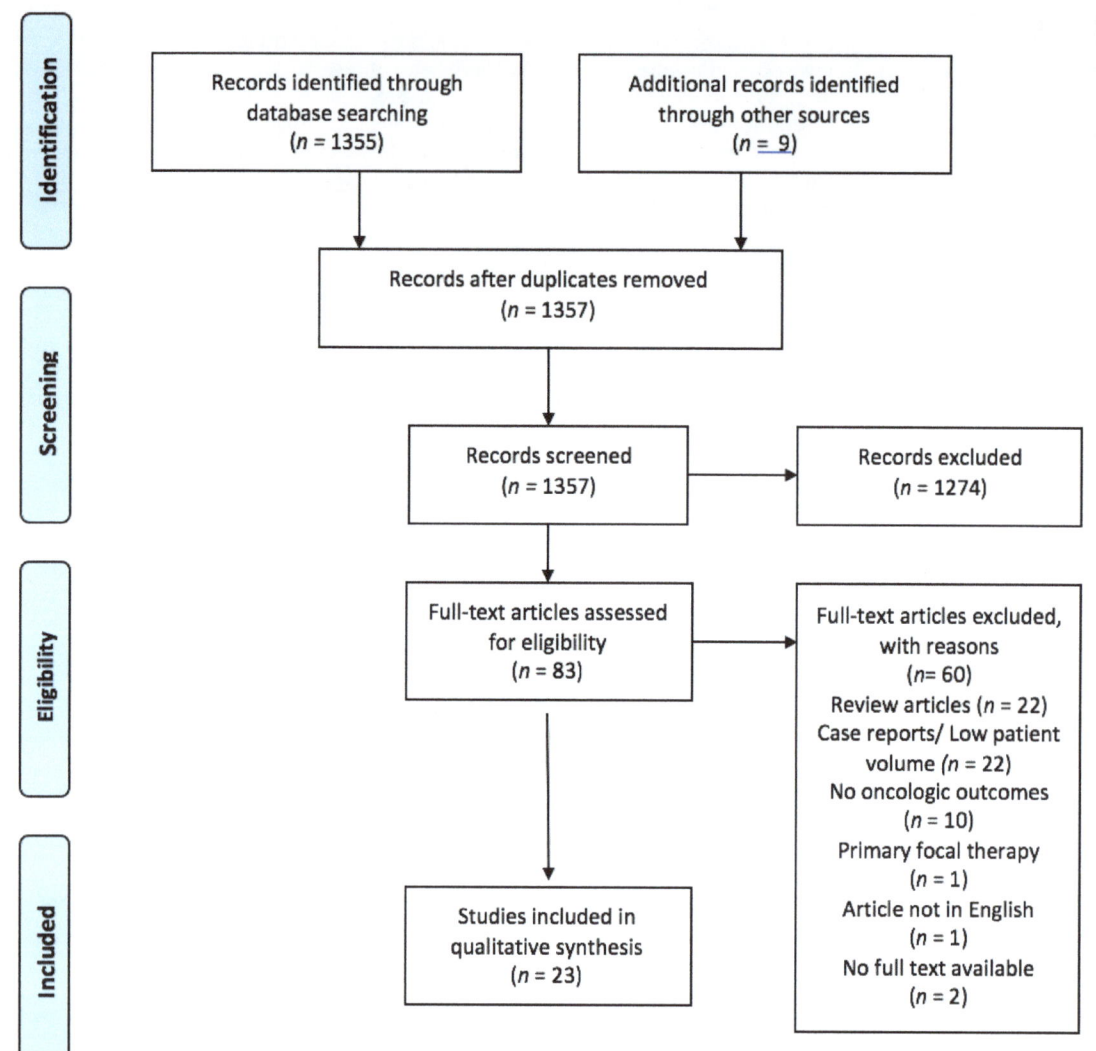

Figure 1. PRISMA flow diagram.

The initial search results have been organized by importing them into the Endnote reference management software (Thomson Reuters (Scientific) LLC, London, UK). Duplicates and irrelevant studies have been removed. Two independent investigators screened the results based on the titles and abstracts to identify ineligible studies, and reasons for exclusions were noted. Additional references were identified from the reference list of each article. Two independent reviewers subjected potentially relevant reports to a full-text review and the relevance of the reports was confirmed after the data extraction process. Both reviewers had to agree on the inclusion of the study in all cases. In cases of disagreement, a third reviewer was consulted for the final decision. After screening 1364 papers, 23 met the inclusion criteria for synthesis (Figure 1).

2.3. Inclusion Criteria

Studies being included had to present data of patients undergoing SRP for radio-recurrent PC, apply a widely accepted qualitative data collection method, and use a well-described methodology.

Criteria for study inclusion took into account the following topics: (1) radio-recurrent PC diagnosis, (2) local recurrence with no evidence of metastatic disease, (3) predictive oncologic factors, (4) surgical approach (open, laparoscopic, or robotic SRP), (5) cancer control, (6) histopathologic outcomes, and (7) functional outcomes.

2.4. Exclusion Criteria

We excluded reviews, letters, editorials, meeting abstracts, replies from authors, and case reports with fewer than 10 patients. In the case of duplicate publications, the higher quality or the most recent publication was selected.

2.5. Data Extraction

Two investigators independently extracted the following information from the included articles: first author's name, publication year, recruitment country, period of patient recruitment, number of patients, age, study design, initial PSA, PSA at SRP, TNM stage, surgical technique, oncological outcome, functional outcomes, predictive oncologic factors, and follow-up duration.

2.6. Missing Data

In case data could not be acquired, only available data were analyzed.

2.7. Statistics

Differences in categorical variables including PSM, organ-confined disease (OCD), T stage, N stage, and usage of laparoscopic/robotic surgery were assessed using Chi-square tests. Continuous variables were analyzed using the t-test. Organ-confined disease was defined as $\leq$pT2 and N0 disease. All p values were two-sided, and statistical significance was defined as a $p < 0.05$. Statistical analyses were performed using Stata/MP 14.2 statistical software (StataCorp., Collage Station, TX, USA).

3. Results

3.1. Epidemiology

In the absence of RCTs, all 23 studies that reported oncologic outcomes and were included in the analyses were of retrospective design (19 single center [12,17–34] and four multi center [5,35–37]). The studies were published between 1988 and 2020. These studies comprised data of 2323 patients in total. The median age was reported in all but five studies [5,22,24,30,31]. The median age of the patients at the time of SRP was 65 years (overall interquartile range (IQR) 63.5–65.5). The complete data about primary therapy for localized PC were provided in 18 studies. The percentage of patients receiving ADT as concomitant therapy with RT ranged from 2% to 60% across the studies. Overall, 9.6% of the included 2323 patients underwent RT with concomitant ADT, while the rest of the patients received RT only. The type of RT within the different studies can be seen in Table 1. The exact definition of BCR after primary RT differed between the studies. Nevertheless, all of the included patients had a confirmatory biopsy in case of BCR before SRP. The overall median time to SRP was 51 months (IQR 41–69) and overall median total serum PSA at SRP was 6.04 ng/mL (IQR 4.5–9.4). Information on the surgical technique was provided in 12 studies [5,12,18–24,31,32,35], compromising 1277 patients. SRP was performed in open approach in 79.9% of the patients, robotic in 19.0%, and laparoscopic in 1.1%. Comparing the surgical technique between studies published before and after 2010, we found a difference in the usage of the laparoscopic/robotic approach over time (0% (0/119) in studies published before 2010 versus 22.4% (259/1158) in studies published after 2010, $p < 0.0001$). We also observed a difference in time to SRP from primary RT over the last decade. While the median time to SRP was 40 months before 2010, it was 68 months after 2010, $p = 0.0068$.

Table 1. Pathologic outcomes after salvage radical prostatectomy.

First Author/Yr	Nb. of Patients	RT Type, % (RT/BT/COMB or Other Focal)	RT + ADT, %	Median Follow-Up	PSM%	Lymph Node Involvement, %	>pT2 after SRP, %
Onol/2020 [12]	94	60.6/24.5/14.9	25.5	32	17	10.6	50
Vartolomei/2019 [35]	214	-	47.7	25.3	22	18.7	43
Metcalfe/2017 [17]	70	68.6/20/11.4	26	-	20	45.8	61.4
Kenney/2016 [18]	39	61.5/38.5/0	-	-	15.4	12.8	61.5
Mandel/2016 [19]	55	49.1/50.9/0	45	36	27	21.8	50
Bates/2015 [20]	53	62.2/26.4/11.2	-	36	18.9	26.4	51
Pearce/2014 [36]	408	89/11/0	-	-	33.7	6.2	49
Yuh/2014 [21]	51	47.1/43.1/9.8	19.6	36	31.4	78.4	51
Meeks/2013 [22]	206	66/29/5	-	-	14	21	57
Gorin/2011 [23]	24	54/46/0	58	-	45.8	13.3	54.2
Chade/2011 [5]	404	65/19/16	-	-	25	16	45
Eandi/2010 [24]	18	-	2.2	18	28	20	50
Pisters/2009 [25]	42	92.9/7.1/0	0	96	-	-	-
Leonardo/2009 [26]	32	100/0/0	0	35	34.4	0	46.9
Paparel/2008 [27]	146	-	-	45	16	13	63
Sanderson/2006 [28]	51	59/23/18	18	84	35.5	15.7	44
Bianco/2005 [37]	100	29/42/29	16	60	21	9	65
Amling/1999 [29]	108	98/2/0	0	-	36	18	61
Tefilli/1998 [30]	27	-	-	34	18.5	-	33
Lerner/1995 [31]	79	90/10/0	-	50	40	8	61
Rogers/1995 [32]	40	35/65/0	2.5	39	37	5	80
Zincke/1992 [33]	32	100/0/0	0	48	-	-	-
Rainwater/1988 [34]	30	-	-	80	-	-	-

Yr = year, Nb = number, RT = radiotherapy, BT = brachytherapy, Comb = Combination therapies or other focal therapies, ADT = androgen deprivation therapy, PSM = positive surgical margins, SRP = salvage radical prostatectomy.

3.2. Oncological Outcomes

The studies with the largest number of patients were retrospective and of multicenter design [5,36]. The median follow-up within all studies ranged from 18 to 96 months (overall median follow-up 37.5 months, IQR 35.5–52.5), which may explain the wide variety of findings in oncologic survival outcomes. The definition of BCR after SRP varied between the different publications, although a PSA rise > 0.2ng/mL was the most widely used definition. The five-year BCR-free survival was reported in 10 out of 23 studies and ranged from 34% to 83% [5,12,17,19,22,25,27,33,35,37]. The 10-year BCR-free survival was available in two studies with 31% [23] and 37% [5]. The clinical progression-free survival was reported in only one study [28] with 47% at five years. The CSS was reported in three studies ranging from 88.7% to 98% at five years [5,19,25] and from 72% to 83% [5,31] at 10 years. The reported OS ranged from 64% to 95% at five years [17,25,28,31] and from 65% to 72% at 10 years [28,29,31], respectively.

None of the studies evaluated differences in oncologic SRP outcomes after RT and after brachytherapy (BT) or between distinct RT techniques or RT dose. At the time of SRP none of the included patients was on ADT. Data evaluating the effect of neoadjuvant or concomitant ADT were poorly described, if at all. Overall, no effect for concomitant ADT at the time of RT was shown on oncologic outcomes after SRP. One study evaluated the impact of concomitant ADT on oncologic outcomes after SRP [31] but found no difference in CSS.

3.3. Histopathological Outcomes

The pathologic characteristics after SRP were reported in all but three studies [25,33,34]. Among these studies, several differences in the pathologic outcomes were found. Overall 847 of the 2323 patients (36.5%) undergoing SRP had a PSM. The PSM-rate ranged from 14% to 45.8%. Pathologic OCD was reported from 20% to 57% and the rate of pathologic > T2 disease ranged from 37% to 80%. Pathologic lymph node (LN) involvement after SRP was reported to be between 0% and 78.4%. Comparing histopathological outcomes between studies published before and after 2010, we could not find a difference in the rate of overall PSM (27.3% vs. 23.9%, $p = 0.11$). Nevertheless, we found a difference in overall pathological LN disease (11.5% in studies before 2010 versus 17.3% in studies published after 2010, $p = 0.0009$) and in the rate of overall ≤pT2-disease after SRP (62.9% in studies before 2010 and 47.4% in studies published after 2010, $p < 0.0001$). Comparing open versus laparoscopic/robotic SRP, there was also no difference in the overall PSM-rate (26.8% vs. 21.8%, $p = 0.13$) and in the pathologic stage after SRP (≤pT2 48.2% vs. 50.5%, $p = 0.55$), but the rate of pathologic N1 disease was higher in the laparoscopic/robotic (31.5%) vs. open cases (15.6%), $p < 0.0001$.

3.4. Functional Outcomes

Although the oncologic outcomes of SRP seem to be accurate, sexual and urinary dysfunction after the surgery are directly influencing the patients' quality of life. Overall, 13 studies (four robotic (216 patients overall) [12,20,21,24], nine open (370 patients overall) [19,23,26,28,30–34]) could be identified reporting on oncologic and functional outcomes after SRP. The outcome measurements and definitions for EF after SRP varied between the different studies: (1) "Sexual Health Inventory for Men" Questionnaire [12,20], (2) IIEF-5-Score [19], (3) "erection sufficient for penetration without PDE-5 inhibitors" [21], (4) "ability to have sexual intercourse with or without the use of PDE-5 inhibitors in >50% of the attempts" [23], (5) "normal erections during intercourse with or without PDE-5 inhibitor" [26]. EF before SRP was already poor with a great variability (two studies did not report on EF-rate before SRP [20,26]) ranging from 25.5% to 40.9%. However, the post-SRP EF-rate dropped significantly and from 0% to 13.1% in five studies [12,19,21,23,26]. One study reported an EF of 31.5% three years after SRP, although the pre-EF-rate was not available [20].

The urinary continence rate after SRP ranged from 21.9% to 90% at one year. Again, here, the definition of urinary continence was not uniform. The definition used most often for urinary continence after SRP was the usage of 0–1 pads/day in eight studies [19–21,24,28,31–33] and ranged from 27% to 76.9%. Three further studies defined 0 pad/day as urinary continent [23,26,30] and the rate was reported to be between 21.9% and 65%. Onol et al [12] ivided their definition into fully continent (0 pad/day: 73%) and social continent (0–1 pad/day: 39.2%). The study with the highest rate of urinary continence of 90% was published by Rainwater et al. [34], but they did not report their used definition.

3.5. Prognostic Risk Factors

Overall, 15 studies could be identified that evaluated both clinical and pathologic predictive factors of oncologic outcomes after SRP [5,17,19–21,23,27–29,31,32,34–37]. One included study could not find any association of clinicopathologic factors with oncologic outcome after SRP [20]. Pre-surgical PSA, the pre-surgery Gleason Score (GS) and the pathologic stage including LN status after SRP seemed to be the strongest prognostic factors. Overall, eight studies found an association of pre-surgical PSA with pathologic and oncologic outcomes. A high pre-surgical PSA correlated with BCR in five studies [5,21,27,32,37], with clinical progression and CSS in one study [5], with OS in three studies [27,28,37], and with PSM-rate in one study [36]. Another important pre-operative predictor was the biopsy GS, as it was associated with the BCR [5,17,19,35,37], clinical progression [5], CSS [5,35], and OS [27,28,35,37]. Further pre-operative factors found to be significant were pre-operative clinical stage in two studies [5,28] and the number of positive cores in one study [17]. Concerning post-operative factors, the pathological stage after SRP was associated with BCR in five studies [19,21,23,35,37], with clinical progression in one study [19], with CSS in one study [37] and with OS in two studies [5,28]. Pathologic LN involvement was found to be associated with BCR [19,35,37], clinical progression [5,19], CSS [35], and with OS [5]. Furthermore, pathologic GS was associated with CSS [5,37] and BCR [37].

Another pathologic prognostic risk factor in SRP specimens in older published studies (all before 2000) was DNA ploidy for BCR [29] and CSS [31,34].

4. Discussion

Radio-recurrent PC after primary RT with curative intent remains a challenging clinical scenario for physicians given the lack of consensus on patient selection and the fact that standard imaging tools, such as CT and bone scans, are not accurate enough to distinguish between locoregional only, distant recurrence, or both [38]. This is changing with the more widespread use of novel imaging tools such as PSMA-PET imaging in the BCR setting [13]. Due to its superior detection rates (sensitivity) also at lower PSA levels, PSMA-PET allows a more individualized salvage therapy decision making with a potential for cure in cases of locoregional recurrence only [39,40]. This is also the reason why SRP and other potentially curative local treatments are becoming more interesting for the management of radio-recurrent PC, again [41]. Furthermore, as shown by Marra et al., recurrences are frequently high grade, with 27% having a GS ≥ 9 compared to 90% having a GS of ≤ 7 at initial PC diagnosis. This discrepancy is likely largely related to treatment induced changes and selection of resistant clones, altering the natural history of PC towards adverse features [42]. Nevertheless, potential risks and side effects and patient selection are still a matter of debate for SRP. The aim of SRP is to cure, to delay progression, to delay the need for systemic therapies, and to prevent local complications. Despite improved early detection of the site of recurrence and despite improved surgical techniques, such as the robot-assisted approach [12], the currently most used treatment for radio-recurrent PC is ADT, which leads to significant morbidity (e.g., bone fractures, diabetes, etc.) in addition to excluding the opportunity for cure [43]. Because of the lack of studies that directly compare SRP to ADT and SRP to nonsurgical local salvage therapies in the case of radio-recurrent PC, we aimed to conduct an updated systematic review of the literature concerning histopathologic and oncologic outcomes for SRP with the aim of identifying predictors of response.

In this systematic review, oncologic outcomes varied among the included studies for the synthesis. Considering a wide range of different follow-up times (from 18 to 96 months) the BCR-free rate ranged from 34% to 83% at five years, meaning that oncological outcomes are promising in the medium term and a significant proportion of men remain free of disease at five years follow-up. The two studies with the largest cohorts [5,36] and the longest follow-up showed a 10-year BCR-free survival of 31% and 37%, respectively. A systematic review and meta-analysis on nonsurgical salvage focal therapies for radio recurrent PC published in 2020 showed comparable results, but patient selection may account for this [41]. The overall pooled prevalence of BCR-free survival was 64%, with a large heterogeneity within the different studies. In a subgroup analysis, the prevalence of biochemical control was the lowest for patients treated with HIFU (58%) and highest for patients treated with BT (69%) and salvage EBRT (69%). Nevertheless, one has to mention that, in this included meta-analysis, the median follow-up time was comparably shorter, and many patients received adjuvant ADT in addition to salvage nonsurgical focal therapy for radio-recurrent PC. Therefore, a direct comparison is not possible considering the studies included in our work, since none of the patients was on concomitant ADT while undergoing SRP. A meta-regression analysis published in 2016 also compared oncologic outcomes of SRP vs. nonsurgical therapies for radio-recurrent PC [44]. The authors concluded that the oncologic outcomes were comparable between SRP and the nonsurgical salvage modalities. However, SRP was associated with a higher rate of urinary incontinence. In addition, the higher rate of given ADT in the nonsurgical studies prevents a fair direct comparison within the investigated treatment modalities.

Similar oncologic results were published by Valle et al., who compared local salvage modalities (SRP, HIFU, cryotherapy, stereotactic body radiotherapy (SBRT), low-dose-rate (LDR) brachytherapy, and high-dose-rate (HDR) brachytherapy) for radiorecurrent disease. Adjusted 5-yr RFS ranged from 50% after cryotherapy to 60% after HDR brachytherapy and SBRT, with no evidence of large differences in 5-yr RFS outcomes for surgical, non-radiotherapeutic ablative, and radiotherapeutic salvage of radiorecurrent PC. As discussed above, this meta-analysis also included studies with significant heterogeneity between studies and within each modality [45].

Furthermore, the published series on nonsurgical salvage therapies are relatively small and consequently, this treatment should be offered in experienced centers only. Therefore, nonsurgical salvage focal therapies are not recommended by the guidelines, except within a clinical trial setting or well-designed prospective study cohorts [1].

Additionally, we found that CSS in the studies included in our review ranged from 88.7% to 98% at five years and from 72% to 83% at 10 years after SRP. OS ranged from 64% to 95% at five years and from 65% to 72% at 10 years, respectively. Despite these outstanding results, most of the patients with local recurrence after primary RT with curative intent are referred to systemic ADT [1]. Interestingly, one randomized prospective trial showed an 86% vs. 79% OS advantage at 10 years for ADT in this setting [46]. In contrast, most studies did not find any differences between early vs. delayed, or no ADT [47]. Moreover, there are studies showing an even unfavorable effect of ADT on survival due to its long-term risks and side-effect [48]. Nevertheless, some high-risk patients seem to benefit most from early ADT, given a life expectancy of more than ten years [49]. Considering these results, SRP seems to be superior to ADT, concerning survival rates and long-term side effects in well-selected patients in case of radio-recurrent PC after primary RT. ADT should be offered to those patients at highest risk of disease progression since there is supporting data on the improvement of survival [46]. However, these patients are likely to be excluded from SRP with the use of modern scanning such as PSMA-PET nowadays [14].

The overall PSM-rate was 36.5% with a range of 14% to 45.8%. The range of OCD on final SRP pathology ranged from 20% to 57% and the rate of pathologic > T2-disease ranged from 37% to 80%. Overall, 0 –78.4% had pathologic positive LN at the time of SRP. Two of the multi-institutional studies including the highest number of patients [5,36] showed a PSM of 33.7% and 25%, OCD in 50.9% and 53%, and LN involvement in 6.2% and 16%. A systematic review published in 2012 showed similar results [11]. Here, the rate of PSM and of OCD ranged from 0% to 70% and 22% to 81%, respectively. This variety among histopathological findings may be explained due to the long period of time and different centers reporting on SRP outcomes. Because surgical techniques improved over time [50] and the robot-assisted laparoscopic approach became the new standard of care [12] (as we could also show an increased use over the last decade: 0% before 2010, 22.4% after 2010, $p < 0.0001$), we compared the histopathological outcomes in studies published before and after the year 2010. Although we could not find a difference in the rate of overall PSM-rate ($p = 0.105$), there was a difference in overall pathological N1 disease ($p = 0.0009$) and in the rate of overall ≤pT2-disease ($p < 0.0001$) in studies before 2010 compared to those published after 2010. The finding that clinical stage and LN involvement increases over time in SRP specimen can possibly be explained by the introduction and increased use of active surveillance in low-risk PC recurrence and a higher awareness of life expectancy and competing health risks [51]. We also compared the histopathological outcomes of open versus laparoscopic/robotic SRP and found no difference in PSM-rate ($p = 0.13$) and in the pathologic stage after SRP ($p = 0.55$). Nevertheless, the rate of pathologic N1 disease was higher in the laparoscopic/robotic (31.5%) vs. open cases (15.6%), $p < 0.0001$. One has to mention that a limitation of the latter analysis is the scarce available data reporting on outcomes of open vs. laparoscopic/robotic SRP in the literature. One possible explanation for this finding might be the fact that attitudes toward lymphadenectomy changed considerably during the period analyzed [52].

Moreover, the functional outcomes differed between the included studies of this systematic review. While the patients had a relatively poor EF before SRP (25.5% to 40.9%), the EF after SRP was reported from 0% to 13.1% in five studies [12,19,21,23,26]. One study reported an EF of 31.5% after three years, but without reporting on the EF before surgery [20]. Clearly, the different definitions and measurements of EF have to be taken into account while interpreting these results. Therefore, the informative value on overall EF after SRP is limited. Concerning urinary continence, we also found a wide range of outcomes. While the used definition was identical in eight studies (0–1 pad/day), we found urinary continence rates ranging from 21.9% to 90% among the 13 included studies. Here, the caveats of heterogeneous outcomes definition are mentionable, as e.g., the study with the highest urinary continence rate [34] did not report on their used definition. Furthermore, functional outcomes are also dependent on the surgeon's experience and expertise.

As shown above, several clinical and pathologic risk factors are associated with oncologic outcomes of SRP patients. Since careful patient selection for SRP is crucial, several studies addressed this question in detail. According to the findings of our review, the most important pre-operative prognostic factors seem to be the PSA-level and the biopsy GS before SRP, while after SRP, the pathological stage and pathologic positive LN were also of significance for oncologic outcomes. All four, i.e., a high pre-surgical PSA, the biopsy GS, the pathological stage, and LN involvement after SRP, correlated with PSM-rate, BCR-rates, clinical progression, CSS, and OS. Although the conclusions of those findings resulted from a few retrospective studies with sometimes small patient cohorts, these factors seem to be important for ideal patient selection in case of attempted local surgery with curative intent. This may also imply that performing an extended LN dissection is mandatory while performing SRP. This is in accordance with the review published in 2012 by Chade et al. [11]. The PSA and pre-SRP biopsy GS were also the strongest predictors for oncologic outcomes in their assessment. However, in contrast to our work, the pathologic stage and pathologic positive LNs were not identified as such significant factors for the prognosis after SRP. This is likely due to studies in the last eight years which showed such an association specifically.

Several limitations weaken the informative value of our study. First of all, reporting, selection, and publication biases must be considered. Furthermore, between-study heterogeneity and the lack of standardized reporting of oncologic and functional outcomes have also to be mentioned. There are currently no randomized and only a few retrospective trials addressing the role and outcomes of SRP (for the matter of fact also for nonsurgical procedures) in the case of radio-recurrent PC. The median follow-up of recently published studies is still limited, making the results subject to follow-up bias. We did not have original data sets from each series available. Nevertheless, the overall findings suggest that SRP is a feasible and effective treatment option regarding oncologic and histopathological outcomes in well-selected patients with radio-recurrent PC.

5. Conclusions

In this systematic review, we found that SRP is an effective local treatment option for this heterogeneous patient cohort with acceptable oncologic, histopathologic, and functional outcomes. Pre-surgical PSA and the biopsy GS seem to be the strongest pre-SRP prognostic factors for ideal patient selection. Pathologic stage and LN status after SRP are also associated with oncologic prognosis. Despite efforts, there is still a need for high quality data from prospective well-designed studies to help strengthen our understanding of the best standard management of patients with radio-recurrent PC.

Author Contributions: B.G.: Conceptualization, Data curation, Formal analysis, Writing–original draft; V.J.: Data curation, Writing–original draft; S.B.: Writing, Review & editing; F.Q.: Methodology, Formal analysis; K.M.: Methodology, Formal analysis; A.H.: Validation, Writing–review & editing; A.B.: Validation, Writing–review & editing; D.T.: Validation, Writing–review & editing; S.F.S.: Conceptualization, Review & editing, Supervision. All authors have read and agreed to the published version of the manuscript.

Funding: No funding or other financial support was received.

Institutional Review Board Statement: Not applicable.

Informed Consent Statement: For this type of study formal consent is not required. Internal Review Board approval for the present study and for retrospective data collection was obtained according to the policy set by each participant institution, when required.

Data Availability Statement: Not applicable.

Conflicts of Interest: The authors declare no conflict of interest.

References

1. Cornford, P.; Bellmunt, J.; Bolla, M.; Briers, E.; Santis, M.D.; Gross, T.; Henry, A.M.; Joniau, S.; Lam, T.B.; Mason, M.D.; et al. EAU-ESTRO-SIOG Guidelines on Prostate Cancer. Part II: Treatment of Relapsing, Metastatic, and Castration-Resistant Prostate Cancer. *Eur. Urol.* **2017**, *71*, 630–642. [CrossRef]
2. Agarwal, P.K.; Sadetsky, N.; Konety, B.R.; Resnick, M.I.; Carroll, P.R. (CaPSURE) C of the PSURE. Treatment failure after primary and salvage therapy for prostate cancer: Likelihood, patterns of care, and outcomes. *Cancer* **2008**, *112*, 307–314. [CrossRef]
3. Shariat, S.F.; Kattan, M.W.; Vickers, A.J.; Karakiewicz, P.I.; Scardino, P.T. Critical review of prostate cancer predictive tools. *Future Oncol.* **2009**, *5*, 1555–1584. [CrossRef]
4. Walz, J.; Gallina, A.; Perrotte, P.; Jeldres, C.; Trinh, Q.-D.; Hutterer, G.C.; Traumann, M.; Ramírez, A.; Shariat, S.F.; McCormack, M.; et al. Clinicians are poor raters of life-expectancy before radical prostatectomy or definitive radiotherapy for localized prostate cancer. *BJU Int.* **2007**, *100*, 1254–1258. [CrossRef]
5. Chade, D.C.; Shariat, S.F.; Cronin, A.M.; Savage, C.J.; Karnes, R.J.; Blute, M.L.; Briganti, A.; Montorsi, F.; van der Poel, H.G.; Van Poppel, H.; et al. Salvage Radical Prostatectomy for Radiation-recurrent Prostate Cancer: A Multi-institutional Collaboration. *Eur. Urol.* **2011**, *60*, 205–210. [CrossRef] [PubMed]
6. Heidenreich, A.; Richter, S.; Thüer, D.; Pfister, D. Prognostic Parameters, Complications, and Oncologic and Functional Outcome of Salvage Radical Prostatectomy for Locally Recurrent Prostate Cancer after 21st-Century Radiotherapy. *Eur. Urol.* **2010**, *57*, 437–445. [CrossRef] [PubMed]
7. Gotto, G.T.; Yunis, L.H.; Vora, K.; Eastham, J.A.; Scardino, P.T.; Rabbani, F. Impact of Prior Prostate Radiation on Complications After Radical Prostatectomy. *J. Urol.* **2010**, *184*, 136–142. [CrossRef] [PubMed]
8. Moschini, M.; Zaffuto, E.; Karakiewicz, P.; Mattei, A.; Gandaglia, G.; Fossati, N.; Montorsi, F.; Briganti, A.; Shariat, S.F. The effect of androgen deprivation treatment on subsequent risk of bladder cancer diagnosis in male patients treated for prostate cancer. *World J. Urol.* **2018**, *37*, 1127–1135. [CrossRef] [PubMed]
9. Gandaglia, G.; Sun, M.; Popa, I.; Schiffmann, J.; Trudeau, V.; Shariat, S.F.; Trinh, Q.-D.; Graefen, M.; Widmer, H.; Saad, F.; et al. Cardiovascular Mortality in Patients With Metastatic Prostate Cancer Exposed to Androgen Deprivation Therapy: A Population-Based Study. *Clin. Genitourin. Cancer* **2015**, *13*, e123–e130. [CrossRef]
10. Kluth, L.A.; Shariat, S.F.; Kratzik, C.; Tagawa, S.; Sonpavde, G.; Rieken, M.; Scherr, D.; Pummer, K. The hypothalamic–pituitary–gonadal axis and prostate cancer: Implications for androgen deprivation therapy. *World J. Urol.* **2013**, *32*, 669–676. [CrossRef]
11. Chade, D.C.; Eastham, J.; Graefen, M.; Hu, J.C.; Karnes, R.J.; Klotz, L.; Montorsi, F.; van Poppel, H.; Scardino, P.T.; Shariat, S.F. Cancer Control and Functional Outcomes of Salvage Radical Prostatectomy for Radiation-recurrent Prostate Cancer: A Systematic Review of the Literature. *Eur. Urol.* **2012**, *61*, 961–971. [CrossRef] [PubMed]
12. Onol, F.F.; Bhat, S.; Moschovas, M.; Rogers, T.; Ganapathi, H.; Roof, S.; Rocco, B.; Patel, V. Comparison of outcomes of salvage robot-assisted laparoscopic prostatectomy for post-primary radiation vs focal therapy. *BJU Int.* **2020**, *125*, 103. [CrossRef] [PubMed]
13. Jansen, B.H.; van Leeuwen, P.J.; Wondergem, M.; van der Sluis, T.M.; Nieuwenhuijzen, J.A.; Knol, R.J.; van Moorselaar, R.J.; van der Poel, H.G.; Oprea-Lager, D.-E.; Vis, A.N. Detection of Recurrent Prostate Cancer Using Prostate-specific Membrane Antigen Positron Emission Tomography in Patients not Meeting the Phoenix Criteria for Biochemical Recurrence After Curative Radiotherapy. *Eur. Urol. Oncol.* **2020**, in press. [CrossRef] [PubMed]
14. Grubmüller, B.; Baltzer, P.; D'Andrea, D.; Korn, S.; Haug, A.; Hacker, M.; Grubmüller, K.H.; Goldner, G.M.; Wadsak, W.; Pfaff, S.; et al. 68Ga-PSMA 11 ligand PET imaging in patients with biochemical recurrence after radical prostatectomy–diagnostic performance and impact on therapeutic decision-making. *Eur. J. Nucl. Med. Mol. Imaging* **2017**, *49*, 1374–1378. [CrossRef]
15. Mohler, J.L.; Antonarakis, E.S.; Armstrong, A.J.; D'Amico, A.V.; Davis, B.J.; Dorff, T.; Eastham, J.A.; Enke, C.A.; Farrington, T.A.; Higano, C.S.; et al. Prostate Cancer, Version 2.2019, NCCN Clinical Practice Guidelines in Oncology. *JNCCN* **2019**, *17*, 479–505. [CrossRef] [PubMed]
16. Liberati, A.; Altman, D.G.; Tetzlaff, J.; Mulrow, C.; Gøtzsche, P.C.; Ioannidis, J.P.A.; Clarke, M.; Devereaux, P.J.; Kleijnen, J.; Moher, D. The PRISMA statement for reporting systematic reviews and meta-analyses of studies that evaluate health care interventions: Explanation and elaboration. *J. Clin. Epidemiol.* **2009**, *62*, e1-34. [CrossRef]
17. Metcalfe, M.J.; Troncoso, P.; Guo, C.C.; Chen, H.-C.; Bozkurt, Y.; Ward, J.F.; Pisters, L.L. Salvage prostatectomy for post-radiation adenocarcinoma with treatment effect: Pathological and oncological outcomes. *Can. Urol. Assoc. J.* **2017**, *11*, E277–E284. [CrossRef] [PubMed]
18. Kenney, P.A.; Nawaf, C.B.; Mustafa, M.; Wen, S.; Wszolek, M.F.; Pettaway, C.A.; Ward, J.; Davis, J.W.; Pisters, L.L. Robotic-assisted laparoscopic versus open salvage radical prostatectomy following radiotherapy. *Can. J. Urol.* **2016**, *23*, 8271–8277. [PubMed]

19. Mandel, P.; Steuber, T.; Ahyai, S.; Kriegmair, M.; Schiffmann, J.; Boehm, K.; Heinzer, H.; Michl, U.; Schlomm, T.; Haese, A.; et al Salvage radical prostatectomy for recurrent prostate cancer: Verification of European Association of Urology guideline criteria *BJU Int.* **2015**, *117*, 55–61. [CrossRef]
20. Bates, A.S.; Samavedi, S.; Kumar, A.; Mouraviev, V.; Rocco, B.; Coelho, R.; Palmer, K.; Patel, V.R. Salvage robot assisted radical prostatectomy: A propensity matched study of perioperative, oncological and functional outcomes. European journal of surgical oncology. *EJSO* **2015**, *41*, 1540–1546. [CrossRef] [PubMed]
21. Yuh, B.; Ruel, N.; Muldrew, S.; Mejia, R.; Novara, G.; Kawachi, M.; Wilson, T. Complications and outcomes of salvage robot-assisted radical prostatectomy: A single-institution experience. *BJU Int.* **2014**, *113*, 769–776. [CrossRef] [PubMed]
22. Meeks, J.J.; Walker, M.; Bernstein, M.; Eastham, J.A. Seminal vesicle involvement at salvage radical prostatectomy. *BJU Int.* **2013**, *111*, E342–E347. [CrossRef] [PubMed]
23. Gorin, M.A.; Manoharan, M.; Shah, G.; Eldefrawy, A.; Soloway, M.S. Urological Oncology Salvage open radical prostatectomy after failed radiation therapy: A single center experience. *Cent. Eur. J. Urol.* **2011**, *64*, 144–147. [CrossRef]
24. Eandi, J.A.; Link, B.A.; Nelson, R.A.; Josephson, D.Y.; Lau, C.; Kawachi, M.H.; Wilson, T.G. Robotic Assisted Laparoscopic Salvage Prostatectomy for Radiation Resistant Prostate Cancer. *J. Urol.* **2010**, *183*, 133–137. [CrossRef] [PubMed]
25. Pisters, L.L.; Leibovici, D.; Blute, M.; Zincke, H.; Sebo, T.J.; Slezak, J.M.; Izawa, J.; Ward, J.; Scott, S.M.; Madsen, L.; et al. Locally Recurrent Prostate Cancer After Initial Radiation Therapy: A Comparison of Salvage Radical Prostatectomy Versus Cryotherapy *J. Urol.* **2009**, *182*, 517–527. [CrossRef]
26. Leonardo, C.; Simone, G.; Papalia, R.; Franco, G.; Guaglianone, S.; Gallucci, M. Salvage radical prostatectomy for recurrent prostate cancer after radiation therapy. *Int. J. Urol. Off. J. Jpn. Urol. Assoc.* **2009**, *16*, 584–586. [CrossRef]
27. Paparel, P.; Cronin, A.M.; Savage, C.; Scardino, P.T.; Eastham, J.A. Oncologic Outcome and Patterns of Recurrence after Salvage Radical Prostatectomy. *Eur. Urol.* **2009**, *55*, 404–410. [CrossRef] [PubMed]
28. Sanderson, K.M.; Penson, D.; Cai, J.; Groshen, S.; Stein, J.P.; Lieskovsky, G.; Skinner, D.G. Salvage Radical Prostatectomy: Quality of Life Outcomes and Long-Term Oncological Control of Radiorecurrent Prostate Cancer. *J. Urol.* **2006**, *176*, 2025–2032. [CrossRef]
29. Amling, C.L.; E Lerner, S.; Martin, S.K.; Slezak, J.M.; Blute, M.L.; Zincke, H. Deoxyribonucleic acid ploidy and serum prostate specific antigen predict outcome following salvage prostatectomy for radiation refractory prostate cancer. *J. Urol.* **1999**, *161* 857–862. [CrossRef]
30. Tefilli, M.V.; Gheiler, E.L.; Tiguert, R.; Banerjee, M.; Forman, J.; Pontes, J.; Wood, D.P. Salvage surgery or salvage radiotherapy for locally recurrent prostate cancer. *Urology* **1998**, *52*, 224–229. [CrossRef]
31. E Lerner, S.; Blute, M.L.; Zincke, H. Critical evaluation of salvage surgery for radio-recurrent/resistant prostate cancer. *J. Urol* **1995**, *154*, 1103–1109. [CrossRef]
32. Rogers, E.; Ohori, M.; Kassabian, V.S.; Wheeler, T.M.; Scardino, P.T. Salvage Radical Prostatectomy. *J. Urol.* **1995**, *153*, 104–110 [CrossRef] [PubMed]
33. Zincke, H. Radical Prostatectomy and Exenterative Procedures for Local Failure after Radiotherapy with Curative Intent Comparison of Outcomes. *J. Urol.* **1992**, *147*, 894–899. [CrossRef]
34. Rainwater, L.M.; Zincke, H. Radical Prostatectomy After Radiation Therapy for Cancer of the Prostate: Feasibility and Prognosis *J. Urol.* **1988**, *140*, 1455–1459. [CrossRef]
35. Vartolomei, M.D.; D'Andrea, D.; Chade, D.C.; Soria, F.; Kimura, S.; Foerster, B.; Abufaraj, M.; Mathieu, R.; Moschini, M.; Rouprêt M.; et al. Role of serum cholinesterase in patients treated with salvage radical prostatectomy. *Urol. Oncol. Semin. Orig. Invest* **2019**, *37*, 123–129. [CrossRef]
36. Pearce, S.M.; Richards, K.; Patel, S.G.; Pariser, J.; Eggener, S.E. Population-based analysis of salvage radical prostatectomy with examination of factors associated with adverse perioperative outcomes. *Urol. Oncol. Semin. Orig. Invest.* **2015**, *33*, 163.e1–163.e6 [CrossRef] [PubMed]
37. Bianco, F.J.; Scardino, P.T.; Stephenson, A.J.; Diblasio, C.J.; Fearn, P.A.; Eastham, J.A. Long-term oncologic results of salvage radical prostatectomy for locally recurrent prostate cancer after radiotherapy. *Int. J. Radiat. Oncol.* **2005**, *62*, 448–453. [CrossRef]
38. Rouvière, O.; Vitry, T.; Lyonnet, D. Imaging of prostate cancer local recurrences: Why and how? *Eur. Radiol.* **2010**, *20*, 1254–1266 [CrossRef]
39. Luiting, H.B.; Van Leeuwen, P.J.; Busstra, M.B.; Brabander, T.; Van Der Poel, H.G.; Donswijk, M.; Vis, A.N.; Emmett, L. Stricker, P.D.; Roobol, M.J. Use of gallium-68 prostate-specific membrane antigen positron-emission tomography for detecting lymph node metastases in primary and recurrent prostate cancer and location of recurrence after radical prostatectomy: An overview of the current literature. *BJU Int.* **2019**, *125*, 206–214. [CrossRef]
40. Oehus, A.-K.; Kroeze, S.G.C.; Schmidt-Hegemann, N.-S.; Vogel, M.M.E.; Kirste, S.; Becker, J.; Burger, I.A.; Derlin, T.; Bartenstein P.; Eiber, M.; et al. Efficacy of PSMA ligand PET-based radiotherapy for recurrent prostate cancer after radical prostatectomy and salvage radiotherapy. *BMC Cancer* **2020**, *20*, 362–369. [CrossRef]
41. Ingrosso, G.; Becherini, C.; Lancia, A.; Caini, S.; Ost, P.; Francolini, G.; Høyer, M.; Bottero, M.; Bossi, A.; Zilli, T.; et al. Nonsurgical Salvage Local Therapies for Radiorecurrent Prostate Cancer: A Systematic Review and Meta-analysis. *Eur. Urol. Oncol.* **2020**, *3* 183–197. [CrossRef]
42. Marra, G.; Karnes, R.J.; Calleris, G.; Oderda, M.; Alessio, P.; Palazzetti, A.; Battaglia, A.; Pisano, F.; Munegato, S.; Munoz, F.; et al Oncological outcomes of salvage radical prostatectomy for recurrent prostate cancer in the contemporary era: A multicenter retrospective study. *Urol. Oncol. Semin. Orig. Invest.* **2021**, *39*, 296.e21–296.e29. [CrossRef]

43. Alibhai, S.M.; Gogov, S.; Allibhai, Z. Long-term side effects of androgen deprivation therapy in men with non-metastatic prostate cancer: A systematic literature review. *Crit. Rev. Oncol.* **2006**, *60*, 201–215. [CrossRef] [PubMed]
44. Philippou, Y.; Parker, R.A.; Volanis, D.; Gnanapragasam, V.J. Comparative Oncologic and Toxicity Outcomes of Salvage Radical Prostatectomy Versus Nonsurgical Therapies for Radiorecurrent Prostate Cancer: A Meta–Regression Analysis. *Eur. Urol. Focus* **2016**, *2*, 158–171. [CrossRef] [PubMed]
45. Valle, L.F.; Lehrer, E.J.; Markovic, D.; Elashoff, D.; Levin-Epstein, R.; Karnes, R.J.; Reiter, R.E.; Rettig, M.; Calais, J.; Nickols, N.G.; et al. A Systematic Review and Meta-analysis of Local Salvage Therapies After Radiotherapy for Prostate Cancer (MASTER). *Eur. Urol.* **2020**, in press. [CrossRef] [PubMed]
46. Duchesne, G.M.; Woo, H.H.; Bassett, J.K.; Bowe, S.; D'Este, C.; Frydenberg, M.; King, M.; Ledwich, L.; Loblaw, A.; Malone, S.; et al. Timing of androgen-deprivation therapy in patients with prostate cancer with a rising PSA (TROG 03.06 and VCOG PR 01-03 [TOAD]): A randomised, multicentre, non-blinded, phase 3 trial. *Lancet Oncol.* **2016**, *17*, 727–737. [CrossRef]
47. Payne, H.; Khan, A.; Chowdhury, S.; Davda, R. Hormone therapy for radiorecurrent prostate cancer. *World J. Urol.* **2012**, *31*, 1333–1338. [CrossRef]
48. Siddiqui, S.A.; Boorjian, S.A.; Inman, B.; Bagniewski, S.; Bergstralh, E.J.; Blute, M.L. Timing of Androgen Deprivation Therapy and its Impact on Survival After Radical Prostatectomy: A Matched Cohort Study. *J. Urol.* **2008**, *179*, 1830–1837, discussion 1837. [CrossRef] [PubMed]
49. Boorjian, S.A.; Thompson, R.H.; Tollefson, M.K.; Rangel, L.J.; Bergstralh, E.J.; Blute, M.L.; Karnes, R.J. Long-Term Risk of Clinical Progression After Biochemical Recurrence Following Radical Prostatectomy: The Impact of Time from Surgery to Recurrence. *Eur. Urol.* **2011**, *59*, 893–899. [CrossRef]
50. Brassetti, A.; Bollens, R. Laparoscopic radical prostatectomy in 2018: 20 years of worldwide experiences, experimentations, researches and refinements. *Minerva Chir.* **2019**, *74*, 37–53. [CrossRef]
51. Klotz, L. Active surveillance for prostate cancer: For whom? *J. Clin. Oncol.* **2005**, *23*, 8165–8169. [CrossRef] [PubMed]
52. Fossati, N.; Willemse, P.-P.M.; den Broeck, T.V.; van den Bergh, R.C.N.; Yuan, C.Y.; Briers, E.; Bellmunt, J.; Bolla, M.; Cornford, P.; Santis, M.D.; et al. The Benefits and Harms of Different Extents of Lymph Node Dissection During Radical Prostatectomy for Prostate Cancer: A Systematic Review. *Eur. Urol.* **2017**, *72*, 84–109. [CrossRef] [PubMed]

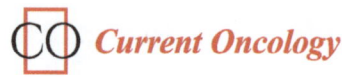 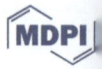

Case Report

Diagnostic and Therapeutic Challenges in a Patient with Synchronous Very High-Risk Prostate Adenocarcinoma and Anal Carcinoma

Jonathan Wallach *, Irini Youssef, Andrea Leaf and David Schwartz

Veterans Affairs New York Harbor Healthcare System, State University of New York-Downstate Medical Center, New York, NY 11209, USA; Irini.Youssef@Downstate.edu (I.Y.); Andrea.Leaf@va.gov (A.L.); David.Schwartz3@va.gov (D.S.)
* Correspondence: Jonathan.Wallach@va.gov

Abstract: A 79-year-old HIV-negative Caucasian man with a medical history of smoking 20 pack-years (quit 40 years prior), early-stage non-small cell lung cancer status post-lobectomy 13 years earlier at an outside hospital without evidence of recurrence, and benign prostatic hypertrophy was diagnosed with synchronous very high-risk prostate adenocarcinoma and early-stage anal basaloid squamous cell carcinoma. He proceeded to undergo concurrent treatment for these tumors, consisting of androgen deprivation therapy, external beam radiation therapy, and a brachytherapy boost for the prostate adenocarcinoma; for the anal carcinoma, he was treated with definitive chemoradiation. Over 3.5 years since the completion of radiotherapy, he remains in clinical and biochemical remission.

Keywords: prostate adenocarcinoma; anal carcinoma; synchronous cancers

Citation: Wallach, J.; Youssef, I.; Leaf, A.; Schwartz, D. Diagnostic and Therapeutic Challenges in a Patient with Synchronous Very High-Risk Prostate Adenocarcinoma and Anal Carcinoma. *Curr. Oncol.* **2022**, *29*, 377–382. https://doi.org/10.3390/curroncol29010033

Received: 30 November 2021
Accepted: 22 December 2021
Published: 15 January 2022

Publisher's Note: MDPI stays neutral with regard to jurisdictional claims in published maps and institutional affiliations.

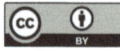

Copyright: © 2022 by the authors. Licensee MDPI, Basel, Switzerland. This article is an open access article distributed under the terms and conditions of the Creative Commons Attribution (CC BY) license (https://creativecommons.org/licenses/by/4.0/).

1. Introduction

Case Description

A 79-year-old HIV-negative Caucasian man with a medical history of smoking 20 pack-years (quit 40 years prior), early-stage non-small cell lung cancer (subtype unknown) status post-lobectomy 13 years earlier at an outside hospital without evidence of recurrence, and benign prostatic hypertrophy began demonstrating accelerating prostate specific antigen (PSA) values, prompting a prostate biopsy by his urologist. His previously stable PSA had increased from 4.3 ng/mL to 6.1 ng/mL three months later, confirmed by repeat laboratory drawing. On physical examination, his prostate was estimated as 45 g and was smooth, without any nodularity appreciated; however, there was also a course lesion along the posterior anal canal. He proceeded with a 12-core ultrasound-guided biopsy, which demonstrated 7/12 cores with tumor, including one core with Gleason 5 + 5 = 10 (grade group 5), one core with Gleason 4 + 5 = 9 (grade group 5), one core with Gleason 5 + 3 = 8 (grade group 4), one core with Gleason 4 + 3 = 7 (grade group 3), and three cores with Gleason 3 + 3 = 6 (grade group 1); there was no perineural invasion or lymphovascular invasion.

A flexible sigmoidoscopy revealed that the anal lesion measured 2 cm and was the only lesion of concern. A biopsy of the anal mass demonstrated grade 3 basaloid squamous cell carcinoma, positive for human papilloma virus (HPV) subtypes 16/18 and negative for HPV subtypes 6/11 and 31/33.

He underwent a bone scan, demonstrating a non-specific focus within the left lateral 10th rib, representing a healed fracture versus a metastasis. A CT-chest/abdomen/pelvis with contrast did not demonstrate any lymphadenopathy or osseous lesions; his bladder measured 5.9 × 5.4 cm, indenting the bladder base; the anal lesion was poorly visualized. He underwent a PET/CT, demonstrating normal uptake within the lungs, a significantly enlarged prostate, no lymphadenopathy, no metabolically active lesions within the bones and focal intense activity within the anal region (consistent with the recent biopsy). An MRI-prostate was deferred at that time because of concern for potential incompatibility of a prosthesis with the magnetic field. Therefore, his diagnosis was synchronous very high-risk prostate adenocarcinoma cT1cN0M0 (grade group 5, pre-treatment PSA = 6.1 ng/mL, stage IIIC) concurrent with cT1N0M0 stage I anal basaloid squamous cell carcinoma, per the AJCC 8th Edition staging system.

The patient's case was discussed at a multidisciplinary tumor board. Per the recommendations, he was started on bicalutamide 50 mg daily, followed by leuprolide acetate 22.5 mg every 3 months after 3 weeks on bicalutamide. The patient underwent prophylactic radiotherapy to his breast buds, consisting of 12 Gy over 4 fractions with 6 MeV en face electrons to prevent gynecomastia. The patient started volumetric modulated arc therapy (VMAT) to the prostate, seminal vesicles, anus, pelvic lymph nodes, and inguinal lymph nodes, as seen in Figure 1, at the radiotherapy doses described in Table 1; radiotherapy was concurrent with two cycles of 5-fluorouracil 1000 mg/m^2/day on days 1–4 and 29–32 and mitomycin-C 10 mg/m^2 on days 1 and 29.

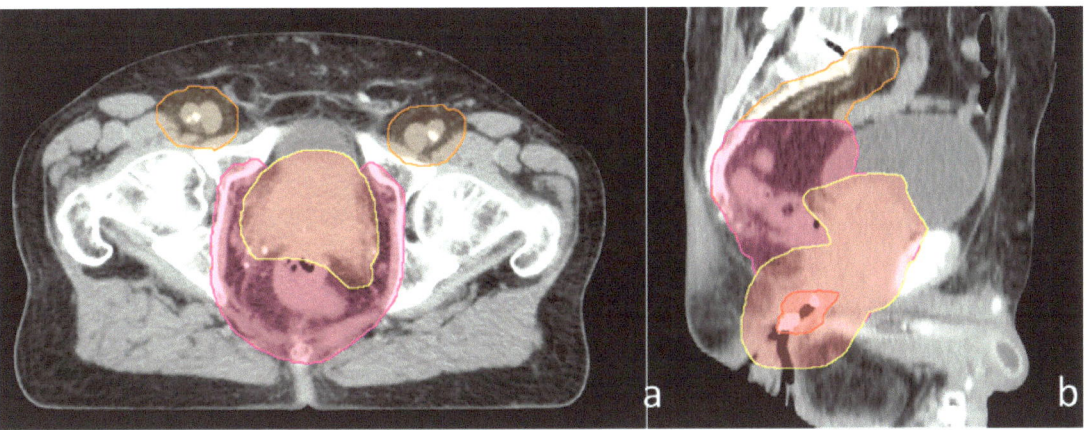

Figure 1. (**a**) Axial view, (**b**) sagittal view.

Table 1. Treatment Schema.

Structure	Region 1	Region 2	Region 3	Fractionation	Figure 1
PTV 36	Common iliac LNs, inguinal LNs	External iliac LNs, internal iliac LNs, obturator LNs	Prostate, seminal vesicles, anus/peri-anal region	36 Gy/18 fractions	Orange
PTV 45		External iliac LNs, internal iliac LNs, obturator LNs	Prostate, seminal vesicles, anus/peri-anal region	45 Gy/25 fractions	Magenta
PTV 50.4			Prostate, seminal vesicles, anus/peri-anal region	50.4 Gy/28 fractions	Yellow (anus in red)

The patient tolerated treatment with some difficulties, as he did experience CTCAE grade 3 dehydration (requiring inpatient intravenous hydration), grade 2 neutropenia treated with filgrastim, grade 2 diarrhea treated with loperamide 2 mg 3x/day PRN, grade 2 urinary frequency treated with tamsulosin 0.4 mg qhs, and grade 1 fatigue. From consultation to the end of this part of treatment, he lost 4.2 kg, which was 5.0% of his initial weight (grade 1 weight loss), while his International Prostate Symptom Score (IPSS) increased from 7 to 11 on tamsulosin 0.4 mg.

He remained on bicalutamide 50 mg daily and leuprolide acetate 22.5 mg q3 months and underwent planning for prostate brachytherapy. Two months later, he returned for low dose rate (LDR) brachytherapy with hydrogel placement between the prostate and the rectum. The I-125 implant consisted of 60 seeds and delivered a 108 Gy boost. He tolerated the procedures well without any complications; the dosimetry was as follows: prostate D90 = 118.88 Gy, prostate V100 = 97.85%, rectum V100 = 0.00 cc, and urethra V150 = 0.00 cc.

Following the brachytherapy implant, the patient continued to receive leuprolide acetate and bicalutamide for a total duration of three years, given his very high-risk disease. He has continued to follow up with urology, radiation oncology, medical oncology, pulmonology, and the surgical service, given his history of three malignancies and emphysema.

With regard to his surveillance, the patient most recently followed up with the surgical service at 3 years and 3 months after the completion of radiotherapy, with no evidence of any anal tumor on physical examination. An MRI-prostate was performed at 2 years 10 months after his radiotherapy, ordered by the surgical service because of painless rectal bleeding for 1 day; the MRI demonstrated no evidence of prostate malignancy, anal malignancy, lymphadenopathy, or osseous lesions. PSAs performed at 2 years 10 months, 3 years 5 months, and 3 months 8 months were 0.02 ng/mL, 0.04 ng/mL, and 0.05 ng/mL, respectively, demonstrating biochemical control.

Of note, the patient did experience increased lower urinary tract symptoms that required botulinum injection twice during post-radiotherapy year 3, and he briefly had a urinary catheter. However, his last IPSS evaluation at 3 years 8 months post-radiotherapy demonstrated an IPSS score of 0/1/4/0/5/3/1 = 14 on tamsulosin 0.4 mg × 2 daily. In addition, during post-radiotherapy year 2, he experienced minor rectal bleeding, which self-resolved.

Additionally, a PET/CT at 3 years 5 months post-radiotherapy demonstrated no evidence of the prostate or anal malignancy but did reveal a new PET-avid pleural-based nodule at the right hemi-diaphragm. A right lower lobe core biopsy demonstrated poorly differentiated lung adenocarcinoma, consistent with a new lung primary. He proceeded with stereotactic body radiation therapy to this focus consisting of 50 Gy over 4 fractions, which he tolerated very well without any acute toxicities.

2. Discussion

Anal cancer is a relatively rare malignancy in the United States, accounting for approximately 2% of all gastrointestinal malignancies [1,2], and is estimated to have been diagnosed in 8590 Americans in 2020 [3]. However, its incidence is increasing because of two major factors: longer survival of patients infected with HIV as a result of successful use of HAART, as well as an increase in the rate of sexually transmitted HPV [4]. Generally, the management of anal cancer includes concurrent chemoradiation (CCRT), with surgery reserved for persistent or recurrent disease [2].

Prostate adenocarcinoma is the most common non-skin cancer in American men, with about 1 in 9 men diagnosed with prostate cancer during their lifetimes [5]. The management paradigm for prostate cancer differs by National Comprehensive Cancer Network (NCCN) risk group, with radical prostatectomy and radiotherapy as the main treatment options, while men with very low-risk, low-risk, and potentially favorable intermediate-risk prostate cancer can pursue active surveillance [6]. For men with at least unfavorable intermediate-risk prostate adenocarcinoma, androgen deprivation therapy is generally added to radiotherapy after taking into consideration co-morbidities and side effects [6].

Additionally, when treating these more aggressive tumors with radiotherapy, the NCCN recommends the consideration of a brachytherapy boost [6]. The ASCENDE-RT trial demonstrated that compared with dose-escalated EBRT to 78 Gy, men who received a boost with LDR brachytherapy were twice as likely to be free of biochemical failure at a median follow-up of 6.5 years [7]. However, despite this category A evidence, as well as numerous prospective and retrospective studies showing improved outcomes with a brachytherapy boost, an analysis of the National Cancer Database from the years 2004–2012 reported a significant decline in the use of prostate brachytherapy at both academic and non-academic institutions, from 15% to 8%, and from 19% to 11%, respectively [8]. For this patient, we chose an LDR brachytherapy boost (instead of a high dose rate [HDR] boost) to be consistent with the ASCENDE-RT trial [7]. The use of brachytherapy with the hydrogel spacer allowed delivery of a boost dose to the prostate while minimizing the dose to the anus after the completion of anal CCRT.

Because of the rarity of synchronous presentations of anal and prostate malignancies, there is almost no available literature on an optimal simultaneous treatment strategy. In one case report by Miles et al. of a 68-year-old man with synchronous unfavorable intermediate-risk prostate and anal cancers, the authors initially utilized a 3D-conformal approach to treat the primary diseases and draining lymph nodes with conedown fields to the anus to a dose of 50.4 Gy, followed by an IMRT boost to 73.8 Gy to the prostate and proximal seminal vesicles, with neoadjuvant and concurrent androgen deprivation therapy [1]. Another case report by Tubin et al. demonstrated the use of definitive IMRT with a simultaneous integrated boost in the management of a 68-year-old Caucasian male with synchronous anal cancer with nodal metastases and intermediate-risk prostate cancer through the use of four planning-treatment volumes: the uninvolved inguinal lymph nodes up to 36 Gy, uninvolved pelvic lymph nodes up to 45 Gy, involved pelvic lymph nodes and primary anal tumor up to 59.4 Gy, and the prostate up to 69.3 Gy [9]. The inguinal lymph nodes were included as a low-dose region, despite being negative on imaging, per the landmark protocol RTOG 05–29 [10].

An important decision for patients diagnosed with synchronous malignancies is whether both tumors require definitive management. Given that our patient had very high-risk prostate cancer, active surveillance was not an option, as men in this risk group have poor outcomes even with very aggressive treatment, with a cancer-specific survival of 62% at 10 years [11]. Additionally, given his age and comorbidities, he was not medically optimal for surgical resection.

Our approach to the management of this patient combined elements from the standard of care for both malignancies. It was necessary to dose the prostate to at least 78 Gy on the basis of randomized trials demonstrating prostate cancer mortality benefits [12] as well as lower biochemical failure and distant metastatic rates [13]. The doses used to treat anal cancer are thus insufficient for prostate cancer control. Additionally, taking both the anus and prostate to such high doses would result in significant anal toxicity. In order to overcome this issue, we delivered a maximum dose of 50.4 Gy to the prostate, seminal vesicles, and anus/perianal regions, with concurrent mitomycin/5-fluorouracil as the standard of care; we added a brachytherapy boost to the prostate to a dose of 108 Gy using the I-125 isotope. This modality allowed treatment of both malignancies to the recommended doses while sparing normal tissue.

Additionally, based on this patient's risk of lymph node involvement of 31% using the MSKCC nomogram [14], we decided to include the pelvic lymph nodes in the treatment volume, regardless of whether the patient had a synchronous anal malignancy. Fortunately, this allowed us to combine pelvic volumes for both the prostate and anal carcinomas. Finally, we incorporated androgen deprivation therapy into his management strategy on the basis of several randomized trials showing a benefit to 2–3 years of androgen deprivation in combination with radiation for high-risk patients [15–17]. With this dual treatment approach, the patient was able to tolerate treatment well, with manageable acute toxicity and long-term toxicity.

3. Conclusions

In summary, there is almost no medical literature on the optimal treatment strategy for patients with synchronous prostate and anal cancers, especially because of the rarity of anal cancer. After it was determined that each malignancy warranted definitive management, we determined that a combined radiation approach, especially one utilizing brachytherapy because of its rapid dose fall-off, in addition to sensitizing chemotherapy, was the most effective strategy. Our experience suggests that this was a well-tolerated and effective strategy for this patient and can be replicated in similar clinical scenarios. Additionally, this case report of a patient with four synchronous/metachronous tumors in three separate organs reinforces the premise that a patient who develops a malignancy is at an elevated risk for developing additional malignancies, both because of systemic genetic derangements and environmental exposures; consideration of genetic counseling and behavior modifications (e.g., tobacco and alcohol cessation) should be considered in appropriate circumstances.

Author Contributions: Conceptualization, J.W. and D.S.; methodology, J.W., I.Y., A.L. and D.S.; writing, J.W., I.Y., A.L. and D.S.; original draft preparation, J.W., I.Y., A.L. and D.S.; writing—review and editing, J.W., I.Y., A.L. and D.S. All authors have read and agreed to the published version of the manuscript.

Funding: This research received no external funding.

Institutional Review Board Statement: Not applicable.

Informed Consent Statement: Informed consent was obtained from all subjects involved in the study.

Data Availability Statement: The data presented in this study are available on request from the corresponding author.

Conflicts of Interest: The authors of this manuscript affirm that they do not have relationships with pharmaceutical companies or employment contracts, consultancy, advisory boards, speaker bureaus, membership of boards of directors, or stock ownership that could represent a financial conflict of interest.

References

1. Miles, F.E.; Jacimore, L.L.; Nelson, J.W. Metachronous anal canal and prostate cancers with simultaneous definitive therapy: A case report and review of the literature. *Case Rep. Oncol. Med.* **2011**, *2011*, 864371. [CrossRef] [PubMed]
2. National Comprehensive Cancer Network. Anal Carcinoma (Version 2.2020). Available online: https://www.nccn.org/professionals/physician_gls/pdf/anal.pdf (accessed on 28 December 2020).
3. American Cancer Society. Key Statistics for Anal Cancer. 2020. Available online: https://www.cancer.org/cancer/anal-cancer/about/what-is-key-statistics.html (accessed on 28 December 2020).
4. Nelson, V.M.; Benson, A.B., 3rd. Epidemiology of Anal Canal Cancer. *Surg. Oncol. Clin. N. Am.* **2017**, *26*, 9–15. [CrossRef] [PubMed]
5. American Cancer Society. Key Statistics for Prostate Cancer. Available online: https://www.cancer.org/cancer/prostate-cancer/about/key-statistics.html (accessed on 28 December 2020).
6. National Comprehensive Cancer Network. Prostate Cancer (Version 3.2020). Available online: https://www.nccn.org/professionals/physician_gls/pdf/prostate.pdf (accessed on 28 December 2020).
7. Morris, W.J.; Tyldesley, S.; Rodda, S.; Halperin, R.; Pai, H.; McKenzie, M.; Duncan, G.; Morton, G.; Hamm, J.; Murray, N. Androgen Suppression Combined with Elective Nodal and Dose Escalated Radiation Therapy (the ASCENDE-RT Trial): An Analysis of Survival Endpoints for a Randomized Trial Comparing a Low-Dose-Rate Brachytherapy Boost to a Dose-Escalated External Beam Boost for High- and Intermediate-risk Prostate Cancer. *Int. J. Radiat. Oncol. Biol. Phys.* **2017**, *98*, 275–285. [PubMed]
8. Orio, P.F., 3rd; Nguyen, P.L.; Buzurovic, I.; Cail, D.W.; Chen, Y.W. The decreased use of brachytherapy boost for intermediate and high-risk prostate cancer despite evidence supporting its effectiveness. *Brachytherapy* **2016**, *15*, 701–706. [CrossRef] [PubMed]
9. Tubin, S.; Wolfgang, R. A Definitive IMRT-SIB with Concomitant Chemotherapy for Synchronous Locally Advanced Anal Canal Cancer and Prostate Cancer. *Case Rep. Oncol. Med.* **2018**, *2018*, 6101759.
10. Kachnic, L.A.; Winter, K.; Myerson, R.J.; Goodyear, M.D.; Willins, J.; Esthappan, J.; Haddock, M.G.; Rotman, M.; Parikh, P.J.; Safran, H.; et al. RTOG 0529: A Phase 2 Evaluation of Dose-Pained Intensity Modulated Radiation Therapy in Combination With 5-Fluorouracil and Mitomycin-C for the Reduction of Acute Morbidity in Carcinoma of the Anal Canal. *Int. J. Radiat. Oncol. Biol. Phys.* **2013**, *86*, 27–33. [CrossRef] [PubMed]
11. Sundi, D.; Wang, V.M.; Pierorazio, P.M.; Han, M.; Bivalacqua, T.J.; Ball, M.W.; Antonarakis, E.S.; Partin, A.W.; Schaeffer, E.M.; Ross, A.E. Very-high-risk localized prostate cancer: Definition and outcomes. *Prostate Cancer Prostatic Dis.* **2014**, *17*, 57–63. [CrossRef] [PubMed]

12. Pasalic, D.; Kuban, D.A.; Allen, P.K.; Tang, C.; Mesko, S.M.; Grant, S.R.; Augustyn, A.A.; Frank, S.J.; Choi, S.; Hoffman, K.E. Dose Escalation for Prostate Adenocarcinoma: A Long-Term Update on the Outcomes of a Phase 3, Single Institution Randomized Clinical Trial. *Int. J. Radiat. Oncol. Biol. Phys.* **2019**, *104*, 790–797. [CrossRef] [PubMed]
13. Michalski, J.M.; Moughan, J.; Purdy, J.; Bosch, W.; Bruner, D.W.; Bahary, J.P.; Lau, H.; Duclos, M.; Parliament, M.; Morton, G.; et al. Effect of Standard vs Dose-Escalated Radiation Therapy for Patients With Intermediate-Risk Prostate Cancer: The NRG Oncology RTOG 0126 Randomized Clinical Trial. *JAMA Oncol.* **2018**, *4*, e180039. [CrossRef] [PubMed]
14. Memorial Sloan Kettering Cancer Center. Pre-Radical Prostatectomy. Prostate Cancer Nomograms. Available online: https://www.mskcc.org/nomograms/prostate/pre_op (accessed on 29 December 2020).
15. Horwitz, E.M.; Bae, K.; Hanks, G.E.; Porter, A.; Grignon, D.J.; Brereton, H.D.; Venkatesan, V.; Lawton, C.A.; Rosenthal, S.A.; Sandler, H.M.; et al. Ten-year follow-up of radiation therapy oncology group protocol 92-02: A phase III trial of the duration of elective androgen deprivation in locally advanced prostate cancer. *J. Clin. Oncol.* **2008**, *26*, 2497–2504. [CrossRef] [PubMed]
16. Bolla, M.; Collette, L.; Blank, L.; Warde, P.; Dubois, J.B.; Mirimanoff, R.O.; Storme, G.; Bernier, J.; Kuten, A.; Sternberg, C.; et al. Long-term results with immediate androgen suppression and external irradiation in patients with locally advanced prostate cancer (an EORTC study): A phase III randomised trial. *Lancet* **2002**, *360*, 103–106. [CrossRef]
17. Bolla, M.; de Reijke, T.M.; Van Tienhoven, G.; Van den Bergh, A.C.; Oddens, J.; Poortmans, P.M.; Gez, E.; Kil, P.; Akdas, A.; Soete, G.; et al. Duration of androgen suppression in the treatment of prostate cancer. *N. Engl. J. Med.* **2009**, *360*, 2516–2527. [PubMed]

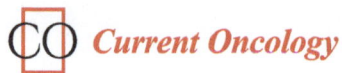

Article

Comparative Prospective and Longitudinal Analysis on the Platelet-to-Lymphocyte, Neutrophil-to-Lymphocyte, and Albumin-to-Globulin Ratio in Patients with Non-Metastatic and Metastatic Prostate Cancer

Stefano Salciccia [1], Marco Frisenda [1], Giulio Bevilacqua [1], Pietro Viscuso [1], Paolo Casale [2], Ettore De Berardinis [1], Giovanni Battista Di Pierro [1], Susanna Cattarino [1], Gloria Giorgino [1], Davide Rosati [1], Francesco Del Giudice [1], Antonio Carbone [3], Antonio Pastore [3], Benjamin I. Chung [4], Michael L. Eisenberg [4], Riccardo Autorino [5], Simone Crivellaro [6], Flavio Forte [7], Alessandro Sciarra [1,*], Gianna Mariotti [1] and Alessandro Gentilucci [1]

[1] Department of "Materno Infantile e Scienze Urologiche, 'Sapienza' University of Rome, Policlinico Umberto I Hospital, 00161 Rome, Italy
[2] Department of Urology, Humanitas, 20089 Milan, Italy
[3] Unit of Urology, ICOT Hospital Latina, Sapienza University, 04100 Latina, Italy
[4] Department of Urology, Stanford University School of Medicine, Stanford, CA 94305, USA
[5] Department of Urology, Rush University Medical Center, Chicago, IL 60612, USA
[6] Department of Urology, University of Illinois Hospital e Camp, Health Sciences System, Chicago, IL 60612, USA
[7] Urology Department, M.G. Vannini Hospital, 00177 Rome, Italy
* Correspondence: alessandro.sciarra@uniroma1.it

Citation: Salciccia, S.; Frisenda, M.; Bevilacqua, G.; Viscuso, P.; Casale, P.; De Berardinis, E.; Di Pierro, G.B.; Cattarino, S.; Giorgino, G.; Rosati, D.; et al. Comparative Prospective and Longitudinal Analysis on the Platelet-to-Lymphocyte, Neutrophil-to-Lymphocyte, and Albumin-to-Globulin Ratio in Patients with Non-Metastatic and Metastatic Prostate Cancer. *Curr. Oncol.* **2022**, *29*, 9474–9500. https://doi.org/10.3390/curroncol29120745

Received: 4 November 2022
Accepted: 1 December 2022
Published: 3 December 2022

Publisher's Note: MDPI stays neutral with regard to jurisdictional claims in published maps and institutional affiliations.

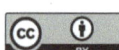

Copyright: © 2022 by the authors. Licensee MDPI, Basel, Switzerland. This article is an open access article distributed under the terms and conditions of the Creative Commons Attribution (CC BY) license (https://creativecommons.org/licenses/by/4.0/).

Abstract: Purpose: To prospectively evaluate the albumin/globulin ratio (AGR), neutrophil/lymphocyte ratio (NLR), and platelet/lymphocyte ratio (PLR) diagnostic and prognostic predictive value in a stratified population of prostate cancer (PC) cases. Methods: Population was divided based on the clinical and histologic diagnosis in: Group A: benign prostatic hyperplasia (BPH) cases (494 cases); Group B: all PC cases (525 cases); Group B1: clinically significant PC (426 cases); Group B2: non-metastatic PC (416 cases); Group B3: metastatic PC (109 cases). NLR, PLR, and AGR were obtained at the time of the diagnosis, and only in cases with PC considered for radical prostatectomy, determinations were also repeated 90 days after surgery. For each ratio, cut-off values were determined by receiver operating characteristics curve (ROC) analysis and fixed at 2.5, 120.0, and 1.4, respectively, for NLR, PLR, and AGR. Results: Accuracy in predictive value for an initial diagnosis of clinically significant PC (csPC) was higher using PLR (0.718) when compared to NLR (0.220) and AGR (0.247), but, despite high sensitivity (0.849), very low specificity (0.256) was present. The risk of csPC significantly increased only according to PLR with an OR = 1.646. The percentage of cases with metastatic PC significantly increased according to high NLR and high PLR. Accuracy was 0.916 and 0.813, respectively, for NLR and PLR cut-off, with higher specificity than sensitivity. The risk of a metastatic disease increased 3.2 times for an NLR > 2.5 and 5.2 times for a PLR > 120 and at the multivariate analysis. Conclusion: PLR and NLR have a significant predictive value towards the development of metastatic disease but not in relation to variations in aggressiveness or T staging inside the non-metastatic PC. Our results suggest an unlikely introduction of these analyses into clinical practice in support of validated PC risk predictors.

Keywords: albumin-to-globulin ratio; neutrophil-to-lymphocyte ratio; metastatic; platelet-to-lymphocyte ratio; prostatic neoplasm; radical prostatectomy

1. Introduction

Prostate cancer (PC) is an extremely heterogeneous tumor and clinical decisions continue to depend upon serum prostate-specific antigen (PSA) levels, tumor stage, risk classes, and Gleason score [1,2]. Predictive nomograms mainly including these clinical parameters are also used to evaluate the risk of advanced stage, undifferentiated tumors, and progression after treatments [3,4].

Different research sustains the hypothesis that chronic inflammation and the immune environment can condition carcinogenesis and tumor progression. The neutrophil-to-lymphocyte ratio (NLR) and platelet-to-lymphocyte ratio (PLR) can be easily obtained from routine blood counts and they have been proposed as markers of the relationship between inflammation or immune responses and tumor growth or progression [5,6]. Low lymphocyte counts and increased platelet counts have been associated with adverse prognostic features for different diseases, including PC [7]. Additionally, hypoalbuminemia can be associated with systemic inflammation in patients with cancer [8]. Inflammatory reaction and immunity are influenced by serum albumin and globulin; hypoalbuminemia and hyperglobulinemia are considered indicators of chronic inflammation in oncologic patients [8,9]. Albumin can reflect the body's nutritional status, globulin the immunological and inflammatory status, and their ratio can be evaluated as albumin divided by total protein minus albumin value in serum [10].

A prognostic role for NLR and PLR has been underlined for several solid tumors [8]. In PC the significance of NLR or PLR has been investigated in different settings, more frequently in advanced metastatic PC submitted to systemic therapies. Most clinical trials on NLR and PLR in PC are retrospective and different meta-analysis [9–11] showed a high level of heterogeneity of results among populations and studies, suggesting that either a high PLR or a high NLR are correlated with poor prognosis in PC [9,10]. Similarly, most clinical trials on AGR in PC are retrospective and different meta-analyses [8,10] showed contrasting results regarding a predictive value for low preoperative AGR in terms of poor prognosis in PC.

Now there has been relevant interest in NLR, PLR, and AGR in PC but data still remain controversial, with mainly retrospective analysis on advanced disease and heterogeneous non-stratified populations.

Aim and Objectives

The aim of the present analysis is to prospectively evaluate and compare the AGR, NLR, and PLR diagnostic and prognostic predictive value in a population of PC cases in comparison with benign prostatic hyperplasia (BPH) patients. In particular, we compared the predictive value of the three ratios either in terms of initial diagnosis of PC or in terms of advanced local staging, systemic metastases, or undifferentiated ISUP grading. Moreover, in a subpopulation of non-metastatic PC cases considered for radical prostatectomy (RP), we longitudinally analyzed AGR, PLR, and NLR variations after surgery and in relation to PSA progression.

2. Materials and Methods

2.1. Study Design

This is a prospective, longitudinal, and mono-center study. From January 2021 to August 2022, patients were consecutively enrolled as outpatients referred to our clinic for the management of prostatic diseases. A real-life situation is analyzed, and all diagnostic and therapeutic procedures reflected our routine clinical practice in a department at high volume for the management of PC disease following recommendations of the European Association of Urology (EAU) guidelines. The protocol was approved by our internal ethical committee and all patients gave their informed consensus for each analysis. In all cases, AGR, NLR, and PLR determination were obtained at baseline when the diagnosis was defined. In non-metastatic cases considered for radical prostatectomy (RP), after discussion of treatment options and presentation to the patient, the ratios were obtained either at baseline or after RP.

2.2. Population

The population was divided based on the clinical and histologic diagnosis in: Group A BPH cases; Group B: PC cases; Group B1: clinically significant PC; Group B2: non-metastatic PC; Group B3: metastatic PC.

Inclusion criteria were: Group A: new histologic diagnosis of BPH and/or clinical diagnosis of BPH without evidence or suspicious for PC; prostate volume > 30 cc, IPSS > 7, PSA level ≤ 2.5 ng/mL or if >2.5 ng/mL not suspicious (PIRADS 1–2) for PC at multiparametric magnetic resonance (mMR) and no evidence for PC at biopsy; Group B: new histologic diagnosis of prostatic adenocarcinoma at biopsy; Group B1: new histologic diagnosis of prostatic adenocarcinoma at biopsy, clinically significant as defined by ISUP grading > 1 Group B2: new histologic diagnosis of prostatic adenocarcinoma at biopsy, no evidence of distant metastasis at systemic imaging; Group B3: new histologic diagnosis of prostatic adenocarcinoma at biopsy, at least one distant metastasis at systemic imaging, stratified in oligometastatic (less than four distant metastasis) and poli-metastatic (four or more distant metastasis).

Exclusion criteria were previous or actual androgen deprivation therapies, chemotherapies, immunotherapies, pelvic radiation therapies, treatments with other agents that could influence prostate growth and immune system, and actual diagnosis of infections, and inflammation or immunity disorders.

2.3. Methods

All cases were submitted to diagnostic and therapeutic practices reflecting our routine clinical activity and following EAU guidelines for the initial diagnosis and management of BPH and PC cases. In particular, either in BPH or in PC cases, prostate volume was assessed using the ellipsoid evaluation at ultrasonography. In cases with suspicion of PC mMR was performed, a PIRADS v2 score was defined and in cases with PIRADS score 3–5, a standard 12-core random biopsy was associated with targeted samples on the sites indicated by mMR. In cases with a histologic diagnosis of PC at biopsy, clinical staging and risk category (D'Amico and EAU classification) assessment was homogeneously performed following EAU guidelines. In particular, local staging was obtained at mMR and systemic staging using bone scan and CT scan or PET-CT scan.

2.3.1. Treatment Choice in Prostate Cancer Cases

In all cases with a new PC diagnosis, treatment decision was considered on the basis of risk classes determination and staging according to EAU guidelines after discussion of the different options with the patient. In particular, in patients considered for RP, every procedure was performed using a standard robotic-assisted (RARP) or laparoscopic (LRP) intraperitoneal approach consistent with best practice. Extended lymph node dissection (eLND) was performed in all cases with high risk or intermediate risk and more than 5% expected risk for positive lymph nodes at Briganti nomogram, including bilateral removal of the nodes overlying the external iliac artery and vein, the nodes within obturator fossa and the nodes medial and lateral to the internal iliac artery.

2.3.2. Pathologic Evaluation

All histologic specimens from prostatic biopsy and RP were analyzed by a uropathologist with a long experience in the PC field. Prostatic adenocarcinoma diagnosis was associated with the determination of ISUP grading, percentage of positive samples for PC, and maximal percentage of PC tissue per core at biopsy and prostate tumor volume pathologic T and N staging, surgical margin status, presence of perineural invasion (PNI) cribriform, and intraductal (IDC) differentiation at RP.

2.3.3. Neutrophil-to-Lymphocyte, Platelet-to-Lymphocyte, and Albumin-to-Globulin Ratio Determination

In all cases for each Group, NLR, PLR, and AGR were obtained at baseline at the time of the diagnosis of BPH or PC using results from routine blood count and proteinogram. Only in cases with PC considered for RP, NLR, PLR, and AGR determinations were repeated 90 days after surgery, using a post-operative laboratory routine control.

For each ratio, cut-off values were determined by receiver operating characteristics curve (ROC) analysis using Youden's index [12], and the optimal cut-off in our population was 2.5, 120.0, and 1.4, respectively, for NLR, PLR, and AGR, so as to distinguish low and high rate cases in each Group.

2.4. Statistical Analysis

Calculations were accomplished using Stata version 1.7 (Stata Corporation, College Station, TX, USA) with all tests being two-sided, and statistical significance set at <0.05.

For the comparison of quantitative data and pairwise intergroup comparisons of variables, a Mann–Whitney test was performed. For the comparison of qualitative data, Fisher's Exact test and chi-square test were used. Pearson correlation analysis was also performed. Univariate and multivariate Cox proportional analyses considering clinical and pathological parameters were used. We tested and compared the accuracy of the AGR, NLR, and PLR for predicting either the initial diagnosis of PC or its staging and aggressiveness. Regression coefficients were used to calculate the risk according to each model and the discrimination accuracy of these models was quantified using the area under the receiver operating characteristic (ROC) curve (AUC). Sensitivity, specificity, positive predictive value (PPV), and negative predictive value (NPV) of the different ratios in predicting PC diagnosis and adverse staging or grading were evaluated. HRs and corresponding 95% CI at univariate and multivariate analysis were considered to evaluate the importance and independency of the prognostic value for the different ratios.

3. Results

A total of 1019 consecutive cases responded to our inclusion and exclusion criteria and were enrolled in the analysis. Table 1 shows the clinical and pathological characteristics of our population stratified into different groups. In particular, 494 cases were enrolled in Group A as BPH cases and 525 cases in Group B as PC cases. PC cases were further stratified into clinically significant (426 cases in Group B1), non-metastatic (416 cases in Group B2), and metastatic (109 cases in Group B3).

Table 1. Characteristics of the whole population included in the study. Group A = patients with diagnosis of benign prostatic hyperplasia (BPH). Group B = patients with diagnosis of prostate cancer (PC), clinically significant in Group B1, non-metastatic (nmPC) in Group B2, and metastatic (mPC) in Group B3. Mean ± SD, median, (range). Number of cases (%).

Parameter	Group A (BPH)	Group B (all PC)	Group B1 (Clinically Significant PC)	Group B2 (nmPC)	Group B3 (mPC)	p Value 1 = A vs. B 2 = A vs. B1 3 = A vs. B2 4 = A vs. B3 5 = B2 vs. B3
Number of cases	494	525	426	416	109	\
Age (years)	66.3 ± 9.2; 68.0: (23–87)	66.6 ± 8.5; 67.0: (40–89)	65.1 ± 8.5; 67.0 (44–84)	65.3 ± 8.4; 67.0 (40–87)	71.2 ± 8.4; 67.0 (52–89)	1. 0.591 2. 0.044 3. 0.086 4. <0.0001 5. <0.0001
BMI	25.2 ± 8.7; 25.0: (16.9–45.6)	26.0 ± 3.3; 25.3 (16.9–39.4)	27.1 ± 7.6; 25.4 (20.4–39.4)	26.1 ± 3.3; 25.4 (16.9–39.4)	25.4 ± 3.3; 25.3 (22.7–29.7)	1. 0.0504 2. 0.0007 3. 0.0367 4. 0.8301 5. 0.0259
Metabolic syndrome %						
0 (absent)	83.6%	64.8%	66%	63.9%	65.1%	1. <0.0001 2. <0.0001 3. <0.0001 4. <0.0001 5. <0.0001
1 (mild)	8.7%	17.3%	16.7%	19.6%	10.7%	
2 (complete)	7.7%	17.9%	17.3%	16.5%	24.2%	
Baseline NLR	2.2 ± 1.2; 2.1: (0.5–17.8) (data on 459 cases)	2.5 ± 1.1; 2.2: (0.1–9.6) (data on 455 cases)	2.4 ± 1.1; 2.2: (0.1–8) (data on 371 cases)	2.5 ± 1.1; 2.2: (0.1–9.6) (data on 355 cases)	2.6 ± 1.5; 2.2 (0.6–4.6) (data on 100 cases)	1. 0.0005 2. 0.0053 3. 0.0038 4. 0.0019 5. 0.1528
Low (2.5)	327 (71.2%)	259 (56.9%)	205 (55.2%)	220 (61.6%)	39 (40.7%)	
High (2.5)	132 (28.8%)	196 (43.1%)	166 (44.8%)	135 (38.4%)	61 (59.3%)	
Baseline PLR	117.3 ± 51.3; 113.0: (28.3–369.5) (data on 456 cases)	132.8 ± 49.3; 116.0: (1.92–439.0) (data on 455 cases)	129.2 ± 49.3; 116.3: (1.92–439.0) (data on 297 cases)	127.8 ± 49.3; 116.3: (1.9–439.0) (data on 355 cases)	149.6 ± 49.5; 116.3 (58.8–255.4) (data on 100 cases)	1. <0.0001 2. <0.0001 3. <0.0001 4. <0.0001 5. <0.0001
Low (<120.0)	289 (63.3%)	193 (42.4%)	149 (50.1%)	173 (49.1%)	20 (19.4%)	
High (120.0)	167 (36.7%)	262 (57.6%)	148 (49.9%)	182 (50.9%)	80 (80.6%)	

Table 1. Cont.

Parameter	Group A (BPH)	Group B (all PC)	Group B1 (Clinically Significant PC)	Group B2 (nmPC)	Group B3 (mPC)	p Value 1 = A vs. B 2 = A vs. B1 3 = A vs. B2 4 = A vs. B3 5 = B2 vs. B3
Baseline AGR	1.5 ± 0.3; 1.5: (0.7–2.1) (data on 239 cases)	1.5 ± 0.3; 1.5: (0.8–5.6) (data on 420 cases)	1.5 ± 0.3; 1.5: (0.9–5.6) (data on 344 cases)	1.5 ± 0.3; 1.5: (0.9–5.6) (data on 327 cases)	1.5 ± 0.3; 1.5 (0.8–1.9) (data on 93 cases)	1. 0.1923 2. 0.4036 3. 0.2164 4. 0.2499 5. 0.7587
Low (≤1.4)	52 (21.7%)	149 (35.4%)	127 (36.9%)	129 (39.8%)	20 (20.8%)	
High (>1.4)	187 (78.3%)	271 (64.6%)	217 (63.1%)	198 (60.2%)	73 (79.2%)	
Prostate volume (cc)	51.5 ± 18.9; 46.0: (25–200)	46.0 ± 18.7; 45.0: (14–104)	42.8 ± 20.3; 45.0 (14–86)	45.1 ± 20.2; 45.0 (14–104)	50.0 ± 20.3; 45.0 (32–90)	1. <0.0001 2. <0.0001 3. <0.0001 4. 0.4669 5. 0.0217
total PSA (ng/mL)	3.2 ± 12.5; 3.2: (0.2–7.3)	13.3 ± 11.7; 4.6: (1.7–106.0)	14.7 ± 11.8; 4.7 (1.7–86.0)	9.3 ± 11.8; 4.7 (1.7–86.0)	26.5 ± 11.9; 4.5 (0.2–106.0)	1. <0.0001 2. <0.0001 3. <0.0001 4. <0.0001 5. <0.0001
PSAD	0.05 ± 0.03; 0.04: (0.004–0.09)	0.36 ± 0.24; 0.08: (0.0025–2.2)	0.34 ± 0.24; 0.08 (0.01–1.56)	0.22 ± 0.24; 0.08 (0.01–1.56)	0.54 ± 0.24; 0.08 (0.01–2.20)	1. <0.0001 2. <0.0001 3. <0.0001 4. <0.0001 5. <0.0001
mMR PIRADS score	/	(data on 257)	(data on 194)	(data on 252)		1. / 2. / 3. / 4. / 5. /
PIRADS 2		12 (4.5%)	9 (4.7%)	12 (4.8%)	-	
PIRADS 3		36 (14.3%)	24 (12.3%)	35 (13.9%)	-	
PIRADS 4		153 (59.0%)	115 (59.3%)	151 (59.9%)	-	
PIRADS 5		56 (22.2%)	46 (23.7%)	54 (21.4%)	-	

Table 1. *Cont.*

Parameter	Group A (BPH)	Group B (all PC)	Group B1 (Clinically Significant PC)	Group B2 (nmPC)	Group B3 (mPC)	p Value 1 = A vs. B 2 = A vs. B1 3 = A vs. B2 4 = A vs. B3 5 = B2 vs. B3
Prostate tumor size (mm) at MR	/	12.3 ± 4.8; 12.0: (4–35)	12.7 ± 4.9; 12.0 (4–52)	12.2 ± 4.9; 12.0 (4–35)	15.8 ± 5.0; 12.0 (18–25)	1. / 2. / 3. / 4. / 5. <0.0001
Clinical T staging	/					1. / 2. / 3. / 4. / 5. <0.0001
T2		454 (86.5%)	356 (83.6%)	365 (88.1%)	89 (80%)	
T3a		62 (11.8%)	62 (14.6%)	42 (9.9%)	20 (20%)	
T3b		9 (12.7%)	8 (1.8%)	9 (2%)	0 (0%)	
Clinical N staging	/					1. / 2. / 3. / 4. / 5. <0.0001
N0		447 (85.1%)	350 (82.1%)	390 (94.2%)	57 (51.7%)	
N1		78 (14.9%)	76 (17.9%)	26 (5.8%)	52 (48.3%)	
M staging	/					1. <0.0001 2. / 3. / 4. / 5. <0.0001
M0		413 (78.6%)	314 (73.7%)	416 (100%)	0 (0%)	
M1 oligometastatic (<4)		106 (20.2%)	106 (24.8%)	0 (0%)	103 (94.6%)	
M1 polimetastatic (≥4)		6 (1.2%)	6 (1.5%)	0 (0%)	6 (5.4%)	
Biopsy outcomes	/					1. / 2. / 3. / 4. / 5. 0.0097
% positive samples PC		35.4 ± 26.2; 28.0: (4.0–100.0)	40.2 ± 26.3; 28.0: (4.0–100.0)	34.4 ± 26.3; 28.0 (4.0–100.0)	41.7 ± 26.3; 28.0 (50.0–100.0)	
Max% PC tissue per core		40.2 ± 25.8; 35.0: (2.0–94.0)	43.9 ± 25.9; 35.0: (4.0–94.0)	35.0 ± 25.9; 35.0: (2.0–94.0)	63.2 ± 26.1; 35.0 (32.0–94.0)	

Table 1. Cont.

Parameter	Group A (BPH)	Group B (all PC)	Group B1 (Clinically Significant PC)	Group B2 (nmPC)	Group B3 (mPC)	p Value 1 = A vs. B 2 = A vs. B1 3 = A vs. B2 4 = A vs. B3 5 = B2 vs. B3
ISUP grading at biopsy						
1		98 (18.6%)	0 (0%)	98 (23.7%)	0 (0%)	1. /
2	/	171 (32.6%)	170 (39.9%)	170 (40.9%)	1 (1.8%)	2. /
3		107 (20.4%)	107 (25.1%)	77 (18.7%)	30 (26.8%)	3. /
4		113 (21.5%)	113 (26.6%)	46 (10.7%)	67 (61.6%)	4. /
5		36 (6.9%)	36 (8.4%)	25 (6%)	11 (9.8%)	5. 0.08
Risk Class (D'Amico)						
Low risk		104 (19.8%)	17 (3.9%)	104 (25.2%)	-	
Intermediate risk	/	219 (41.8%)	210 (49.3%)	219 (52.8%)	-	/
High risk		202 (38.4%)	199 (46.8%)	93 (22%)	-	
Radical prostatectomy		(Data on 371)	(Data on 281)	(Data on 371)		
Laparoscopic	/	223 (60.1%)	166 (59%)	223 (60.1%)	/	/
Robotic-assisted		148 (39.9%)	115 (41%)	148 (39.9%)		
Pathological stage (T)		(Data on 371)	(Data on 281)	(Data on 371)		
pT2		190 (51.2%)	112 (39.9%)	190 (51.2%)		
pT3a	/	141 (38%)	130 (46.3%)	141 (38%)	/	/
pT3b		40 (10.8%)	39 (13.8%)	40 (10.8%)		
pT4		0 (0%)	0 (0%)	0 (0%)		
Pathological stage (N)						
N0	/	284 (94%)	213 (92.2%)	284 (94%)	/	/
N+		18 (6%)	18 (1.8%)	18 (6%)		

Table 1. Cont.

Parameter	Group A (BPH)	Group B (all PC)	Group B1 (Clinically Significant PC)	Group B2 (nmPC)	Group B3 (mPC)	p Value 1 = A vs. B; 2 = A vs. B1; 3 = A vs. B2; 4 = A vs. B3; 5 = B2 vs. B3
ISUP grading at surgery		(data on 371)	(data on 281)	(data on 371)		/
1		64 (17.4%)	4 (1.4%)	64 (17.3%)		
2	/	163 (43.9%)	140 (49.8%)	163 (43.9%)		
3		85 (23%)	79 (28.2%)	85 (23%)		
4		23 (6.2%)	23 (8.1%)	23 (6.3%)		
5		36 (9.5%)	35 (12.4%)	36 (9.5%).		
Surgical margin (R)						/
Negative	/	280 (78.2%)	209 (74.3%)	280 (78.2%)	/	
Positive		91 (21.8%)	72 (25.7%)	91 (21.8%)		
PNI at surgery						/
Positive	/	258 (62.2%)	213 (75.8%)	258 (62.2%)	/	
Negative		113 (37.8%)	68 (24.2%)	113 (37.8%)		
Cribriform/IDC at surgery						/
Positive	/	68 (16.4%)	57 (20.2%)	68 (16.5%)	/	
Negative		303 (83.6%)	224 (79.8%)	303 (83.5%)		
Postoperative total PSA (ng/mL)	/	0.2 ± 0.9; 0.02: (0.01–10)	0.2 ± 0.9; 0.02: (0.01–10)	0.2 ± 0.9; 0.02: (0.01–10)	/	/
Biochemical progression (number of cases and %)	/	46 (12.3%)	41 (14.5%)	46 (12.3%)	/	/

3.1. Comparative Analysis among the Different Groups

Table 1 shows the distribution of the different variables according to the different groups examined and Figure 1 shows the distribution of low and high ratios according to the diagnosis in the different groups.

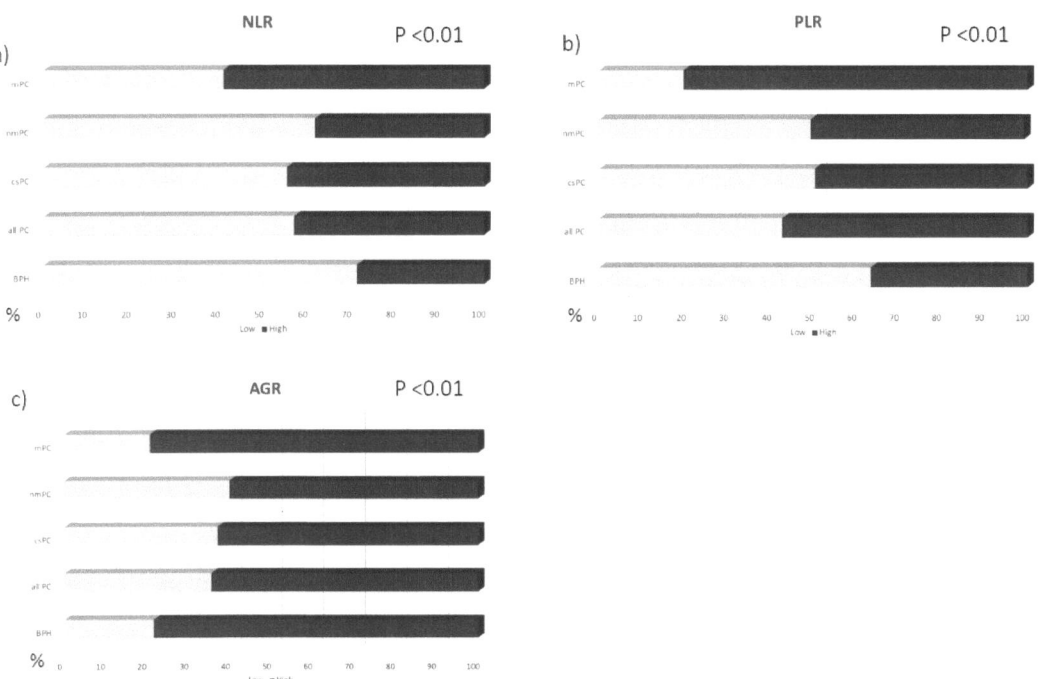

Figure 1. Percentage of cases with low or high NLR (**a**), PLR (**b**), and AGR (**c**) according to the diagnosis in the different groups.

3.1.1. Benign Prostatic Hyperplasia versus Prostate Cancer Cases

No significant differences ($p = 0.591$) were found between Group A (BPH cases) and Group B (PC cases) in terms of age, whereas total PSA was significantly higher ($p < 0.001$) in Group B than in Group A. Mean values of NLR and PLR were significantly ($p < 0.001$) lower in Group A (2.23 ± 1.22 and 117.30 ± 51.3, respectively) than in Group B (2.49 ± 1.14 and 132.8 ± 49.3, respectively) and the percentage of cases with high NLR and PLR according to the cut-off, was higher in Group B (43.1% and 57.6%, respectively) than in Group A (28.8% and 36.7%, respectively). On the contrary, no significant differences ($p = 0.1923$) in mean values of AGR were found between Group A (1.52 ± 0.29) and Group B (1.49 ± 0.28) but the percentage of cases with low AGR was higher in Group B (35.4%) than in Group A (21.7%) (Table 1).

Considering Group B1 (clinically significant PC), mean values of NLR and PLR (2.45 ± 1.15 and 129.19 ± 49.32, respectively) were significantly ($p = 0.0053$) higher when compared with Group A and the percentage of cases with high NLR and PLR was higher in Group B1 (44.8% and 49.9%, respectively) than in Group A (Table 1). On the contrary, no significant differences ($p = 0.4036$) in mean values of AGR were found between Group B1 (1.50 ± 0.28) and Group A but the percentage of cases with low AGR was higher in Group B1 (36.9%) than in Group A (Table 1).

3.1.2. Non-Metastatic versus Metastatic Prostate Cancer Cases

In Group B3, 94.6% of cases were oligometastatic and only 5.4% were poli-metastatic. Mean values of PLR were significantly ($p < 0.001$) higher in metastatic (Group B3: 149.63 ± 49.46) than in non-metastatic (Group B2: 127.79 ± 49.32) cases. On the contrary, no significant differences ($p > 0.05$) between Group B2 and Group B3 were found in terms of mean values of PLR and AGR (Table 1). The percentage of cases with high NLR and PLR according to the cut-off was higher in Group B3 (59.3% and 80.6%, respectively) than in Group B2 (38.4% and 50.9%, respectively) whereas no significant variations between Group B2 and Group B3 were found in terms of low AGR distribution (Table 1).

3.2. Results on the Basis of Neutrophil-to-Lymphocyte, Platelet-to-Lymphocyte, and Albumin-to-Globulin Ratio Stratification (Low versus High)

Tables 2 and 3 show the distribution of the different clinical and pathological variables according to the stratification of cases on the basis of NLR, PLR, and AGR cut-offs.

Table 2. Characteristics of the population stratified on the basis of NLR, PLR, and AGR. Mean ± SD, median, (range). Number of cases (%).

Parameter	Low NLR (<2.5)	High NLR (≥2.5)	Low PLR (<120.0)	High PLR (≥120.0)	Low AGR (<1.4)	High AGR (≥1.4)	p Value 1. NLR 2. PLR 3. AGR
Number of cases	586	328	482	429	201	458	/
Age (years)	66.1 ± 8.7 66.0 (40–89)	66.8 ± 7.9 68.0 (44–85)	66.2 ± 8.7 67.0 (40–89)	66.4 ± 8.3 67.5 (23–85)	67.9 ± 6.9 68.4 (48.84)	65.7 ± 8.4 67.3 (23–87)	1. 0.2347 2. 0.7246 3. 0.0856
BMI	25.7 ± 3.4 26.4 (16.9–45.6)	25.5 ± 2.9 25.4 (16.9–41.5)	25.9 ± 3.6 25.5 (17.0–45.6)	25.3 ± 2.8 25.2 (16.9–41.5)	26.2 ± 3.7 25.6 (18.5–41.5)	25.8 ± 3.0 25.5 (16.9–36.3)	1. 0.3099 2. 0.0044 3. 0.1263
Metabolic syndrome							
0 (absent)	432 (73.72%)	237 (72.26%)	346 (71.78%)	320 (74.59%)	127 (63.18%)	326 (71.18%)	1. 0.522 2. 0.890 3. 0.350
1 (mild)	77 (13.14%)	44 (13.41%)	64 (13.28%)	57 (13.29%)	37 (18.41%)	60 (13.10%)	
2 (complete)	77 (13.14%)	47 (14.33%)	72 (14.94%)	52 (12.12%)	37 (18.41%)	72 (15.72%)	
Prostate volume (cc)	50.0 ± 22.0 46 (14–274)	47.9 ± 17.5 45 (14–165)	50.5 ± 23.3 45 (14–274)	47.8 ± 16.8 45 (14–165)	49.9 ± 21.2 45 (15–165)	50.0 ± 22.3 47 (14–274)	1. 0.1304 2. 0.0515 3. 0.9228
Total PSA (ng/mL)	7.6 ± 11.3 4.2 (0.05–106.0)	10.4 ± 12.8 5.8 (0.06–97.0)	6.9 ± 10.7 3.9 (0.05–105.0)	10.4 ± 12.9 6.0 (0.06–106.0)	10.3 ± 10.9 6.8 (0.4–81.0)	10.4 ± 13.7 6.0 (0.04–106.0)	1. 0.0009 2. <0.0001 3. 0.8766
PSAD	0.15 ± 0.22 0.07 (0.001–2.21)	0.23 ± 0.28 0.12 (0.001–2.06)	0.14 ± 0.20 0.07 (0.001–1.69)	0.24 ± 0.29 0.13 (0.001–2.21)	0.23 ± 0.25 0.14 (0.01–1.69)	0.22 ± 0.28 0.1 (0.001–2.21)	1. <0.0001 2. <0.0001 3. 0.6631
mMR PIRADS score	(data on 149)	(data on 88)	(data on 113)	(data on 124)	(data on 71)	(data on 129)	
PIRADS 2	9 (6.05%)	4 (4.54%)	5 (4.43%)	8 (6.45%)	2 (2.82%)	7 (5.43%)	1. 0.447 2. 0.891 3. 0.393
PIRADS 3	23 (15.44%)	11 (12.5%)	20 (17.70%)	14 (11.29%)	10 (14.08%)	19 (14.73%)	
PIRADS 4	84 (56.36%)	56 (63.64%)	61 (53.98%)	79 (63.70%)	45 (63.38%)	72 (55.81%)	
PIRADS 5	33 (22.15%)	17 (19.32%)	27 (23.89%)	23 (18.55%)	14 (19.72%)	31 (24.03%)	
Diagnosis							
BPH	327 (55.8%)	132 (40.2%)	289 (59.9%)	167 (38.9%)	52 (25.8%)	187 (40.8%)	1. 0.021 2. 0.034 3. 0.045
All PC	259 (44.2%)	196 (59.7%)	193 (40%)	262 (61.%)	149 (74.1%)	271 (59.1%)	
Clinical significant PC	205 (34.9%)	166 (50.6%)	149 (30.9%)	148 (34.5%)	127 (63.1%)	217 (47.3%)	
nmPC	220 (37%)	135 (41.1%)	173 (35.8%)	182 (41.7%)	129 (61.1%)	198 (42.5%)	
mPC	39 (7.1%)	61 (18.5%)	20 (4.1%)	80 (19.3%)	20 (9.9%)	73 (16.5%)	

Table 3. Characteristics of the non-metastatic prostate cancer (nmPC) population stratified on the basis of NLR, PLR, and AGR score. Mean ± SD, median, (range). Number of cases (%).

Parameter	Low NLR (<2.5)	High NLR (≥2.5)	Low PLR (<120.0)	High PLR (≥120.0)	Low AGR (<1.4)	High AGR (≥1.4)	p Value 1. NLR 2. PLR 3. AGR
Number of cases with available ratios	220 (62.0%)	135 (38.0%)	173 (67.8%)	182 (32.2%)	129 (39.4%)	198 (61.6%)	/
Age (years)	64.7 ± 8.7; 66.0: (40–87)	64.9 ± 6.6 66.0: (44–78)	65.9 ± 6.7 66.0: (47–87)	64.0 ± 6.9 65.0: (40–78)	66.2 ± 6.2 67.0: (48–84)	64.4 ± 6.7 65.0: (47–81)	1. 0.836 2. 0.010 3. 0.014
Total PSA (ng/mL)	10.1 ± 9.1; 4.3: (1.7–86.0)	8.1 ± 4.7 7.0:(0.06–30.0)	10.4 ± 10.3 7.4: (0.05–86.0)	8.5 ± 6.3 7.0: (0.06–58.0)	9.3 ± 6.7 7.7: (1.7–48.0)	10.0 ± 10.5 7.1: (0.04–86.0)	1. 0.022 2. 0.031 3. 0.471
PSAD	0.23 ± 0.18; 0.07: (0.02–1.56)	0.22 ± 0.19 0.16: (0.01–1.48)	0.23 ± 0.24 0.08: (0.01–1.56)	0.35 ± 0.24 0.08: (0.01–2.20)	0.24 ± 0.20 0.08: (0.04–1.48)	0.23 ± 0.24 0.08: (0.01–1.56)	1. 0.619 2.<0.0001 3. 0.694
mMR PIRADS score	Data on 141 cases	Data on 85 cases	Data on 107 cases	Data on 111 cases	Data on 69 cases	Data on 129 cases	
PIRADS 2	7 (5%)	3 (3%)	3 (3%)	6 (5%)	1 (1%)	7 (5%)	1. 0.787 2. 0.256 3. 0.394
PIRADS 3	20 (14%)	11 (13%)	18 (17%)	11 (10%)	10 (15%)	19 (15%)	
PIRADS 4	82 (58%)	55 (65%)	60 (56%)	72 (65%)	45 (65%)	72 (56%)	
PIRADS 5	32 (23%)	16 (19%)	26 (24%)	22 (20%)	13 (19%)	31 (24%)	
Prostate tumor size (mm) at mMR	12.6 ± 5.0; 12.0: (5.0–26.0)	12.8 ± 5.6 12: (4.0–35.0)	13.52 ± 6.12 12: (4.0–38.0)	13.22 ± 5.95 12: (4.0–47.0)	12.06 ± 5.0 12: (4.0–38.0)	13.64 ± 6.10 12.0: (4.0–47.0)	1. 0.727 2. 0.639 3. 0.214
Clinical T staging							
T2	196 (89%)	118 (87%)	153 (88%)	161 (88%)	116 (90%)	171 (86%)	1. 0.871 2. 0.477 3. 0.349
T3a	19 (9%)	13 (10%)	14 (8%)	18 (10%)	12 (9%)	21 (11%)	
T3b	5 (2%)	4 (3%)	6 (4%)	3 (2%)	1 (1%)	6 (3%)	
Clinical N staging							
N0	205 (93%)	129 (96%)	163 (94%)	171 (94%)	120 (93%)	187 (94%)	1. 0.357 2. 0.916 3. 0.600
N1	15 (7%)	6 (4%)	10 (6%)	11 (6%)	9 (7%)	11 (6%)	
Biopsy outcomes							
% positive samples PC	39.7 ± 25.9; 28.0: (12.0–100.0)	30.4 ± 23.9; 28.0: (4.0–87.0)	30.1 ± 19.2; 25: (12.0–100.0)	41.4 ± 30.7; 32.5: (4.0–100.0)	30.2 ± 23.2; 25.0: (4.0–95.0)	35.3 ± 24.8; 32.0 (4.0–100.0)	1. 0.0008 2.<0.0001 3. 0.062
Max% PC tissue per core	36.9 ± 24.3; 32.0: (2.0–94.0)	34.8 ± 24.0; 30.0: (4.0–90.0)	36.3 ± 20.2; 33.0; (4.0–83.0)	35.8 ± 25.4; 32.0: (2.0–94.0)	31.5 ± 20.2; 25.2: (4.0–77.0)	38.8 ± 23.5; 35.0: (4.0–94.0)	1. 0.427 2. 0.809 3. 0.004
ISUP grading at biopsy							
1	54 (24%)	29 (22%)	44 (25%)	39 (21%)	21 (16%)	54 (27%)	1. 0.621 2. 0.549 3. 0.140
2	95 (43%)	53 (39%)	75 (43%)	73 (40%)	59 (46%)	72 (36%)	
3	37 (17%)	31 (23%)	31 (18%)	37 (20%)	26 (20%)	38 (19%)	
4	24 (11%)	14 (10%)	17 (10%)	21 (12%)	14 (11%)	25 (13%)	
5	10 (5%)	8 (6%)	6 (4%)	12 (7%)	9 (7%)	9 (5%)	
Risk Class (D'Amico)							
Low risk	54 (24%)	32 (24%)	42 (24%)	44 (24%)	24 (19%)	50 (25%)	1. 0.980 2. 0.917 3. 0.354
Intermediate risk	120 (55%)	74 (55%)	96 (56%)	98 (54%)	75 (58%)	103 (52%)	
High risk	46 (21%)	29 (21%)	35 (20%)	40 (22%)	30 (23%)	45 (23%)	
Radical prostatectomy	Data on 203 cases	Data on 124 cases	Data on 154 cases	Data on 173 cases	Data on 120 cases	Data on 187 cases	1. 0.696 2. 0.875 3. 0.0001
Laparoscopic	120 (59%)	76 (61%)	93 (60%)	103 (60%)	91 (76%)	101 (54%)	
Robotic-assisted	83 (41%)	48 (39%)	61 (40%)	70 (40%)	29 (24%)	86 (46%)	
Pathological stage (T)							
pT2	101 (50%)	59 (48%)	75 (49%)	85 (49%)	54 (45%)	95 (51%)	1. 0.690 2. 0.532 3. 0.417
pT3a	82 (40%)	49 (39%)	59 (38%)	72 (42%)	54 (45%)	70 (37%)	
pT3b	20 (10%)	16 (13%)	20 (13%)	16 (9%)	12 (10%)	22 (12%)	

Table 3. Cont.

Parameter	Low NLR (<2.5)	High NLR (≥2.5)	Low PLR (<120.0)	High PLR (≥120.0)	Low AGR (<1.4)	High AGR (≥1.4)	p Value 1. NLR 2. PLR 3. AGR
Pathological stage (N)							1. 0.457 2. 0.997 3. 0.985
N0	191 (94%)	119 (96%)	146 (95%)	164 (95%)	113 (94%)	176 (94%)	
N+	12 (6%)	5 (4%)	8 (5%)	9 (5%)	7 (6%)	11 (6%)	
ISUP grading at surgery							1. 0.103 2. 0.916 3. 0.186
1	37 (18%)	19 (15%)	29 (19%)	27 (16%)	16 (13%)	37 (20%)	
2	95 (47%)	50 (40%)	69 (45%)	76 (44%)	56 (47%)	77 (41%)	
3	39 (19%)	37 (30%)	33 (21%)	43 (25%)	26 (22%)	43 (23%)	
4	10 (5%)	10 (8%)	9 (6%)	11 (6%)	6 (5%)	16 (9%)	
5	22 (11%)	8 (7%)	14 (9%)	16 (9%)	16 (13%)	14 (7%)	
Surgical margin (R)							1. 0.841 2. 0.131 3. 0.890
Negative	151 (74%)	91 (73%)	108 (70%)	134 (77%)	89 (74%)	140 (75%)	
Positive	52 (26%)	33 (27%)	46 (30%)	39 (23%)	31 (26%)	47 (25%)	
PNI at surgery							1. 0.012 2. 0.365 3. 0.049
Positive	136 (67%)	99 (80%)	107 (69%)	128 (74%)	91 (76%)	122 (65%)	
Negative	67 (33%)	25 (20%)	47 (31%)	45 (26%)	29 (24%)	65 (35%)	
Cribriform/IDC at surgery							1. 0.740 2. 0.836 3. 0.445
Positive	39 (19%)	22 (18%)	28 (18%)	33 (19%)	24 (20%)	31 (17%)	
Negative	164 (81%)	102 (82%)	126 (82%)	140 (81%)	96 (80%)	156 (83%)	
Postoperative total PSA (ng/mL)	0.21 ± 0.96; 0.02: (0.01–10)	0.25 ± 0.87 0.03: (0.01–7)	0.28 ± 1.22 0.02: (0.01–10)	0.17 ± 0.47 0.03: (0.01–2.9)	0.13 ± 0.34 0.03: (0.01–2.34)	0.29 ± 1.20 0.02: (0.01–10.0)	1. 0.705 2. 0.273 3. 0.155
Biochemical progression (number of cases and %)	22 (11%)	18 (15%)	20 (13%)	20 (12%)	18 (15%)	19 (10%)	1. 0.247 2. 0.645 3. 0.172

3.2.1. Benign Prostatic Hyperplasia versus Prostate Cancer Diagnosis (Group A versus B)

Neutrophil-to-Lymphocyte Ratio

A total of 586 cases showed low NLR and 328 cases high NLR according to the cut-off 2.5. No significant differences ($p > 0.05$) were found in terms of age, prostate volume, and PIRADS score between the two groups, whereas in the high NLR group the mean values of total PSA were significantly ($p = 0.0009$) higher (10.36 ± 12.82) when compared to low NLR (7.63 ± 11.33). Cases with a low NLR showed a higher percentage of BPH diagnosis (55.8%) than cases with a high NLR (40.2%). Cases with a high NLR showed a higher percentage of clinically significant (50.6%) and metastatic PC (18.5%) than cases with low NLR (34.9% and 7.1%, respectively) (Table 2).

Platelet-to-Lymphocyte RATIO

A total of 482 cases showed low PLR and 429 cases with high PLR according to the cut-off 120.0. No significant differences ($p > 0.05$) were found in terms of age, prostate volume, or PIRADS score between the two groups, whereas in high PLR group mean values of total PSA were significantly ($p < 0.0001$) higher (10.39 ± 12.89) when compared to low PLR (6.99 ± 10.72). Cases with a low PLR showed a higher percentage of BPH diagnosis (59.9%) than cases with high PLR (38.9%). Cases with a high PLR showed a higher percentage of clinically significant (34.5%) and metastatic PC (19.3%) than cases with low PLR (30.9% and 4.1%, respectively) (Table 2).

Albumin-to-Globulin Ratio

A total of 201 cases showed low AGR and 458 cases high AGR according to the cut-off 1.4. No significant differences ($p > 0.05$) were found in terms of age, prostate volume, total

PSA, and PIRADS score between the two groups. Cases with a high AGR showed a higher percentage of BPH diagnosis (40.8%) than cases with a low AGR (25.8%). Cases with a low AGR showed a higher percentage of clinically significant (63.1%) but lower of metastatic PC (9.9%) than cases with high AGR (47.3% and 16.5%, respectively) (Table 2).

3.2.2. Non-Metastatic Prostate Cancer (Group B2)

Neutrophil-to-Lymphocyte Ratio

In the non-metastatic PC group, 62% showed low NLR and 38% high NLR according to the cut-off 2.5. No significant differences ($p > 0.05$) were found in terms of T staging, ISUP grading, and biochemical progression after RP. The percentage of PNI at final pathology was significantly ($p = 0.012$) higher in the high (80%) than in the low (67%) NLR group (Table 3).

Platelet-to-Lymphocyte Ratio

A total of 67.8% showed low PLR and 32.2% high PLR according to the cut-off of 120.0. No significant differences ($p > 0.05$) were found in terms of T staging, ISUP grading, other pathologic variables, and biochemical progression (Table 3).

Albumin-to-Globulin Ratio

A total of 61.6% showed high AGR and 39.4% low AGR according to the cut-off 1.4. No significant differences ($p > 0.05$) were found in terms of T stage, ISUP grading, and biochemical progression. The percentage of PNI at final pathology was significantly ($p = 0.049$) higher in the low (76%) than in the high (65%) AGR group (Table 3).

3.3. Variation in Neutrophil-to-Lymphocyte, Platelet-to-Lymphocyte, and Albumin-to-Globulin Ratio According to Radical Prostatectomy Procedure

A total of 371 cases with PC diagnosis were submitted to radical prostatectomy. After surgery, mean NLR, PLR, and AGR values significantly ($p < 0.0001$) varied when compared to pre-surgical values (Figure 2). In particular, NLR mean values (pre: 2.47 ± 1.15 and post: 10.77 ± 6.93) and AGR mean values (pre: 1.50 ± 0.28 and post: 1.65 ± 0.20) significantly increased, whereas PLR (pre: 128.04 ± 49.29 and post: 107.75 ± 62.07) significantly reduced after RP. These significant variations after RP were mainly maintained also after the stratification of cases on the basis of pT stage, ISUP grading, and risk classes (Table 4).

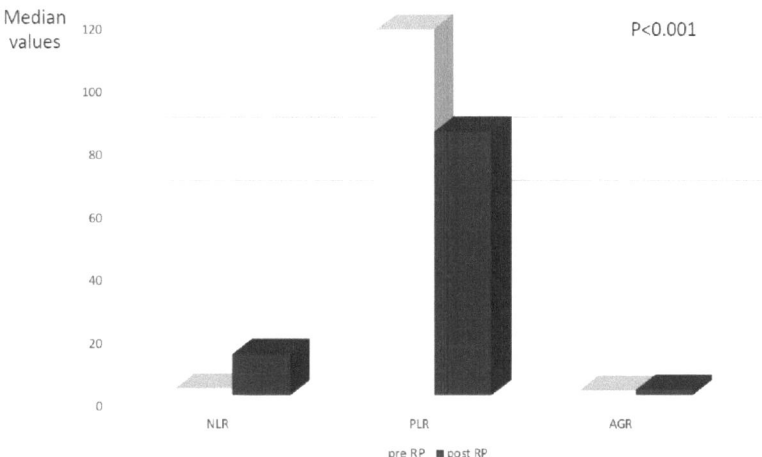

Figure 2. Variation in median values of NLR, PLR, and AGR after radical prostatectomy (RP) in patients with non-metastatic prostate cancer.

Table 4. Changes in NLR, PLR, and AGR from pre-RP to post RP determination. Mean ± SD, median (range).

PC Cases Submitted to RP	NLR Pre-RP	NLR Ratio Post-RP	PLR Pre-RP	PLR Post-RP	AGR Pre-RP	AGR Post-RP	p Value 1. NLR 2. PLR 3. AGR
All cases (371)	2.47 ± 1.15; 2.18: (0.09–9.60)	10.77 ± 6.93; 13.19: (1.08–26.90)	128.04 ± 49.29; 116.31: (1.92–439.09)	107.75 ± 62.07; 83.7: (33.13–330.0)	1.50 ± 0.28; 1.50: (0.92–5.60)	1.65 ± 0.20; 1.70: (1.13–2.10)	1. <0.0001 2. <0.0001 3. <0.0001
pT2 (190)	2.52 ± 1.15; 2.18: (1.07–9.60)	11.82 ± 6.98; 13.47: (1.08–26.95)	128.81 ± 49.32; 116.31: (53.68–300.0)	102.61 ± 61.83; 83.70: (46.90–261.90)	1.49 ± 0.28; 1.50: (0.92–2.11)	1.59 ± 0.20; 1.70: (1.16–2.0)	1. <0.0001 2. <0.0001 3. 0.0001
pT3 (181)	2.41 ± 1.15; 2.18: (30.09–6.11)	9.0 ± 6.93; 13.19: (1.50–22.0)	126.77 ± 49.26; 116.31: (1.92–439.09)	113.20 ± 62.07; 83.76: (33.13–330.0)	1.50 ± 0.28; 1.50: (0.98–5.60)	1.63 ± 0.20; 1.7: (1.13–2.10)	1. <0.0001 2. 0.0218 3. <0.0001
ISUP 1–2 (227)	2.48 ± 1.15; 2.18: (0.90–9.60)	12.09 ± 6.98; 13.47: (1.08–26.90)	126.79 ± 49.32; 116.31: (40.95–439.09)	98.68 ± 61.83; 83.78: (46.90–261.90)	1.49 ± 0.28; 1.50: (0.92–5.60)	1.62 ± 0.18; 1.7: (1.50–2.0)	1. <0.0001 2. <0.0001 3. <0.0001
ISUP 3–5 (144)	2.43 ± 1.15; 2.18: (0.09–5.78)	8.69 ± 6.97; 13.16: (1.50–22.03)	129.31 ± 49.26; 116.31: (33.13–330.0)	118.82 ± 62.07; 83.74: (33.13–330.0)	1.50 ± 0.28; 1.50: (0.98–2.19)	1.60 ± 0.20; 1.7: (1.13–2.10)	1. <0.0001 2. 0.1133 3. 0.0006
Low risk (90)	2.73 ± 1.15; 2.18: (1.24–9.60)	11.25 ± 6.95; 13.47: (1.47–26.95)	128.21 ± 49.36; 116.31: (71.15–300.0)	92.12 ± 62.90; 82.85: (33.13–228.86)	1.46 ± 0.28; 1.50: (0.92–2.04)	1.62 ± 0.20; 1.70: (1.60–2.10)	1. <0.0001 2. <0.0001 3. <0.0001
Intermediate risk (197)	2.39 ± 1.17; 2.12: (0.77–7.45)	10.03 ± 7.02; 13.19: (1.08–23.24)	126.37 ± 49.68; 115: (40.95–439.09)	117.10 ± 61.83; 83.78: (46.94–330.0)	1.50 ± 0.28; 1.50: (0.98–5.60)	1.54 ± 0.20; 1.70: (1.50–1.80)	1. <0.0001 2. 0.1017 3. 0.1036
High risk (84)	2.32 ± 1.22; 2.09: (0.09–5.78)	10.91 ± 7.04; 13.77: (1. 78–22.03)	129.38 ± 50.16; 112.20: (1.92–371.0)	100.20 ± 55.73; 82.85: (58.86–209.0)	1.50 ± 0.29; 1.50: (0.98–2.19)	1.56 ± 0.20; 1.70: (1.13–2.0)	1. <0.0001 2. 0.0005 3. 0.1204

3.4. Correlation among Neutrophil-to-Lymphocyte, Platelet-to-Lymphocyte, Albumin-to-Globulin Ratio, and Other Clinical and Pathological Variables

We investigated significant correlations among each ratio and the clinical and pathological variables of our population, as described in Table 5. A significant correlation was found between NLR and PLR values (r = 0.590765385; p < 0.0001), but not between NLR or PLR and AGR (p > 0.05).

Table 5. Pearson correlation coefficients among NLR, PLR, AGR, and the different pathological and clinical variables.

Correlation	Coefficient	p Value
NLR–PLR	0.590765385	**<0.0001**
NLR–AGR	−0.056808466	0.233
PLR–AGR	−0.032381744	0.495
NLR–age	−0.003393898	0.949
NLR BMI	−0.043542716	0.360
NLR metabolic syndrome	−0.011263298	0.814
NLR–prostate volume	0.012090362	0.798
NLR–risk class	−0.031727259	0.509
NLR–preoperative PSA	0.060700932	0.196
NLR–PSAD	0.084847705	0.070
NLR–PIRADS score	−0.019247647	0.686
NLR–diagnosis PC	0.119796458	**0.000324**
NLR–prostate tumor size	−0.057921656	0.224
NLR–percentage positive core at biopsy	−0.117607299	**0.012**

Table 5. *Cont.*

Correlation	Coefficient	*p* Value
NLR–T stage	−0.0530888	0.259
NLR–N stage	−0.045416757	0.338
NLR–M stage	0.089695182	0.056
NLR–ISUP grading	0.022020966	0.639
NLR–surgical margins	−0.013402868	0.782
NLR–PNI	0.065605296	0.162
NLR–cribriform/IDC	−0.041355254	0.382
NLR–postoperative PSA	0.00894501	0.849
NLR–biochemical progression	−0.009564575	0.848
PLR–age	−0.041847787	0.388
PLR–BMI	−0.095185293	**0.045**
PLR–metabolic syndrome	−0.045276738	0.344
PLR–prostate volume	−0.0306643	0.528
PLR–risk class	0.12076586	**0.010**
PLR–preoperative PSA	0.112118686	**0.018**
PLR–PSAD	0.138732191	**0.003**
PLR–PIRADS score	−0.006489868	0.899
PLR–diagnosis PC	0.16085218	**<0.0001**
PLR–prostate tumor size	−0.055344287	0.247
PLR–percentage positive core at biopsy	0.153215834	**0.0012**
PLR–T stage	−0.0143615	0.768
PLR–N stage	−0.022325927	0.643
PLR–M stage	0.186703018	**0.000076**
PLR–ISUP grading	0.00920659	0.846
PLR–surgical margins	−0.031205866	0.514
PLR–PNI	0.078362099	0.099
PLR–cribriform/IDC	−0.018649791	0.705
PLR–postoperative PSA	−0.004990327	0.933
PLR–biochemical progression	−0.001641053	0.983
AGR–age	−0.189983803	**0.000096**
AGR–BMI	−0.039096382	0.424
AGR–metabolic syndrome	−0.054469657	0.268
AGR–prostate volume	−0.031335926	0.525
AGR–risk class	0.025717996	0.599
AGR–preoperative PSA	−0.039384808	0.424
AGR–PSAD	−0.046284517	0.346
AGR–PIRADS score	0.001454159	0.977
AGR–diagnosis PC	−0.051833904	0.195
AGR–prostate tumor size	0.070965303	0.146
AGR–percentage positive core at biopsy	−0.117692213	**0.016**

Table 5. *Cont.*

Correlation	Coefficient	p Value
AGR–T stage	0.041302814	0.397
AGR–N stage	0.026190226	0.593
AGR–M stage	−0.023100814	0.637
AGR–ISUP grading	0.013429298	0.783
AGR–Risk classes	0.025717996	0.599
AGR–surgical margins	−0.027616388	0.580
AGR–PNI	−0.056143388	0.251
AGR–cribriform/IDC	−0.050339474	0.306
AGR–postoperative PSA	0.05732158	0.240
AGR–biochemical progression	−0.020713105	0.682

The bold in this table can be useful to underline the significant values of *p*-value.

NLR significantly correlated with PC initial diagnosis (r = 0.119796458; $p = 0.000324$) but not with T, N, and M staging, ISUP grading or biochemical progression ($p > 0.05$) (Table 5).

PLR significantly correlated with PC initial diagnosis (r = 0.16085218, $p < 0.0001$) and M stage (r = 0.186703018; $p = 000076$), but not with T or N staging, ISUP grading, or biochemical progression ($p > 0.05$) (Table 5).

No significant ($p > 0.05$) correlations were found between *AGR* and the other variables (Table 5).

3.5. Sensitivity, Specificity, Positive Predictive Value, Negative Predictive Value, and Area under the Curve Results in Predicting Pathologic Features

The analysis was performed considering the optimal cut-off for each ratio of 2.5, 120.0 and 1.4, respectively, for NLR, PLR, and AGR, so as to distinguish low and high rate cases in each group.

3.5.1. Initial Diagnosis of Clinically Significant Prostate Cancer

The performance of the three ratios in predicting clinically significant PC (csPC) at initial diagnosis is reported in Table 6 (A). In our population, PLR cut-off showed the highest sensitivity (0.848) but the lowest specificity (0.256) when compared to NLR (0.000 and 1.000 respectively, for sensitivity and specificity) and AGR (0.087 and 0.974, respectively, for sensitivity and specificity). Accuracy in predictive value was higher using PLR (0.718 when compared to NLR (0.220) and AGR (0.247) and the ROC curves for AUC for the three ratios were similar (Figure 3). Considering a PPV and NPV of 0.801 and 0.323, respectively 80% of cases with high PLR presented a csPC at initial diagnosis and 32% of cases with low PLR were negative for PC.

Table 6. A: sensitivity, specificity, positive predictive value (PPV), negative predictive value (NPV), accuracy, and AUC of the different ratios in predicting diagnosis of clinically significant PC. B: sensitivity, specificity, positive predictive value (PPV), negative predictive value (NPV), accuracy, and AUC of the different ratios in predicting the metastatic M+ stage. C: sensitivity, specificity, positive predictive value (PPV), negative predictive value (NPV), accuracy, and AUC of the different ratios in predicting extracapsular T3 stage. D: sensitivity, specificity, positive predictive value (PPV), negative predictive value (NPV), accuracy, and AUC of the different ratios in predicting ISUP 3–5 grading. E: sensitivity, specificity, positive predictive value (PPV), negative predictive value (NPV), accuracy, and AUC of the different ratios in predicting biochemical progression after RP.

	Sensitivity (CI 95% Range)	Specificity (CI 95% Range)	PPV (CI 95% Range)	NPV (CI 95% Range)	Accuracy	AUC (CI 95% Range)
A						
NLR $\geq$ 2.5	0.000 (0.000–0.033)	1.000 (0.891–1.000)	0.000	0.220	0.220	0.402 (0.307–0.497)
PLR $\geq$ 120.0	0.848 (0.777–0.899)	0.256 (0.145–0.413)	0.801	0.323	0.718	0.493 (0.388–0.599)
AGR $\leq$ 1.4	0.087 (0.061–0.122)	0.974 (0.902–0.998)	0.938	0.190	0.247	0.458 (0.388–0.528)
B						
NLR $\geq$ 2.5	0.500 (0.217–0.783)	0.922 (0.896–0.942)	0.085	0.992	0.916	0.616 (0.332–0.900)
PLR $\geq$ 120.0	0.625 (0.304–0.862)	0.815 (0.781–0.846)	0.047	0.993	0.813	0.669 (0.429–0.908)
AGR $\leq$ 1.4	0.785 (0.690–0.857)	0.321 (0.284–0.361)	0.159	0.901	0.386	0.492 (0.436–0.548)
C						
NLR $\geq$ 2.5	0.574 (0.455–0.684)	0.581 (0.467–0.687)	0.557	0.597	0.577	0.483 (0.386–0.580)
PLR $\geq$ 120.0	0.471 (0.357–0.588)	0.622 (0.507–0.723)	0.533	0.561	0.549	0.493 (0.397–0.589)
AGR $\leq$ 1.4	0.201 (0.146–0.271)	0.880 (0.817–0.923)	0.640	0.510	0.531	0.485 (0.420–0.549)
D						
NLR $\geq$ 2.5	0.574 (0.455–0.684)	0.581 (0.467–0.687)	0.557	0.597	0.577	0.483 (0.386–0.580)
PLR $\geq$ 120.0	0.471 (0.357–0.588)	0.622 (0.507–0.723)	0.533	0.561	0.549	0.493 (0.397–0.589)
AGR $\leq$ 1.4	0.199 (0.144–0.268)	0.881 (0.818–0.924)	0.640	0.508	0.529	0.485 (0.421–0.549)
E						
NLR $\geq$ 2.5	0.727 (0.428–0.905)	0.539 (0.463–0.614)	0.095	0.967	0.551	0.620 (0.447–0.792)
PLR $\geq$ 120.0	0.455 (0.214–0.719)	0.873 (0.812–0.916)	0.192	0.960	0.847	0.604 (0.395–0.814)
AGR $\leq$ 1.4	0.231 (0.125–0.386)	0.869 (0.832–0.900)	0.153	0.917	0.810	0.479 (0.373–0.584)

3.5.2. Metastatic Disease (M+)

The performance of the 3 ratios in predicting a metastatic stage is reported in Table 6 (B). In our population, NLR cut-off showed the lowest sensitivity (0.500) but the highest specificity (0.922) when compared to PLR (0.625 and 0.815, respectively, for sensitivity and specificity) and AGR (0.785 and 0.321, respectively, for sensitivity and specificity). Accuracy in predictive value was higher using NLR (0.916) when compared to PLR (0.813) and AGR (0.386) and the AUC for the three ratios were similar between NLR and PLR and higher when compared to AGR (Figure 4). Considering a PPV and NPV of 0.085 and 0.992, respectively, 8% of cases with high NLR presented a metastatic PC, and 99% of cases with low NLR presented a non-metastatic disease.

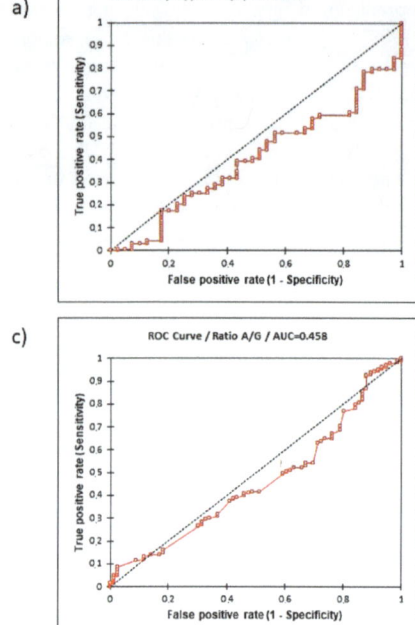
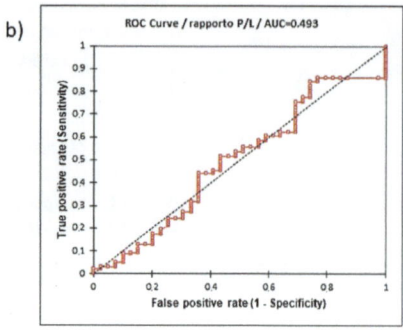

Figure 3. Receiver operating characteristic (ROC) curve and relative area under the curve. (AUC) of PC of NLR (**a**), PLR (**b**), and AGR (**c**) in predicting initial diagnosis.

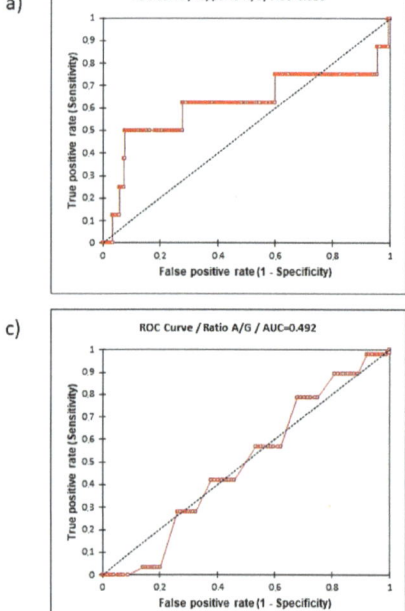
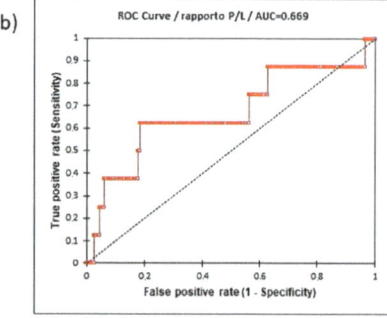

Figure 4. Receiver operating characteristic (ROC) curve and relative area under the curve. (AUC) of NLR (**a**), PLR (**b**), and AGR (**c**) in predicting metastatic stage.

3.5.3. Extraprostatic Disease (T3)

The performance of the three ratios in predicting an extracapsular T3 stage is reported in Table 6 (C). In our population, AGR cut-off showed the lowest sensitivity (0.201) but the highest specificity (0.880) when compared to PLR (0.471 and 0.622, respectively, for sensitivity and specificity) and NLR (0.574 and 0.581, respectively, for sensitivity and specificity). Accuracy in predictive value was similar among the three ratios and also the ROC curves for AUC were similar (Figure 3c). Considering a PPV and NPV of 0.640 and 0.510, respectively, 64% of cases with low AGR presented an extracapsular PC and 51% of cases with high AGR presented a T2 disease.

3.5.4. Aggressive Disease (ISUP 3–5)

The performance of the three ratios in predicting an aggressive ISUP 3–5 PC is reported in Table 6 (D). In our population, NLR cut-off showed the highest sensitivity (0.574) but the lowest specificity (0.581) when compared to PLR (0.471 and 0.622, respectively, for sensitivity and specificity) and AGR (0.199 and 0.881, respectively, for sensitivity and specificity). Accuracy in predictive value was higher using PLR (0.549) when compared to NLR (0.577) and AGR (0.529) and the ROC curves for AUC for the three ratios were similar (Figure 3d). Considering a PPV and NPV of 0.557 and 0.597, respectively, 38% of cases with high NLR presented a ISUP 3–5 PC, and 73% of cases with low NLR presented a ISUP 1–2 disease.

3.5.5. Biochemical Progression

The performance of the three ratios in predicting a biochemical progression is reported in Table 6 (E). In our population, NLR cut-off showed the highest sensitivity (0.727) but the lowest specificity (0.539) when compared to PLR (0.455 and 0.873, respectively, for sensitivity and specificity) and AGR (0.231 and 0.869, respectively, for sensitivity and specificity). Accuracy in predictive value was higher using PLR (0.847) when compared to NLR (0.551) and AGR (0.810) and the ROC curves for AUC were similar between NLR and PLR and higher when compared to AGR (Table 6 (E)). Considering a PPV and NPV of 0.095 and 0.967, respectively, 38% of cases with high NLR presented a biochemical progression, and 73% of cases with low NLR remained without biochemical progression at follow-up.

3.6. Logistic Regression Analysis

Table 7 shows a logistic regression analysis carried out to identify the predictive value of the three ratios in comparison with other clinical and pathological variables in terms of different outcomes. At the univariate analysis, the risk of clinically significant PC at initial diagnosis significantly increased only according to PLR ($p = 0.040$) with an OR 1.646 (95% CI 1.023–2.649) (Table 7 (A)). The risk of a metastatic disease significantly increased according to all three ratios; in particular, it increased 3.2 times for an NLR > 2.5 (95% CI 2.089–4.914), 5.2 times for a PLR > 120 (95% CI 3.182–8.812), and 0.5 times for an AGR < 1.4 (95% 0.340–0.972). In the multivariate analysis, the three ratios maintained an independent predictive value in terms of risk for a metastatic PC ($p < 0.05$), together with ISUP grading ($p < 0.001$) (Table 7 (B)).

On the contrary, neither the risk of an extracapsular PC, nor of an aggressive ISUP 3–5 disease, nor of biochemical progression significantly varied according to the three ratios (Table 7 (C–E)).

Table 7. (**A**): logistic regression analysis to identify predictors for clinically significant prostate cancer diagnosis. Univariate and multivariate analysis. Odds ratio (OR), 95% confidential interval (CI) (**B**): logistic regression analysis to identify predictors for metastatic stage (M+) PC. Univariate and multivariate analysis. Odds ratio (OR), 95% confidential interval (CI). (**C**): logistic regression analysis to identify predictors for extracapsular T stage (T3) PC. Univariate and multivariate analysis. Odds ratio (OR), 95% confidential interval (CI). (**D**): logistic regression analysis to identify predictors for ISUP grading 3–5 PC. Univariate and multivariate analysis. Odds ratio (OR), 95% confidential interval (CI). (**E**): logistic regression analysis to identify predictors for biochemical progression after RP for PC. Univariate and multivariate analysis. Odds ratio (OR), 95% confidential interval (CI).

A					
			Univariable		
		OR	95% CI_Lower	95% CI_Upper	p-Value
Preoperative PSA (ng/mL)	<4	Ref	-	-	-
	>4	0.808	0.367	1.782	0.598
PIRADS score	1–3	Ref	-	-	-
	4–5	1.458	0.722	2.942	0.293
NLR	<2.5	Ref	-	-	-
	≥2.5	1.545	0.943	2.532	0.084
PLR	<120	Ref	-	-	-
	≥120.0	1.646	1.023	2.649	0.040
AGR	>1.4	Ref	-	-	-
	≤1.4 variabile categorica	1.466	0.853	2.519	0.166

B										
			Univariable					Multivariable		
		OR	95% CI_Lower	95% CI_Upper	p-Value	OR	95% CI_Lower	95% CI_Upper	p-Value
Preoperative PSA (ng/mL)	<4	Ref	–	–	–				
	>4	1.411	0.642	3.102	0.391	1.135	1.097	1.174	<0.0001
PIRADS score	1–3	Ref	–	–	–				
	4–5	1.712	0.085	34.589	0.726				
NLR	<2.5	Ref	–	–	–				
	≥2.5	3.204	2.089	4.914	<0.0001	2.241	0.946	5.311	0.067
PLR	<120	Ref	–	–	–				
	≥120.0	5.295	3.182	8.812	<0.0001	2.717	1.010	7.307	0.048
AGR	>1.4	Ref	–	–	–				
	≤1.4	0.575	0.340	0.972	0.039	0.414	0.190	0.901	0.026
T stage	T1–2	Ref	–	–	–				
	T3	1.613	0.915	2.842	0.098				
ISUP grading	1–2	Ref	–	–	–				
	3–5	68.416	4.155	1126.443	0.003	3.339	2.222	5.017	<0.0001

Table 7. Cont.

C

		Univariable			
		OR	95% CI_Lower	95% CI_Upper	p-Value
Preoperative PSA (ng/mL)	<4	Ref	–	–	–
	>4	1.574	0.741	3.343	0.238
PIRADS score	1–3	Ref	–	–	–
	4–5 variabile categorica	-	-	-	-
NLR	<2.5	Ref	–	–	–
	≥2.5	1.062	0.680	1.659	0.790
PLR	<120	Ref	–	–	–
	≥120.0	0.959	0.622	1.479	0.851
AGR	>1.4	Ref	–	–	–
	≤1.4	1.209	0.767	1.906	0.414
T stage	T1–2	Ref	–	–	–
	T3 variabile categorica	-	-	-	-
ISUP grading	1–2	Ref	–	–	–
	3–5	9.836	5.122	18.890	<0.0001

D

		Univariable			
		OR	95% CI_Lower	95% CI_Upper	p-Value
Preoperative PSA (ng/mL)	<4	Ref	–	–	–
	>4	0.810	0.390	1.683	0.572
PIRADS score	1–3	Ref	–	–	–
	4–5 variabile categorica	1.225	0.605	2.478	0.573
NLR	<2.5	Ref	–	–	–
	≥2.5	1.482	0.938	2.340	0.092
PLR	<120	Ref	–	–	–
	≥120.0	1.189	0.760	1.860	0.447
AGR	>1.4	Ref	–	–	–
	≤1.4	0.977	0.613	1.557	0.923
T stage	T1–2	Ref	–	–	–
	T3	8.599	5.278	14.009	<0.0001
ISUP grading	1–2	Ref	–	–	–
	3–5	-	-	-	-

Table 7. Cont.

E

		Univariable			
		OR	95% CI_Lower	95% CI_Upper	p-Value
Preoperative PSA (ng/mL)	<4	Ref	–	–	–
	>4	1.276	0.371	4.384	0.699
PIRADS score	1–3	Ref	–	–	–
	4–5	0.958	0.306	3.002	0.942
NLR	<2.5	Ref	–	–	–
	≥2.5	1.156	0.607	2.202	0.658
PLR	<120	Ref	–	–	–
	≥120.0	0.754	0.396	1.433	0.389
AGR	>1.4	Ref	–	–	–
	≤1.4	1.611	0.830	3.129	0.159
T stage	T1–2	Ref	–	–	–
	T3	3.709	1.817	7.571	0.0001
ISUP grading	1–2	Ref	–	–	–
	3–5	1.851	1.431	2.394	<0.0001

4. Discussion

A prognostic role for NLR, PLR, or AGR has been underlined in several solid tumors [7,8]. For example, in lung cancer, a poorer OS in patients with elevated NLR or PLR values (HR 1.18 and 1.14) has been described as they were associated with a greater risk of lymph node metastases development, poor tumor differentiation, and vascular invasion [9]. The relationships between NLR and PLR with esophageal and breast cancers were also studied and a lower OS and CSS for NLR and PLR values beyond the cut-off (OS: HR 1.55 for NLR and 1.37 for PLR in esophageal cancer and 1.46 for NLR in breast cancer) has been described [10,13]. The serum albumin/globulin ratio (AGR) has been suggested as a prognostic marker for colorectal cancer, lung cancer, breast cancer, and nasopharyngeal carcinoma [13–16].

Hypoalbuminemia was also studied in relation to fibrinogen values in other neoplastic diseases, such as in muscle-invasive bladder tumors [15]. Authors showed that a low ratio was associated with poor differentiation, non-organ-confined disease, and independently predicted time to progression [15].

We recently published two meta-analyses on the prognostic role of these ratios in PC [8,17].

The first meta-analysis on AGR found a very low level of heterogeneity (I^2 = 7.0%) of results among studies. In non-metastatic PC cases, pretreatment AGR was not able to show a significant predictive value either in terms of pathologic features (T and N staging, ISUP grading) or in terms of biochemical progression risk. Considering a random effect model, the pooled risk difference for non-organ confined PC, lymph-node involvement, and BCF between low and high AGR groups was close to 0.00. Only one study (18) analyzed AGR in metastatic PC. In this population, significant results were obtained either in terms of PFS or CSS prediction with a maintained independent (p < 0.01) value for AGR at multivariate analysis. Authors (18) reported 68.0% of patients in the low AGR and 50.9% in the high AGR group experienced tumor progression and a higher percentage of cases in the low AGR (77.0%) than in the high AGR (27.2%) group who died from PC.

The second meta-analysis found a high rate of heterogeneity either among studies on PLR (I^2 = 71.49%; test of group differences $p < 0.001$), or on NLR (I^2 = 95.87%; test of group differences $p = 0.72$) regarding the analysis on tumor stage and aggressiveness, whereas a lower rate of heterogeneity ($I^2 < 50\%$; test of group differences $p > 0.05$) was present in the analysis on progression.

A low predictive value of both NLR and PLR was found in terms of T staging or PC aggressiveness. The pooled risk difference for non-organ confined PC between high NLR and low NLR cases was 0.06 (95% CI: −0.03–0.15) and between high PLR and low PLR increased to 0.30 (95% CI: 0.16–0.43). A higher predictive value was found in terms of risk for progression. In particular, a higher pooled HR for overall mortality in the metastatic PC population was related to a high NLR (1.79 (95% CI:1.44–2.13)) when compared to a high PLR (1.05 (95% CI:0.87–1.24)).

Despite the numerous data present in the literature, most of the works on these three ratios in PC are retrospective, and the few prospective ones lack various analytical data or do not stratify the population. The result is that the research interest in these ratios to date has not been able to transform into clinical indications in the management of PC.

The strength of our study is represented by the prospective design in a situation of normal clinical practice. Furthermore, the population considered is numerically significant, there is a control group with BPH diagnosis, and patients with PC can be stratified into two subgroups with non-metastatic and metastatic disease. In this way, our prospective analysis allows for the first time to compare the three ratios both in terms of initial diagnosis of clinically significant PC and in terms of aggressiveness and staging of tumors. Another novelty related to our study is the longitudinal analysis in patients undergoing radical prostatectomy on the changes in the three ratios induced by surgery. The major limitation of our study lies in the analysis of survival limited to the risk of biochemical progression, given the short follow-up.

As in the present literature, different analyses were performed, distinguishing patients in low and high rate cases on the basis of cut-offs determined by ROC and Youden's index [12]. The optimal cut-offs in our population were 2.5, 120.0, and 1.4 for NLR, PLR, and AGR, respectively, similar to those used in previous studies [18–21].

We also considered the ratios as continuous variables based on the mean and median values, an analysis that is often absent in the literature.

The first data to be underlined is a significant correlation between NLR and PLR values (r = 0.590765385; $p < 0.0001$), but not between NLR or PLR and AGR ($p > 0.05$).

Regarding the initial diagnosis of PC and clinically significant PC, either mean values of NLR and PLR or the percentage of cases with high NLR and PLR significantly ($p < 0.01$) increased between the group without PC and those with PC or csPC. On the contrary, no significant differences were found in terms of AGR. Accuracy in predictive value for csPC was higher using PLR (0.718) when compared to NLR (0.220) and AGR (0.247), but, despite a high sensitivity (0.849), a very low specificity (0.256) was present. A total of 80% of cases with high PLR and only 20% of those with low PLR presented a clinically significant PC at initial diagnosis and the risk of csPC significantly increased only according to PLR ($p = 0.040$) with an OR = 1.646 (95% CI: 1.023–2.649).

Regarding the predictive value of the ratios in terms of aggressiveness and T stage in non-metastatic PC, no significant differences were found either in terms of mean values or in terms of percentage of high or low ratios. The accuracy was particularly low and the risk for an extracapsular T3 disease or a ISUP 3–5 PC did not significantly increase according to none of the three ratios.

The best performance as predictive value, limited to NLR and PLR, was found for the risk of metastatic disease. The percentage of cases with metastatic PC significantly increased according to high NLR (from 7.1% to 18.5%) and high PLR (from 4.1% to 19.3%), and also mean value of PLR was significantly ($p < 0.01$) higher in metastatic (149.6 ± 49.5) than in non-metastatic (127.8 ± 49.3) cases. Accuracy was 0.916 and 0.813, respectively, for NLR and PLR cut-off, with higher specificity than sensitivity for both. In particular, for both NLR and PLR, 99% of cases with a ratio under the cut-off presented a non-metastatic disease whereas only 8% (NLR) and 4% (PLR) of cases with a ratio over the cut-off presented a metastatic PC. The risk of a metastatic disease increased 3.2 times for an NLR > 2.5 (95% CI: 2.089–4.914) and 5.2 times for a PLR > 120 (95% CI: 3.182–8.812) and at the multivariate analysis, the ratios maintained an independent predictive value in terms of risk for a metastatic PC ($p < 0.05$), together with ISUP grading ($p < 0.001$).

Accuracy in predictive value for a biochemical progression was higher using PLR (0.631) when compared to NLR (0.553) and AGR (0.557) and 38% of cases with high NLR presented a biochemical progression and 73% of cases with low NLR remained without biochemical progression at follow-up. The risk of a biochemical progression did not significantly vary according to the ratios, results that could be negatively influenced by a limited follow-up that does not allow a complete survival analysis.

The interpretation of the results obtained through the longitudinal analysis in patients undergoing radical prostatectomy is uncertain. Radical removal of the prostate induces significant changes in all the ratios, regardless of the stratification based on stage, grading and risk classes. However, whereas NLR underwent the greatest increase post-surgery, PLR was significantly reduced. The explanation of a significant but inverse behavior between PLR and NLR after surgery is contrary to the univocity of the results between the two ratios in relation to the other predictive analyses.

5. Conclusions

Our prospective study in the real world allows for the first time the comparison of the three ratios both in terms of initial diagnosis of clinically significant PC, and in terms of prognostic value for the aggressiveness and staging in a large population of non-metastatic and metastatic PC compared to BPH controls.

PLR appears to have the greatest accuracy in predicting an initial diagnosis of csPC but with very low specificity. PLR and NLR have a significant predictive value towards the development of metastatic disease but not in relation to variations in aggressiveness or T staging inside the non-metastatic PC.

These ratios can represent the inflammatory and immunity status of the patient related to several conditions other than PC. The simplicity of the analysis is certainly the major advantage of these ratios, being influenced by a large number of coexisting inflammatory conditions in the patient strongly limits their specific prognostic value for prostate cancer characteristics.

It is possible to hypothesize that in metastatic disease, the systemic involvement of the tumor causes variations in inflammatory and immune indices that can be translated into variations in the ratios, rather than the opposite process. Our results suggest an unlikely introduction of these analyses into clinical practice in support of validated PC risk predictors.

Author Contributions: Conceptualization, A.S. and S.S.; methodology, A.S., S.S. and M.F.; software F.D.G.; validation, E.D.B., G.M. and A.G.; formal analysis, G.B.D.P., S.C. (Susanna Cattarino) and F.F.; investigation, P.V., P.C. and D.R.; resources, G.G. and M.F.; data curation, G.G., B.I.C. and M.L.E.; writing—original draft preparation, S.S., M.F., G.B., P.V., P.C., E.D.B., G.B.D.P., S.C. (Susanna Cattarino), S.C. (Simone Crivellaro), G.G., D.R., F.D.G., A.C., A.P., B.I.C., M.L.E., R.A., F.F., A.S., G.M. and A.G.; writing—review and editing, all authors; visualization, all authors; supervision A.S.; project administration, S.S.; funding acquisition, none. All authors have read and agreed to the published version of the manuscript.

Funding: This research received no external funding.

Institutional Review Board Statement: The prospective study has been evaluated and approved by our Ethics Committee (ref. cod. 6732 Prot. 0355/2022).

Informed Consent Statement: Informed consent was obtained from all subjects involved in the study

Data Availability Statement: The data presented in this study are available on request from the corresponding author. The data are not publicly available to respect patients privacy.

Conflicts of Interest: The authors declare no conflict of interest.

Abbreviations

RP	Radical prostatectomy
PC	Prostate cancer
NLR	Neutrophil-to-lymphocyte ratio
PLR	Platelet-to-lymphocyte ratio
AGR	Albumin-to-globulin ratio
EAU	European Association of Urology
CI	Confidence interval
OR	Odds ratio
HR	Hazard ratio
BCP	Biochemical progression
CSS	Cancer-specific survival
OS	Overall survival

References

1. Mottet, N.; van den Bergh, R.C.N. Prostate Cancer: European Association of Urology (EAU) Guidelines 2022. Available online: https://uroweb.org/guideline/prostate-cancer/ (accessed on 1 October 2022).
2. Shariat, S.F. Critical review of prostate cancer predictive tools. *Future Oncol.* **2009**, *10*, 1555–1584. [CrossRef] [PubMed]
3. Briganti, A.; Larcher, A.; Abdollah, F.; Capitanio, U.; Gallina, A.; Suardi, N.; Bianchi, M.; Sun, M.; Freschi, M.; Salonia, A.; et al. Updated nomogram predicting lymph node invasion in patients with prostate cancer undergoing extended pelvic lymph node dissection: The essential importance of percentage of positive cores. *Eur. Urol.* **2012**, *61*, 480. [CrossRef] [PubMed]
4. Gandaglia, G.; Fossati, N.; Zaffuto, E.; Bandini, M.; Dell'Oglio, P.; Bravi, C.A.; Fallara, G.; Pellegrino, F.; Nocera, L.; Karakiewicz, P.I.; et al. Development and Internal Validation of a Novel Model to Identify the Candidates for Extended Pelvic Lymph Node Dissection in Prostate Cancer. *Eur. Urol.* **2017**, *72*, 632. [CrossRef] [PubMed]
5. Sciarra, A.; Gentilucci, A.; Salciccia, S.; Pierella, F.; Del Bianco, F.; Gentile, V.; Silvestri, I.; Cattarino, S. Prognostic value of inflammation in prostate cancer progression and response to therapeutic: A critical review. *J. Inflamm. (Lond)* **2016**, *13*, 35. [CrossRef] [PubMed]
6. Guo, J.; Fang, J.; Huang, X.; Liu, Y.; Yuan, Y.; Zhang, X.; Zou, C.; Xiao, K.; Wang, J. Prognostic role of neutrophil to lymphocyte ratio and platelet to lymphocyte ratio in prostate cancer: A meta-analysis of results from multivariate analysis. *Int. J. Surg.* **2018**, *60*, 216–223. [CrossRef] [PubMed]
7. Zanaty, M.; Ajib, K.; Alnazari, M.; El Rassy, E.; Aoun, F.; Zorn, K.C.; El-Hakim, A. Prognostic utility of neutrophil-to-lymphocyte and platelets-to-lymphocyte ratio in predicting biochemical recurrence post robotic prostatectomy. *Biomark. Med.* **2018**, *12*, 841–848. [CrossRef] [PubMed]
8. Salciccia, S.; Frisenda, M.; Bevilacqua, G.; Viscuso, P.; Casale, P.; De Berardinis, E.; Di Pierro, G.B.; Cattarino, S.; Giorgino, G.; Rosati, D.; et al. Prognostic Value of Albumin to Globulin Ratio in Non-Metastatic and Metastatic Prostate Cancer Patients: A Meta-Analysis and Systematic Review. *Int. J. Mol. Sci.* **2022**, *23*, 11501. [CrossRef] [PubMed]
9. Gupta, D.; Lis, C.G. Pretreatment serum albumin as a predictor of cancer survival: A systematic review of the epidemiological literature. *Nutr. J.* **2010**, *9*, 69. [CrossRef] [PubMed]
10. Meyer, E.J.; Nenke, M.A.; Rankin, W.; Lewis, J.G.; Torpy, D.J. Corticosteroid-Binding Globulin: A Review of Basic and Clinical Advances. *Horm. Metab. Res.* **2016**, *48*, 359–371. [CrossRef] [PubMed]
11. Guan, Y.; Xiong, H.; Feng, Y.; Liao, G.; Tong, T.; Pang, J. Revealing the prognostic landscape of neutrophil-to-lymphocyte ratio and platelet-to-lymphocyte ratio in metastatic castration-resistant prostate cancer patients treated with abiraterone or enzalutamide: A meta-analysis. *Prostate Cancer Prostatic Dis.* **2020**, *23*, 220–231. [CrossRef] [PubMed]
12. Aydh, A.; Mori, K.; D'Andrea, D.; Motlagh, R.S.; Abufaraj, M.; Pradere, B.; Mostafaei, H.; Laukhtina, E.; Quhal, F.; Karakiewicz, P.I.; et al. Prognostic value of the pre-operative serum albumin to globulin ratio in patients with non-metastatic prostate cancer undergoing radical prostatectomy. *Int. J. Clin. Oncol.* **2021**, *26*, 1729–1735. [CrossRef] [PubMed]
13. Lv, G.Y.; An, L.; Sun, X.D.; Hu, Y.L.; Sun, D.W. Pretreatment albumin to globulin ratio can serve as a prognostic marker in human cancers: A meta-analysis. *Clin. Chim. Acta* **2018**, *476*, 81–91. [CrossRef] [PubMed]
14. Soeters, P.B.; Wolfe, R.R.; Shenkin, A. Hypoalbuminemia: Pathogenesis and Clinical Significance. *J. Parenter. Enter. Nutr.* **2019**, *43*, 181–193. [CrossRef] [PubMed]
15. Claps, F.; Rai, S.; Mir, M.C.; van Rhijn, B.W.G.; Mazzon, G.; Davis, L.E.; Valadon, C.L.; Silvestri, T.; Rizzo, M.; Ankem, M.; et al. Prognostic value of preoperative albumin-to-fibrinogen ratio (AFR) in patients with bladder cancer treated with radical cystectomy. *Urol. Oncol. Semin. Orig. Investig.* **2021**, *39*, 835.e9–835.e17. [CrossRef] [PubMed]

16. Azab, B.N.; Bhatt, V.R.; Vonfrolio, S.; Bachir, R.; Rubinshteyn, V.; Alkaied, H.; Habeshy, A.; Patel, J.; Picon, A.I.; Bloom, S.W. Value of the pretreatment albumin to globulin ratio in predicting long-term mortality in breast cancer patients. *Am. J. Surg.* **2013**, *206*, 764–770. [CrossRef] [PubMed]
17. Salciccia, S.; Frisenda, M.; Bevilacqua, G.; Viscuso, P.; Casale, P.; De Berardinis, E.; Di Pierro, G.B.; Cattarino, S.; Giorgino, G.; Rosati, D.; et al. Prognostic role of platelet-to-lymphocyte ratio and neutrophil-to-lymphocyte ratio in patients with non-metastatic and metastatic prostate cancer: A meta-analysis and systematic review. *Asian J. Urol.*. ahead of print.
18. Sun, Z.; Ju, Y.; Han, F.; Sun, X.; Wang, F. Clinical implications of pretreatment inflammatory biomarkers as independent prognostic indicators in prostate cancer. *J. Clin. Lab. Anal.* **2018**, *32*, e22277. [CrossRef] [PubMed]
19. Nkengurutse, G.; Tian, F.; Jiang, S.; Wang, Q.; Wang, Y.; Sun, W. Preoperative Predictors of Biochemical Recurrence-Free Survival in High-Risk Prostate Cancer Following Radical Prostatectomy. *Front. Oncol.* **2020**, *10*, 1761–1769. [CrossRef] [PubMed]
20. Adhyatma, K.P.; Prapiska, F.F.; Siregar, G.P.; Warli, S.M. Systemic Inflammatory Response in Predicting Prostate Cancer: The Diagnostic Value of Neutrophil-to-Lymphocyte Ratio. *Open Access Maced. J. Med. Sci.* **2019**, *7*, 1628–1630. [CrossRef] [PubMed]
21. Chung, J.W.; Ha, Y.S.; Kim, S.W.; Park, S.C.; Kang, T.W.; Jeong, Y.B.; Park, S.W.; Park, J.; Yoo, E.S.; Kwon, T.G.; et al. The prognostic value of the pretreatment serum albumin to globulin ratio for predicting adverse pathology in patients under-going radical prostatectomy for prostate cancer. *Investig. Clin. Urol.* **2021**, *62*, 545–552. [CrossRef] [PubMed]

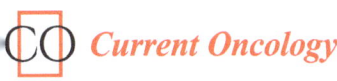

Article

Renal and Salivary Gland Functions after Three Cycles of PSMA-617 Therapy Every Four Weeks in Patients with Metastatic Castration-Resistant Prostate Cancer

Tim Wollenweber [1], Lucia Zisser [1], Elisabeth Kretschmer-Chott [1], Michael Weber [2], Bernhard Grubmüller [3], Gero Kramer [3], Shahrokh F. Shariat [3,4,5,6,7], Markus Mitterhauser [1,8], Stefan Schmitl [1], Chrysoula Vraka [1], Alexander R. Haug [1,9], Marcus Hacker [1], Markus Hartenbach [1] and Sazan Rasul [1,*]

1. Department of Biomedical Imaging and Image-guided Therapy, Division of Nuclear Medicine, Medical University of Vienna, 1090 Vienna, Austria; tim.wollenweber@meduniwien.ac.at (T.W.); lucia.zisser@meduniwien.ac.at (L.Z.); elisabeth.kretschmer-chott@meduniwien.ac.at (E.K.-C.); markus.mitterhauser@meduniwien.ac.at (M.M.); stefan.schmitl@akhwien.at (S.S.); chrysoula.vraka@meduniwien.ac.at (C.V.); alexander.haug@meduniwien.ac.at (A.R.H.); marcus.hacker@meduniwien.ac.at (M.H.); markus.hartenbach@me.com (M.H.)
2. Department of Biomedical Imaging and Image-guided Therapy, Division of General Radiology, Medical University of Vienna, 1090 Vienna, Austria; michael.weber@meduniwien.ac.at
3. Department of Urology, Medical University of Vienna, 1090 Vienna, Austria; bernhard.grubmueller@meduniwien.ac.at (B.G.); gero.kramer@meduniwien.ac.at (G.K.); shahrokh.shariat@meduniwien.ac.at (S.F.S.)
4. Department of Urology, Weill Cornell Medical College, New York, NY 10065, USA
5. Department of Urology, Second Faculty of Medicine, Charles University, 15006 Prague, Czech Republic
6. Institute for Urology and Reproductive Health, I.M. Sechenov First Moscow State Medical University, 119991 Moscow, Russia
7. Department of Urology, University of Texas Southwestern Medical Center, Dallas, TX 75390, USA
8. Ludwig Boltzmann Institute Applied Diagnostics, 1090 Vienna, Austria
9. Christian Doppler Laboratory for Applied Metabolomics (CDL AM), Medical University of Vienna, 1090 Vienna, Austria
* Correspondence: sazan.rasul@meduniwien.ac.at; Tel.: +43-1-40400-58742; Fax: +43-1-40400-55520

Abstract: Background: [^{177}Lu]Lu-PSMA-617 radioligand therapy (PSMA-RLT) could affect kidney and salivary gland functions in metastatic castration-resistant prostate cancer (mCRPC) patients. Methods: We retrospectively analyzed clinical, renal, and salivary scintigraphy data and salivary [^{68}Ga]Ga-PSMA-11 ligand PET scan measures such as metabolic volume and SUVmax values of 27 mCRPC men (mean age 71 ± 7 years) before and 4 weeks after receiving three cycles of PSMA-RLT every 4 weeks. Twenty-two patients additionally obtained renal and salivary scintigraphy prior to each cycle. A one-way ANOVA, post-hoc Scheffé test and Cochran's Q test were applied to assess organ toxicity. Results: In total, 54 PSMA PET scans, 98 kidney, and 98 salivary scintigraphy results were evaluated. There were no significant differences for the ejection fraction, peak time, and residual activity after 5 min for both parotid and submandibular glands prior to each cycle and 4 weeks after the last cycle. Similarly, no significant differences in serum creatinine and renal scintigraphy parameters were observed prior to each cycle and 4 weeks after the last treatment. Despite there being no changes in the metabolic volume of both submandibular glands, SUVmax values dropped significantly ($p < 0.05$). Conclusion: Results evidenced no alterations in renal function and only minimal impairment of salivary function of mCRPC patients who acquired an intense PSMA-RLT regimen every 4 weeks.

Keywords: PSMA; prostate cancer; mCRPC; renal scintigraphy; salivary scintigraphy

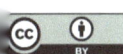

1. Introduction

Prostate cancer is one of the most commonly diagnosed cancers and the second leading cause of tumor-related death in men [1]. Prostate-specific membrane antigen (PSMA) is a class II transmembrane glycoprotein expressed in all types of prostate tissues. Nevertheless, overexpression of PSMA has been found in prostate tumors including its metastatic cells and in metastatic castration-resistant prostate cancer (mCRPC), making it an ideal target for prostate cancer diagnosis and therapy [2–6]. Therefore, various small molecule PSMA ligands have been developed, labeled with either gamma or positron emitters for positron emission tomography (PET) diagnosis or with beta or alpha particles for radionuclide therapy [7–11]. While the initial growth of prostate cancer is still androgen-dependent and can be effectively treated with luteinizing hormone-releasing hormone (LHRH) agonists and antagonists or anti-androgen receptors (ARs), almost all patients eventually advance to mCRPC where these therapies are no longer effective [12–14]. Consequently, [^{177}Lu]Lu-PSMA-617 targeted radionuclide therapy (PSMA-RLT) has shown in numerous studies including TheraP and Vision studies [15,16], promising results in terms of good tolerability, a favorable response rate, and the fewest adverse effects and organ toxicities in treated mCRPC patients [17–20].

However, PSMA is not prostate specific and several other organs such as the kidneys, salivary glands, lacrimal glands, or small intestine also express PSMA [21]. Therefore proximal renal tubules and salivary glands, among others, are considered critical organs in patients receiving PSMA-RLT [22–25]. In this context, it has been shown that a highly standardized therapy regimen of 4–6 therapy cycles at 8–10-week intervals did not exceed the International Commission on Radiological Protection critical dose for critical organs such as kidneys and salivary glands, and no significant nephrotoxicity occurred in 10 patients treated with PSMA-RLT [26]. Indeed, the results of previous studies on the effects of PSMA-RLT on the kidney and salivary gland were largely based on the results of clinical centers offering this treatment to mCRPC patients with different inhomogeneous therapeutic regimens consisting of 1–8 cycles of 2–8 GBq activity per cycle and with an inter-cycle interval of 6–12 weeks [17,27,28]. Previously, we have shown that a more intensive, highly standardized PSMA-RLT protocol applied at our clinical institution with a shorter interval of only four weeks between the cycles has good tolerability and favorable response rates, progression-free survival, and survival rates for patients with mCRPC [29,30]. Therefore, the purpose of this study was to evaluate the renal and salivary glands (parotid and submandibular) toxicity under this unique intensive treatment regimen using clinical and scintigraphy parameters in mCRPC patients who all equally received three cycles of highly standardized PSMA-RLT every 4 weeks.

2. Methods

2.1. Study Population

In this study, patients (n: 61) referred to the Department of Nuclear Medicine, Medical University of Vienna, Vienna General Hospital, between September 2015 and December 2020 to receive PSMA-RLT due to mCRPC were retrospectively evaluated. The therapy was performed in all patients with the recommendation of an interdisciplinary tumor board. The treatments were performed according to §8 of the Austrian Medicines Act (AMG). However, this analysis included only patients with properly and fully performed PSMA PET scans as well as salivary and renal scintigraphy (Figure 1). None of the patients studied underwent radiotherapy to the neck region. The studied patients had acquired a salivary and kidney scintigraphy directly before the first cycle and one month after the last (3rd) cycle of PSMA-RLT. Among them, a subgroup of patients additionally underwent salivary and kidney scintigraphy prior to each of the 3 therapy cycles. In addition, all patients underwent [^{68}Ga]Ga-PSMA-11 ligand ([^{68}Ga]Ga-PSMA) PET scans before the first cycle and 4 weeks after the last (3rd) therapy cycle. Clinical laboratory parameters including serum creatinine levels were measured in all patients before the start of each cycle and 4 weeks after the third cycle of therapy, and patients were requested to answer a questionnaire asking whether they suffer from dry mouth.

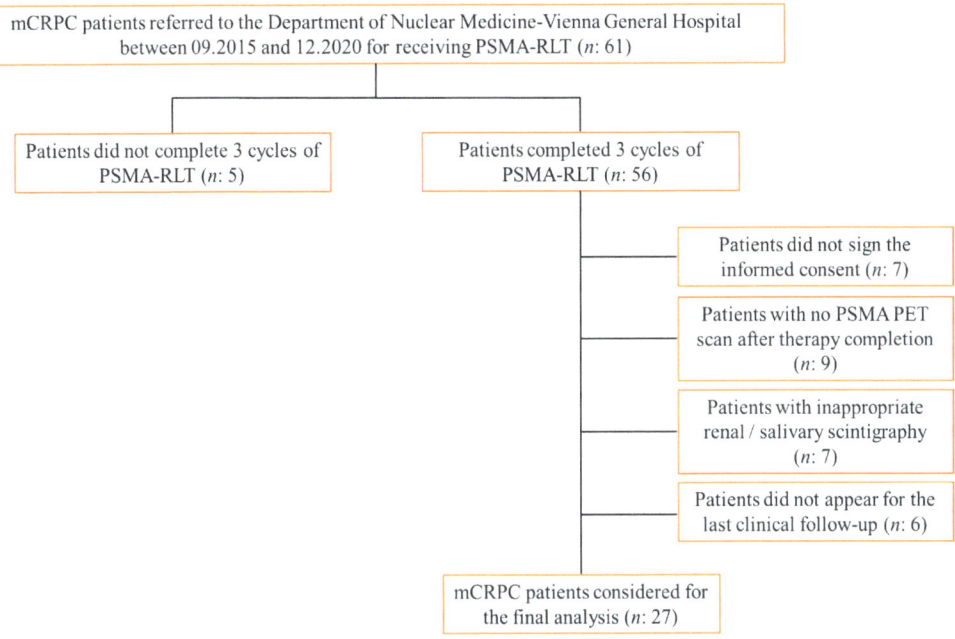

Figure 1. Flowchart for the selected mCRPC patients included in this study.

2.2. [^{177}Lu]Lu-PSMA-617 Radioligand Therapy

The PSMA-617 precursor was obtained from ABX GmbH (Radeberg, Germany) and was labeled with [^{177}Lu]Lutetium following procedures described previously [31]. In all patients, the therapy protocol consisted of 3 cycles of 7361 ± 293 MBq of PSMA-RLT administered intravenously every 4 weeks [30,32]. Prior to and after the slow intravenous administration of PSMA-RLT, each patient received 1000 mL of normal 0.9% saline infusion at 300 mL/h over 30 min. To protect the salivary glands, each patient received cold packs on the salivary glands 30 min before and up to 6 h after the therapy injection (p.i.), which were changed regularly.

2.3. Salivary Gland Scintigraphy

The salivary gland scintigraphy was performed on a double-headed gamma camera (Axis, Philips Medical Systems, Amsterdam, The Netherlands) equipped with a low energy all-purpose parallel hole collimator. The energy window around the 140 keV photopeak of [^{99m}Tc]Technetium was 15%. Dynamic imaging was performed over 30 min after an intravenous administration of 102 ± 13 MBq 99mTc-pertechnetat in a 64 × 64-pixel matrix with 30 s per frame. Twenty minutes of p.i., p.i. = after the therapy injection, each patient received 5 mL lemon juice diluted with water (1:1). Patients were encouraged not to swallow the juice immediately but to hold it in the mouth for as long as possible and then swallow it without moving the head.

The data were analyzed using Hermes Hybrid 3D software (Hermes Medical Solutions, Stockholm, Sweden). For image analysis, a region of interest (ROI) was drawn over each salivary gland (left and right parotid, submandibular gland, oral cavity, and background). Time-activity curves were generated for each region. From these time-activity curves, the ejection fraction (EF) was defined as the percentage of the difference between the maximum count and the minimum count after stimulation divided by the maximum count [33–35]. Peak time was defined as the time after injection when the maximum count was reached.

The residual activity (RA) at peak time plus 5 min was specified as the percentage of counts 5 min after the peak time divided by the maximum counts.

2.4. Kidney Scintigraphy

All kidney scintigraphy were also conducted on a double-headed gamma camera (Axis, Philips Medical Systems, Eindhoven, Nederland) equipped with a low energy all-purpose parallel hole collimator. The energy window around the 140 keV photopeak of [^{99m}Tc]Technetium was 15%. After injection of 95 ± 11 MBq [^{99m}Tc]-Mercaptoacetyltriglycine3 (MAG3), dynamic planar images from dorsal were acquired over 20 min (120 frames, 10 s per frame) in a 128 × 128 matrix. As for salivary gland scintigraphy, the data were analyzed using Hermes Hybrid 3D software (Hermes Medical Solutions, Stockholm, Sweden). For this, ROIs were drawn around each kidney. The background ROIs were then automatically drawn by the software.

From the generated time-activity curves, the relative function of the kidney was determined from the slopes of the right and left Patlak plots [36–38]. Since no blood samples were taken during the renal scintigraphy, the clearance parameters were determined using a camera-based method without blood or urine sampling. Therefore, we determined a measure of clearance similar to the methods that have been previously published [39,40]. Because the counts of the injected activity were not available, we could not express the clearance in terms of percent of uptake. Thus, we normalized the integral from 0.7 to 2 min over the renogram curves to the amount of the injected activity, which should be proportional to the injected counts using the same camera system for every patient.

2.5. PSMA-PET Imaging

Following our therapy protocol, all patients underwent [^{68}Ga]Ga-PSMA PET examination prior to the initiation of the therapy and four weeks after the third treatment cycle. The scan was carried out 60 min after the application of 173.5 ± 16.3 MBq [^{68}Ga]Ga-PSMA. Imaging was performed with four bed positions at 5 min scan time, thoroughly described in [41]. Accordingly, the parotid gland was not fully imaged in PET scans and, thus, a volume of interest (VOI) was generated only for the submandibular gland. To estimate the metabolic volume and the maximum standardized uptake value (SUVmax) of the submandibular glands, a cubic VOI was placed around the submandibular glands and then a threshold value of 10% of the maximum pixel value within the VOI was used for the delineation of the corresponding submandibular gland, as described previously in van Kalmhout et al. study [42].

2.6. Statistical Analysis

Descriptive statistical analysis was conducted with the software IBM SPSS Statistics version 24.0. The Kolmogorov–Smirnov test was applied to check the distribution of the values. Non-normally distributed data were presented as medians and ranges while normally distributed data were expressed as mean ± standard deviation. Other mentioned statistical analysis was performed using MedCalc v19.1 (Ostend, Belgium). One-way analysis of variance (one-way ANOVA) was used to test for statistically significant differences between the means of three or more groups. As a post-hoc test, the Scheffé test was conducted to find out which pairs of means were significant. Cochran's Q test was used for evaluation of the results of the questioner concerning mouth dryness. A p-value lower than 0.05 was considered as statistically significant.

3. Results

3.1. Study Population

A total of 27 patients who underwent a proper [^{68}Ga]Ga-PSMA PET scan as well as salivary and kidney scintigraphy prior to the first cycle and 4 weeks after the third cycle of PSMA-RLT were included in this study. The mean age of the patients was 71 ± 7 years. Prior to therapy, the median and range of creatinine level for all patients was

0.95 (0.71–1.16 mg/dL), respectively and of serum PSA level was 81.03 (5.91–3305 µg/L), respectively. The characteristics of the studied patients are summarized in Table 1. Of these patients, a subset of 24 patients underwent additional salivary and renal scintigraphy immediately before each PSMA-RLT cycle.

Table 1. Clinical characteristics of the entire studied mCRPC patients prior to receiving any PSMA-RLT.

Features	Values
Patients (n)	27
Age (mean ± SD) years	71 ± 7
Weight (mean ± SD) kilogram	85 ± 14
Karnofsky Score (n) % <80% ≥80%	 (9) 33 (18) 66
ECOG-Index (n) % 0 1 2	 (0) (25) 92.5 (2) 7.4
* PSA µg/L	81.03 (5.91–3305)
Hb (mean ± SD) g/dL	12.1 ± 1.6
Leucocyte g/L	6.9 ± 2.5
Thrombocyte (mean ± SD) g/L	242 ± 71
* Creatinine mg/dL	0.95 (0.71–1.16)
Previous treatments (n) % Enzalutamide/Abiraterone Docetaxel/Cabazitaxel Ra-223 (Xofigo®) No chemo- or hormone or Ra-223 (Xofigo®)	 (19) 70 (19) 70 (11) 41 (2) 7
Metastatic lesions (n) % cM1a cM1b cM1c	 (5) 18.5 (16) 59.3 (6) 22.2

n: Number of studied patients; SD: Standard deviation; PSA: Prostate specific antigen; Hb: Hemoglobin; *: Data not normally distributed and presented in median and range.

3.2. Salivary Gland Scintigraphy

In total, 98 salivary scintigraphy were performed. In all patients (n: 27), and as demonstrated in Table 2, there was no significant difference for the EF prior to as well as between each therapy cycle and four weeks after the 3rd PSMA-RLT cycle for the right and left parotid gland as well as for the right and left submandibular gland and for all glands together. Concerning the peak time in salivary scintigraphy prior to as well as between the three therapy cycles and one month after the last therapy cycle, there was no significant difference for the right and left parotid gland, or for the right and left submandibular gland. However, for all salivary glands combined, an ANOVA test yielded significant differences in the values of peak time before the start of therapy compared to the values four weeks after the last third treatment ($p = 0.03$), with the Scheffé test as a post-hoc test then revealing no significant differences in mean values between cycles, as shown in Table 2. In addition, there was no significant difference between the values of RA after 5 min for the left and right parotid glands as well as for the left and right submandibular glands, and for all glands together prior to the initiation of PSMA-RLT and four weeks after the last third cycle, all depicted in Table 2 and Figure 2a.

Table 2. Function of salivary glands directly before each cycle and 4 weeks after receiving 3 cycles of PSMA-RLT.

Parameters Mean ± SD	1st Cycle (n: 27)	2nd Cycle (n: 22)	3rd Cycle (n: 22)	4 Weeks after 3rd Cycle (n: 27)	p-Value
Ejection fraction (%):					
All glands	56.0 ± 12.0	54.6 ± 9.4	56.0 ± 12.1	53.9 ± 12.9	$p = 0.31$
Right parotid	62.0 ± 11.6	59.3 ± 8.3	61.8 ± 10.8	57.1 ± 14.0	$p = 0.28$
Left parotid	58.7 ± 14.1	57.6 ± 10.4	58.5 ± 16.1	54.3 ± 15.9	$p = 0.60$
Right submandibular	51.1 ± 10.9	50.6 ± 9.3	52.4 ± 8.2	51.7 ± 10.6	$p = 0.94$
Left submandibular	52.3 ± 7.2	51.1 ± 6.6	51.4 ± 9.6	52.5 ± 10.3	$p = 0.91$
Peak time (minutes):					
All glands combined	16.9 ± 3.6	16.5 ± 3.9	16.5 ± 4.4	17.9 ± 3.9	$p = 0.03$ *
Right parotid	17.9 ± 2.5	17.8 ± 2.0	17.5 ± 3.8	18.6 ± 2.5	$p = 0.50$
Left parotid	18.2 ± 3.2	17.9 ± 2.8	18.1 ± 3.4	18.9 ± 3.9	$p = 0.68$
Right submandibular	15.7 ± 4.3	15.7 ± 5.1	14.6 ± 5.3	17.3 ± 4.0	$p = 0.23$
Left submandibular	15.9 ± 3.7	14.6 ± 4.3	15.9 ± 4.4	16.8 ± 4.7	$p = 0.33$
RA after 5 min:					
All glands combined	56.9 ± 17.2	59.2 ± 17.0	57.5 ± 18.5	59.0 ± 19.7	$p = 0.64$
Right parotid	47.7 ± 14.9	53.6 ± 17.9	50.2 ± 16.6	54.7 ± 21.0	$p = 0.27$
Left parotid	51.1 ± 17.2	55.1 ± 16.2	52.1 ± 18.0	54.9 ± 20.6	$p = 0.73$
Right submandibular	63.0 ± 13.5	63.3 ± 17.2	62.1 ± 18.8	64.1 ± 18.6	$p = 0.98$
Left submandibular	65.8 ± 16.1	65.0 ± 14.8	65.6 ± 17.0	62.3 ± 17.8	$p = 0.84$

SD: Standard deviation; RA: Residual activity; *: Scheffé-test demonstrated no significant differences between the different cycles.

3.3. Kidney Function and Scintigraphy

There was no significant difference in mean creatinine levels between the 3 cycles of therapy and 4 weeks after the last cycle: (1st cycle 0.98 ± 0.28; 2nd cycle: 0.94 ± 0.27; 3rd cycle: 0.95 ± 0.28; four weeks after 3rd cycle: 1.02 ± 0.35; $p = 0.58$), as shown in Table 3. Furthermore, parameters of relative renal function acquired from renal scintigraphy such as the slopes of the right and left Patlak did not reveal significant differences between the first three therapy cycles and one month after the third cycle in all studied patients (Patlak right: 1st cycle: 47.3 ± 11.9; 2nd cycle: 48.9 ±13.1; 3rd cycle: 51.6 ± 8.0; four weeks after 3rd cycle: 45.4 ± 11.1; $p = 0.28$) and (Patlak left: 1st cycle: 52.7 ± 11.9; 2nd cycle 51.1 ± 13.1; 3rd cycle: 48.4 ± 8.0 four weeks after 3rd cycle: 54.6 ± 11.1; $p = 0.28$). There was also no significant difference for the integral of 0.7 to 2 min over the renogram curves normalized to the injected activity as a measure of clearance, as well as there being no significant difference between the values before the three cycles of therapy and the values four weeks after the third-to-last cycle: (both kidneys combined: 1st cycle: 94.5 ± 46.7; 2nd cycle: 94.3 ± 40.5; 3rd cycle: 101.5 ± 36.5; four weeks after 3rd cycle: 83.1 ± 32.7; $p = 0.16$) (right kidney: 1st cycle: 88.7 ± 42.3; 2nd cycle: 89.1 ± 38.8; 3rd cycle: 100.8 ± 31.7; four weeks after 3rd cycle: 77.0 ± 34.2; $p = 0.20$) and (left kidney: 1st cycle: 100.4 ± 50.5; 2nd cycle: 99.7 ± 43.0; 3rd cycle: 102.2 ± 41.8; four weeks after 3rd cycle: 89.2 ± 30.6; $p = 0.67$) see Table 3 and Figure 2b.

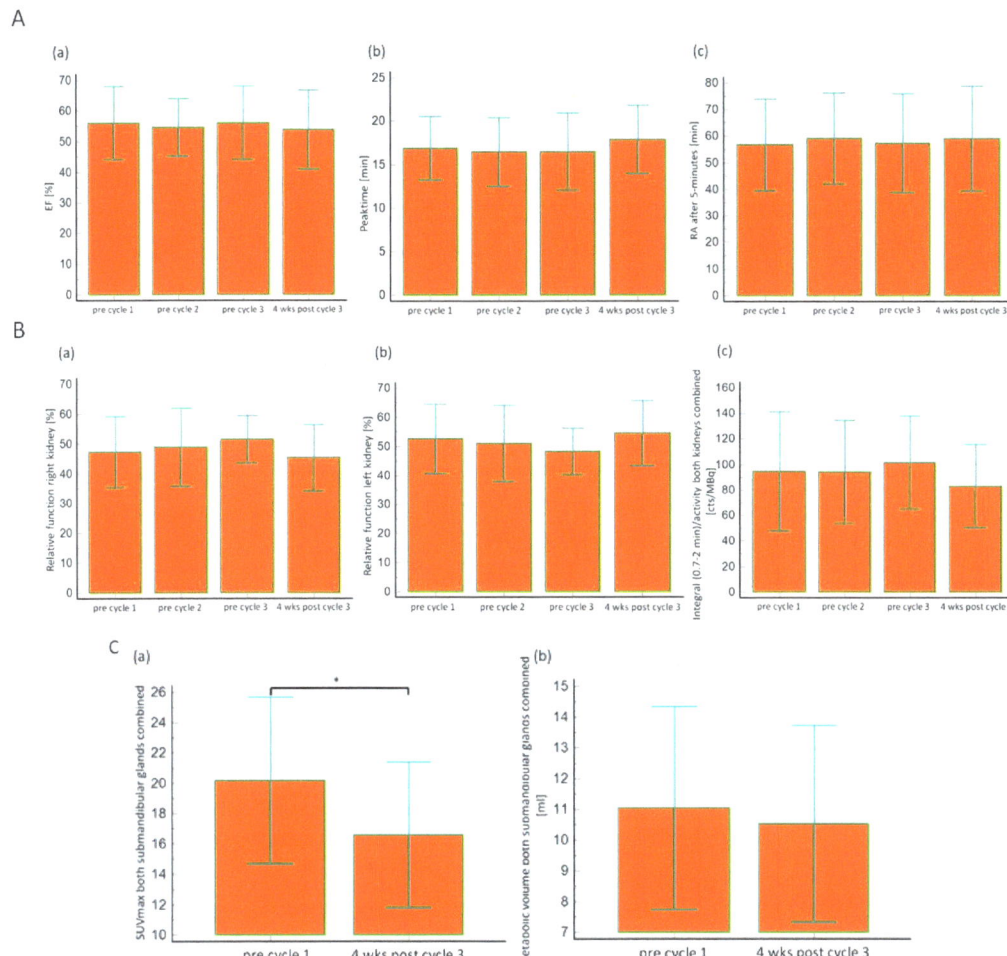

Figure 2. (**A**) Salivary gland scintigraphy prior to each three cycles of PSMA-RLT and four weeks after the third cycle. No significant difference in salivary gland function for percentage of ejection fraction (EF) (a) peak time (b) and RA after 5 min (c) for the whole parotid and submandibular glands prior to each three cycles of therapy and four weeks after the third cycle. wks.: weeks. (**B**) Kidney scintigraphy prior to each three cycles of PSMA-RLT and four weeks after the third cycle. Relative renal function such as slopes of the right (a) and left (b) Patlak as well as the integral of both kidneys combined from 0.7 to 2 min over the renogram curves normalized to the injected activity (c) did not reveal significant differences between the 3 therapy cycles and one month after the third cycle in all studied patients. wks.: weeks. (**C**) Quantification of the [^{68}Ga]Ga-PSMA PET before the first cycle and 4 weeks after the last PSMA-RLT cycle. Significant reduction in values of SUVmax (a) without changes in metabolic volume (b) of the whole submandibular glands after receiving 3 cycles of PSMA-RLT. wks.: weeks.

3.4. [^{68}Ga]Ga-PSMA PET Imaging

Quantification of the [^{68}Ga]Ga-PSMA PET images demonstrated significant difference in the SUVmax values for whole submandibular glands of both sides (20.2 ± 5.5 vs. 16.6 ± 4.8; $p = 0.001$) before the first cycle and 4 weeks after the third therapy cycle. Furthermore, SUVmax values of the left (20.5 ± 5.7 vs. 16.6 ± 4.8; $p = 0.014$) and the right (19.9 ± 5.4 vs. 16.6 ± 4.9; $p = 0.03$) submandibular glands significantly decreased four weeks after the third therapy cycle as compared to the SUVmax values before the therapy start, Table 4.

Table 3. Serum kidney and isotope nephrogram ([^{99}Tc]Tc-MAG$_3$) parameters directly before each cycle and 4 weeks after receiving 3 cycles of PSMA-RLT.

Parameters Mean ± SD	1st Cycle (n: 27)	2nd Cycle (n: 22)	3rd Cycle (n: 22)	4 Weeks after 3rd Cycle (n: 27)	p-Value
Creatinine mg/dL	0.98 ± 0.28	0.94 ± 0.27	0.95 ± 0.28	1.02 ± 0.35	p = 0.58
* Relative function:					
Right	47.3 ± 11.9	48.9 ± 13.1	51.6 ± 8.0	45.4 ± 11.1	p = 0.28
Left	52.7 ± 11.9	51.1 ± 13.1	48.4 ± 8.0	54.6 ± 11.1	p = 0.28
# Integral:					
All	94.5 ± 46.7	94.3 ± 40.5	101.5 ± 36.5	83.1 ± 32.7	p = 0.16
Right	88.7 ± 42.3	89.1 ± 38.3	100.8 ± 31.7	77.0 ± 34.2	p = 0.20
Left	100.4 ± 50.5	99.7 ± 43.0	102.2 ± 41.8	89.2 ± 30.6	p = 0.67

SD: Standard deviation; *: Relative function = (Patlak/Slope Plot) %; #: Integral (0.7–2.0 min)/activity [counts/MBq].

Table 4. [^{68}Ga]Ga-PSMA PET parameters of salivary glands directly before and 4 weeks after receiving 3 cycles of PSMA-RLT.

Parameters Mean ± SD	Prior 1st Cycle (n: 27)	4 Weeks after 3rd Therapy (n: 27)	p-Value
SUVmax.:			
All (both sides submandibular)	20.2 ± 5.5	16.6 ± 4.8	p = 0.001 *
Right submandibular	19.9 ± 5.4	16.6 ± 4.9	p = 0.03 *
Left submandibular	20.5 ± 5.7	16.6 ± 4.8	p = 0.014 *
Metabolic volume:			
All (both sides submandibular	11.1 ± 3.3	10.5 ± 3.2	p = 0.44
Right submandibular	11.3 ± 3.5	10.9 ± 3.3	p = 0.65
Left submandibular	10.8 ± 3.1	10.2 ± 3.2	p = 0.53

SD: Standard deviation; SUVmax: Maximum standard uptake value. *: Significant changes with Scheffé test before and 4 weeks after receiving 3 cycles of PSMA-RLT.

Concerning metabolic volume, on the other hand, results indicated no significant difference between the PSMA scan before and 4 weeks after the last therapy cycle, neither for the right nor for the left side, nor for the whole submandibular gland, see Table 4 and Figure 2c.

3.5. Questionnaire

Of the 27 patients, 21 completed a questionnaire concerning dry mouth prior to obtaining the first cycle, 20 prior to the second cycle, 14 prior to the third cycle, and 19 one month after the third cycle. Of these, four patients answered "yes" (19%) and seventeen (81%) answered "no" to the question about dry mouth before receiving PSMA-RLT. Before the second cycle, three men (15%) answered "yes" and seventeen (85%) answered "no". Before the third cycle, two patients (14%) answered "yes" and twelve (86%) answered "no". Four weeks after the third cycle, seven patients (37%) gave a "yes" response and twelve (63%) gave a "no" response. The results of the Cochran's Q test indicated no significant differences on the question of dry mouth (yes or no) before obtaining each cycle and four weeks after the last third cycle, $p = 0.19$.

4. Discussion

Salivary glands feature a high expression of PSMA receptors and are, consequently, the organ with the highest absorbed radiation dose (1.0 ± 0.6 Gy/GBq) after PSMA-RLT [43]. This study is the first utilizing both salivary gland scintigraphy and [^{68}Ga]Ga-PSMA PET images to assess the effect of an intensive PSMA-RLT regimen of three cycles of 7400 PSMA-RLT every four weeks on salivary gland function. Besides the fact that the values of salivary scintigraphy parameters such as EF, RA after 5 min, and peak time di not change significantly before and after treatment with this therapeutic regimen, there was only a small but statistically non-significant increase from 19% to 37% of patients reporting dry mouth. This is in good agreement with the mild and transient impairment of salivary glands previously noted in other studies under various PSMA-RLT regimens. Ahmadzarfar et al. reported dry lips in merely 20% of patients 2 weeks after receiving a cycle of 4.1–6.1 GBq [^{177}Lu]Lu-PSMA-617 [31]. Other studies have either reported a temporary xerostomia or only a slight percentage of xerostomia (about 8.7%) in men who acquired 1–2 cycles of 4.1–7.1 GBq PSMA-RLT [44,45]. In addition, Scarpa et al. recorded xerostomia in three out of ten patients, which was transient in two patients and permanent in only one patient [46], and Kratochwil and colleagues described relevant xerostomia after three PSMA-RLT cycles in two out of thirty patients [27]. Although it was only mild (i.e., grade 1) or transient functional impairment, other earlier studies detected xerostomia in a large proportion of patients (87%) after up to four cycles of 7.5 GBq PSMA-RLT [43,47]. Hence, for the patients we studied, the mean peak time increased by approximately one minute when we compared values before and four weeks after the third cycle, indicating a slight impairment of salivary gland function after three cycles of therapy.

Furthermore, the results of the quantified [^{68}Ga]Ga-PSMA PET scan displayed a significant decrease in SUVmax for the right and left submandibular glands and for both submandibular glands combined. This is in accordance with the findings of a previous study [46] in which a significant decrease in SUVmax was also evident for the submandibular glands after 2–3 cycles of 6.1 ± 0.3 GBq PSMA-RLT. Indeed, PSMA is known to be expressed on the epithelium of acinar gland cells and not on duct cells [48]. The decline in SUVmax can, thus, probably be explained by cell death resulting from salivary toxicity, which is accompanied by a loss of function. In contrast to Scarpa et al. who found a significant decrease in the volume of the submandibular glands from 7.5 mL to 6.2 mL, we did not find a meaningful change in the metabolic volume, which would have to be associated with an appreciable cell loss. This is also supported by the consideration that assuming an absorbed dose to the salivary glands of 0.8 to 2.5 Gy/GBq [49], the maximum cumulative dose under our therapy regimen of 3 cycles of 7.4 GBq only slightly exceeds the critical dose to the salivary glands of 26–50 Gy [43]. As mentioned in the introduction, PSMA-RLT can also be conducted with alpha emitters, in particular with [^{225}Ac]Actinium. Here, salivary gland toxicity is also an important limiting factor of this therapy [50,51]. Thus, studies comparable to ours with salivary gland scintigraphy would be beneficial to assess the precise impact of such therapies on salivary gland function.

Regarding renal function, there was no significant change in mean creatinine levels during the entire duration of therapy and four weeks after the last cycle. This corresponds well with outcomes of several other studies that used other therapeutic regimens, in which no significant changes in renal function were also reported after PSMA-RLT. Among them is the recent work of Rosar et al. who demonstrated an increase in GFR determined by the MDRD formula after six cycles of PSMA-RLT with a median activity of 6.5 GBq [52]. Some studies described a dose-dependent mild renal function impairment of approximately 4.5% after 2–5 five cycles of PSMA-RLT with a mean cumulative [^{177}Lu]Lutetium dose of 18.8 ± 6.7 GBq at 6–10 week intervals [53,54]. In other earlier studies, such as the study by Yadav et al., no nephrotoxicity was detected in 31 patients after 1.11–5.55 GBq [^{177}Lu]Lu-PSMA-617 [55]. The proportion of patients with elevated cystatin C who had a higher diagnostic sensitivity than serum creatinine and could detect even moderate GFR limitation, increased from 25% at baseline to 58% after treatment in a study by Yordanova et al. [23], which might further indicate a slight reduction of only about 30% from baseline and the low burden of therapy on the renal function of mCRPC patients. Nevertheless, Rahbar et al. found no significant alteration in the median creatinine and median tubular extraction rate in male patients who experienced up to two doses of PSMA-RLT with a mean activity of 5.9 ± 0.5 GBq [56].

Essentially, even under our stricter therapy interval of only 4 weeks, there was no relevant nephrotoxicity, which was also confirmed by the results of renal scintigraphy.

Specifically, the finding that the integral (0.7–2.0 min)/activity, as a surrogate parameter of renal function, did not change significantly suggests that no clinically relevant restriction of renal function occurs after PSMA-RLT. Likewise, the implication of [^{51}Cr]Cr-EDTA GFR in the study of Hofman et al. to evaluate renal toxicity under the effect of PSMA-RLT revealed no renal toxic effects of this therapy on mCRPC patients after obtaining up to 4 cycles with a median activity of 7.5 GBq and a median time between treatment cycles of 6.1 weeks [47]

Despite the use of scintigraphy as a dependable investigation to assess salivary and renal function in a cohort of patients who all obtained a homogeneous therapy protocol with equal activity dose and interval between the cycles, the retrospective design of the study and the small sample size of patients analyzed might limit the findings of this research. Therefore, differences in the patient population concerning their pre PSMA-RLT treatments including chemotherapy, which might negatively affect renal function, and tumor stages could have influenced the incidence of treatment toxicity observed in patients included in this study. In addition, the short follow-up period of only 4 weeks after the last cycle of therapy is another issue that may hinder the conclusions of this present study.

5. Conclusions

Altogether, we concluded that the salivary gland and renal function of mCRPC patients were only slightly affected under the more restrictive treatment regimen of 7.4 GBq per cycle and an interval of only 4 weeks between cycles. This further supports the good tolerability and innocuity of PSMA-RLT in male patients with mCRPC, even though longitudinal studies of salivary gland function after PSMA-RLT might provide a better assessment of the long-term effects of this therapy.

Author Contributions: Data curation, T.W., L.Z., E.K.-C., B.G., G.K. and S.R.; Investigation, T.W. and S.R.; Methodology, M.W., B.G., G.K., S.S., C.V., M.H. (Markus Hartenbach) and S.R.; Writing—original draft, T.W. and S.R.; Writing—review and editing, S.F.S., M.M., A.R.H., M.H. (Marcus Hacker) and M.H. (Markus Hartenbach). All authors have read and agreed to the published version of the manuscript.

Funding: This research received no external funding.

Institutional Review Board Statement: The study was conducted according to the guidelines of the Declaration of Helsinki, and approved by the Ethics Committee of the Medical University of Vienna (EK: 1143/2019).

Informed Consent Statement: Informed consent was obtained from all subjects involved in the study.

Data Availability Statement: The data presented in this study are available on request from the corresponding author.

Conflicts of Interest: All authors declare no conflicts of interest related to this article.

References

1. Sung, H.; Ferlay, J.; Siegel, R.L.; Laversanne, M.; Soerjomataram, I.; Jemal, A.; Bray, F. Global Cancer Statistics 2020: GLOBOCAN Estimates of Incidence and Mortality Worldwide for 36 Cancers in 185 Countries. *CA Cancer J. Clin.* **2021**, *71*, 209–249. [CrossRef] [PubMed]
2. Sweat, S.D.; Pacelli, A.; Murphy, G.P.; Bostwick, D.G. Prostate-specific membrane antigen expression is greatest in prostate adenocarcinoma and lymph node metastases. *Urology* **1998**, *52*, 637–640. [CrossRef]
3. Ghosh, A.; Heston, W.D. Tumor target prostate specific membrane antigen (PSMA) and its regulation in prostate cancer. *J. Cell Biochem.* **2004**, *91*, 528–539. [CrossRef]
4. O'Keefe, D.S.; Bacich, D.J.; Huang, S.S.; Heston, W.D. A Perspective on the Evolving Story of PSMA Biology, PSMA-Based Imaging, and Endoradiotherapeutic Strategies. *J. Nucl. Med.* **2018**, *59*, 1007–1013. [CrossRef] [PubMed]
5. Silver, D.A.; Pellicer, I.; Fair, W.R.; Heston, W.D.; Cordon-Cardo, C. Prostate-specific membrane antigen expression in normal and malignant human tissues. *Clin. Cancer Res.* **1997**, *3*, 81–85. [PubMed]
6. Bostwick, D.G.; Pacelli, A.; Blute, M.; Roche, P.; Murphy, G.P. Prostate specific membrane antigen expression in prostatic intraepithelial neoplasia and adenocarcinoma: A study of 184 cases. *Cancer* **1998**, *82*, 2256–2261. [CrossRef]

7. Hillier, S.M.; Maresca, K.P.; Lu, G.; Merkin, R.D.; Marquis, J.C.; Zimmerman, C.N.; Eckelman, W.C.; Joyal, J.L.; Babich, J.W. 99mTc-labeled small-molecule inhibitors of prostate-specific membrane antigen for molecular imaging of prostate cancer. *J. Nucl. Med.* **2013**, *54*, 1369–1376. [CrossRef] [PubMed]
8. Eder, M.; Schäfer, M.; Bauder-Wüst, U.; Hull, W.-E.; Wängler, C.; Mier, W.; Haberkorn, U.; Eisenhut, M. ^{68}Ga-Complex Lipophilicity and the Targeting Property of a Urea-Based PSMA Inhibitor for PET Imaging. *Bioconjug. Chem.* **2012**, *23*, 688–697. [CrossRef] [PubMed]
9. Weineisen, M.; Schottelius, M.; Simecek, J.; Baum, R.P.; Yildiz, A.; Beykan, S.; Kulkarni, H.R.; Lassmann, M.; Klette, I.; Eiber, M.; et al. ^{68}Ga- and ^{177}Lu-Labeled PSMA I&T: Optimization of a PSMA-Targeted Theranostic Concept and First Proof-of-Concept Human Studies. *J. Nucl. Med.* **2015**, *56*, 1169–1176.
10. Mease, R.C.; Dusich, C.L.; Foss, C.A.; Ravert, H.T.; Dannals, R.F.; Seidel, J.; Prideaux, A.; Fox, J.J.; Sgouros, G.; Kozikowski, A.P.; et al. N-[N-[(S)-1,3-Dicarboxypropyl]Carbamoyl]-4-[^{18}F]Fluorobenzyl-l-Cysteine, [^{18}F]DCFBC: A New Imaging Probe for Prostate Cancer. *Clin. Cancer Res.* **2008**, *14*, 3036–3043. [CrossRef]
11. Kratochwil, C.; Bruchertseifer, F.; Giesel, F.L.; Weis, M.; Verburg, F.A.; Mottaghy, F.; Kopka, K.; Apostolidis, C.; Haberkorn, U.; Morgenstern, A. 225Ac-PSMA-617 for PSMA-Targeted α-Radiation Therapy of Metastatic Castration-Resistant Prostate Cancer. *J. Nucl. Med.* **2016**, *57*, 1941–1944. [CrossRef]
12. Rice, M.; Malhotra, S.V.; Stoyanova, T. Second-Generation Antiandrogens: From Discovery to Standard of Care in Castration Resistant Prostate Cancer. *Front. Oncol.* **2019**, *9*, 801. [CrossRef]
13. Nuhn, P.; De Bono, J.S.; Fizazi, K.; Freedland, S.J.; Grilli, M.; Kantoff, P.W.; Sonpavde, G.; Sternberg, C.N.; Yegnasubramanian, S.; Antonarakis, E.S. Update on Systemic Prostate Cancer Therapies: Management of Metastatic Castration-resistant Prostate Cancer in the Era of Precision Oncology. *Eur. Urol.* **2018**, *75*, 88–99. [CrossRef] [PubMed]
14. Nguyen-Nielsen, M.; Borre, M. Diagnostic and Therapeutic Strategies for Prostate Cancer. *Semin. Nucl. Med.* **2016**, *46*, 484–490. [CrossRef] [PubMed]
15. Hofman, M.S.; Emmett, L.; Sandhu, S.; Iravani, A.; Joshua, A.M.; Goh, J.C.; Pattison, D.A.; Tan, T.H.; Kirkwood, I.D.; Ng, S.; et al. [(^{177})Lu]Lu-PSMA-617 versus cabazitaxel in patients with metastatic castration-resistant prostate cancer (TheraP): A randomised, open-label, phase 2 trial. *Lancet* **2021**, *397*, 797–804. [CrossRef]
16. Novartis Announces Positive Result of Phase III Study with Radioligand Therapy 177Lu-PSMA-617 in Patients with Advanced Prostate Cancer. Available online: https://bit.ly/3ce0zCQ (accessed on 23 March 2021).
17. Rahbar, K.; Ahmadzadehfar, H.; Kratochwil, C.; Haberkorn, U.; Schäfers, M.; Essler, M.; Baum, R.P.; Kulkarni, H.R.; Schmidt, M.; Drzezga, A.; et al. German Multicenter Study Investigating ^{177}Lu-PSMA-617 Radioligand Therapy in Advanced Prostate Cancer Patients. *J. Nucl. Med.* **2017**, *58*, 85–90. [CrossRef] [PubMed]
18. Bräuer, A.; Grubert, L.S.; Roll, W.; Schrader, A.J.; Schäfers, M.; Bögemann, M.; Rahbar, K. ^{177}Lu-PSMA-617 radioligand therapy and outcome in patients with metastasized castration-resistant prostate cancer. *Eur. J. Nucl. Med. Mol. Imaging* **2017**, *44*, 1663–1670. [CrossRef] [PubMed]
19. Kratochwil, C.; Giesel, F.L.; Eder, M.; Afshar-Oromieh, A.; Benešová, M.; Mier, W.; Kopka, K.; Haberkorn, U. [^{177}Lu]Lutetium-labelled PSMA ligand-induced remission in a patient with metastatic prostate cancer. *Eur. J. Nucl. Med. Mol. Imaging* **2015**, *42*, 987–988. [CrossRef] [PubMed]
20. Rahbar, K.; Boegemann, M.; Yordanova, A.; Eveslage, M.; Schäfers, M.; Essler, M.; Ahmadzadehfar, H. PSMA targeted radioligandtherapy in metastatic castration resistant prostate cancer after chemotherapy, abiraterone and/or enzalutamide. A retrospective analysis of overall survival. *Eur. J. Nucl. Med. Mol. Imaging* **2017**, *45*, 12–19. [CrossRef]
21. O'Keefe, D.S.; Bacich, D.J.; Heston, W.D. Comparative analysis of prostate-specific membrane antigen (PSMA) versus a prostate-specific membrane antigen-like gene. *Prostate* **2004**, *58*, 200–210. [CrossRef]
22. Tönnesmann, R.; Meyer, P.T.; Eder, M.; Baranski, A.-C. [^{177}Lu]Lu-PSMA-617 Salivary Gland Uptake Characterized by Quantitative In Vitro Autoradiography. *Pharmaceuticals* **2019**, *12*, 18. [CrossRef] [PubMed]
23. Yordanova, A.; Becker, A.; Eppard, E.; Kürpig, S.; Fisang, C.; Feldmann, G.; Essler, M.; Ahmadzadehfar, H. The impact of repeated cycles of radioligand therapy using [^{177}Lu]Lu-PSMA-617 on renal function in patients with hormone refractory metastatic prostate cancer. *Eur. J. Nucl. Med. Mol. Imaging* **2017**, *44*, 1473–1479. [CrossRef]
24. Delker, A.; Fendler, W.P.; Kratochwil, C.; Brunegraf, A.; Gosewisch, A.; Gildehaus, F.J.; Tritschler, S.; Stief, C.G.; Kopka, K.; Haberkorn, U.; et al. Dosimetry for ^{177}Lu-DKFZ-PSMA-617: A new radiopharmaceutical for the treatment of metastatic prostate cancer. *Eur. J. Nucl. Med. Mol. Imaging* **2015**, *43*, 42–51. [CrossRef] [PubMed]
25. Kabasakal, L.; Abuqbeitah, M.; Aygün, A.; Yeyin, N.; Ocak, M.; Demirci, E.; Toklu, T. Pre-therapeutic dosimetry of normal organs and tissues of ^{177}Lu-PSMA-617 prostate-specific membrane antigen (PSMA) inhibitor in patients with castration-resistant prostate cancer. *Eur. J. Nucl. Med. Mol. Imaging* **2015**, *42*, 1976–1983. [CrossRef] [PubMed]
26. Özkan, A.; Uçar, B.; Seymen, H.; Yarar, Y.Y.; Falay, F.O.; Demirkol, M.O. Posttherapeutic Critical Organ Dosimetry of Extensive ^{177}Lu-PSMA Inhibitor Therapy With Metastatic Castration-Resistant Prostate Cancer: One Center Results. *Clin. Nucl. Med.* **2020**, *45*, 288–291. [CrossRef]
27. Kratochwil, C.; Giesel, F.L.; Stefanova, M.; Benešová, M.; Bronzel, M.; Afshar-Oromieh, A.; Mier, W.; Eder, M.; Kopka, K.; Haberkorn, U. PSMA-Targeted Radionuclide Therapy of Metastatic Castration-Resistant Prostate Cancer with ^{177}Lu-Labeled PSMA-617. *J. Nucl. Med.* **2016**, *57*, 1170–1176. [CrossRef]

28. Yadav, M.P.; Ballal, S.; Sahoo, R.K.; Dwivedi, S.N.; Bal, C. Radioligand Therapy With ^{177}Lu-PSMA for Metastatic Castration-Resistant Prostate Cancer: A Systematic Review and Meta-Analysis. *Am. J. Roentgenol.* **2019**, *213*, 275–285. [CrossRef] [PubMed]
29. Rasul, S.; Hacker, M.; Kretschmer-Chott, E.; Leisser, A.; Grubmüller, B.; Kramer, G.; Shariat, S.; Wadsak, W.; Mitterhauser, M.; Hartenbach, M.; et al. Clinical outcome of standardized ^{177}Lu-PSMA-617 therapy in metastatic prostate cancer patients receiving 7400 MBq every 4 weeks. *Eur. J. Nucl. Med. Mol. Imaging* **2019**, *47*, 713–720. [CrossRef] [PubMed]
30. Rasul, S.; Hartenbach, M.; Wollenweber, T.; Kretschmer-Chott, E.; Grubmüller, B.; Kramer, G.; Shariat, S.; Wadsak, W.; Mitterhauser, M.; Pichler, V.; et al. Prediction of response and survival after standardized treatment with 7400 MBq ^{177}Lu-PSMA-617 every 4 weeks in patients with metastatic castration-resistant prostate cancer. *Eur. J. Nucl. Med. Mol. Imaging* **2020**, *48*, 1650–1657. [CrossRef]
31. Ahmadzadehfar, H.; Rahbar, K.; Kürpig, S.; Bögemann, M.; Claesener, M.; Eppard, E.; Gärtner, F.; Rogenhofer, S.; Schäfers, M.; Essler, M. Early side effects and first results of radioligand therapy with ^{177}Lu-DKFZ-617 PSMA of castrate-resistant metastatic prostate cancer: A two-centre study. *EJNMMI Res.* **2015**, *5*, 114. [CrossRef]
32. Rasul, S.; Wollenweber, T.; Zisser, L.; Kretschmer-Chott, E.; Grubmüller, B.; Kramer, G.; Shariat, S.; Eidherr, H.; Mitterhauser, M.; Vraka, C.; et al. Response and Toxicity to the Second Course of 3 Cycles of ^{177}Lu-PSMA Therapy Every 4 Weeks in Patients with Metastatic Castration-Resistant Prostate Cancer. *Cancers* **2021**, *13*, 2489. [CrossRef] [PubMed]
33. Shizukuishi, K.; Nagaoka, S.; Kinno, Y.; Saito, M.; Takahashi, N.; Kawamoto, M.; Abe, A.; Jin, L.; Inoue, T. Scoring analysis of salivary gland scintigraphy in patients with Sjögren's syndrome. *Ann. Nucl. Med.* **2003**, *17*, 627–631. [CrossRef] [PubMed]
34. Vitali, C.; Bombardieri, S.; Moutsopoulos, H.M.; Coll, J.; Gerli, R.; Hatron, P.Y.; Kater, L.; Konttinen, Y.T.; Manthorpe, R.; Meyer, O. et al. Assessment of the European classification criteria for Sjögren's syndrome in a series of clinically defined cases: Results of a prospective multicentre study. The European Study Group on Diagnostic Criteria for Sjögren's Syndrome. *Ann. Rheum. Dis.* **1996**, *55*, 116–121. [CrossRef]
35. Klutmann, S.; Bohuslavizki, K.H.; Kröger, S.; Bleckmann, C.; Brenner, W.; Mester, J.; Clausen, M. Quantitative salivary gland scintigraphy. *J. Nucl. Med. Technol.* **1999**, *27*, 20–26.
36. Taylor, A.T.; Brandon, D.C.; de Palma, D.; Blaufox, M.D.; Durand, E.; Erbas, B.; Grant, S.F.; Hilson, A.J.; Morsing, A. SNMMI Procedure Standard/EANM Practice Guideline for Diuretic Renal Scintigraphy in Adults With Suspected Upper Urinary Tract Obstruction 1.0. *Semin. Nucl. Med.* **2018**, *48*, 377–390. [CrossRef]
37. Peters, A.M. Graphical analysis of dynamic data: The Patlak-Rutland plot. *Nucl. Med. Commun.* **1994**, *15*, 669–672. [CrossRef] [PubMed]
38. Piepsz, A.; Kinthaert, J.; Tondeur, M.; Ham, H.R. The robustness of the Patlak-Rutland slope for the determination of split renal function. *Nucl. Med. Commun.* **1996**, *17*, 817–821. [CrossRef] [PubMed]
39. Gates, G.F. Glomerular filtration rate: Estimation from fractional renal accumulation of 99mTc-DTPA (stannous). *Am. J. Roentgenol.* **1982**, *138*, 565–570. [CrossRef]
40. Esteves, F.P.; Halkar, R.K.; Issa, M.M.; Grant, S.; Taylor, A. Comparison of camera-based 99mTc-MAG3 and 24-h creatinine clearances for evaluation of kidney function. *Am. J. Roentgenol.* **2006**, *187*, W316–W319. [CrossRef]
41. Grubmüller, B.; Senn, D.; Kramer, G.; Baltzer, P.; D'Andrea, D.; Grubmüller, K.H.; Mitterhauser, M.; Eidherr, H.; Haug, A.R.; Wadsak, W.; et al. Response assessment using (68)Ga-PSMA ligand PET in patients undergoing (^{177}Lu-PSMA radioligand therapy for metastatic castration-resistant prostate cancer. *Eur. J. Nucl. Med. Mol. Imaging* **2019**, *46*, 1063–1072. [CrossRef] [PubMed]
42. Van Kalmthout, L.W.M.; Lam, M.G.E.H.; De Keizer, B.; Krijger, G.C.; Ververs, T.F.T.; De Roos, R.; Braat, A.J.A.T. Impact of external cooling with icepacks on (^{68})Ga-PSMA uptake in salivary glands. *EJNMMI Res.* **2018**, *8*, 56. [CrossRef]
43. Fendler, W.P.; Reinhardt, S.; Ilhan, H.; Delker, A.; Böning, G.; Gildehaus, F.J.; Stief, C.; Bartenstein, P.; Gratzke, C.; Lehner, S.; et al. Preliminary experience with dosimetry, response and patient reported outcome after ^{177}Lu-PSMA-617 therapy for metastatic castration-resistant prostate cancer. *Oncotarget* **2016**, *8*, 3581–3590. [CrossRef]
44. Ahmadzadehfar, H.; Eppard, E.; Kürpig, S.; Fimmers, R.; Yordanova, A.; Schlenkhoff, C.D.; Gartner, F.; Rogenhofer, S.; Essler, M. Therapeutic response and side effects of repeated radioligand therapy with ^{177}Lu-PSMA-DKFZ-617 of castrate-resistant metastatic prostate cancer. *Oncotarget* **2016**, *7*, 12477–12488. [CrossRef]
45. Rahbar, K.; Bode, A.; Weckesser, M.; Avramovic, N.; Claesener, M.; Stegger, L.; Bögemann, M. Radioligand Therapy With ^{177}Lu-PSMA-617 as A Novel Therapeutic Option in Patients With Metastatic Castration Resistant Prostate Cancer. *Clin. Nucl. Med.* **2016**, *41*, 522–528. [CrossRef]
46. Scarpa, L.; Buxbaum, S.; Kendler, D.; Fink, K.; Bektic, J.; Gruber, L.; Decristoforo, C.; Uprimny, C.; Lukas, P.; Horninger, W.; et al. The (^{68})Ga/(^{177})Lu theragnostic concept in PSMA targeting of castration-resistant prostate cancer: Correlation of SUV(max) values and absorbed dose estimates. *Eur. J. Nucl. Med. Mol. Imaging* **2017**, *44*, 788–800. [CrossRef]
47. Hofman, M.S.; Violet, J.; Hicks, R.J.; Ferdinandus, J.; Thang, S.P.; Akhurst, T.; Iravani, A.; Kong, G.; Kumar, A.R.; Murphy, D.G. et al. [(^{177})Lu]-PSMA-617 radionuclide treatment in patients with metastatic castration-resistant prostate cancer (LuPSMA trial): A single-centre, single-arm, phase 2 study. *Lancet Oncol.* **2018**, *19*, 825–833. [CrossRef]
48. Wolf, P.; Freudenberg, N.; Bühler, P.; Alt, K.; Schultze-Seemann, W.; Wetterauer, U.; Elsässer-Beile, U. Three conformational antibodies specific for different PSMA epitopes are promising diagnostic and therapeutic tools for prostate cancer. *Prostate* **2010**, *70*, 562–569. [CrossRef] [PubMed]

49. Taïeb, D.; Foletti, J.-M.; Bardiès, M.; Rocchi, P.; Hicks, R.J.; Haberkorn, U. PSMA-Targeted Radionuclide Therapy and Salivary Gland Toxicity: Why Does It Matter? *J. Nucl. Med.* **2018**, *59*, 747–748. [CrossRef] [PubMed]
50. Sathekge, M.M.; Bruchertseifer, F.; Vorster, M.; Morgenstern, A.; Lawal, I.O. Global experience with PSMA-based alpha therapy in prostate cancer. *Eur. J. Nucl. Med. Mol. Imaging* **2021**, *26*, 1–7.
51. Filippi, L.; Chiaravalloti, A.; Schillaci, O.; Bagni, O. The potential of PSMA-targeted alpha therapy in the management of prostate cancer. *Expert Rev. Anticancer. Ther.* **2020**, *20*, 823–829. [CrossRef]
52. Rosar, F.; Kochems, N.; Bartholomä, M.; Maus, S.; Stemler, T.; Linxweiler, J.; Khreish, F.; Ezziddin, S. Renal Safety of [^{177}Lu]Lu-PSMA-617 Radioligand Therapy in Patients with Compromised Baseline Kidney Function. *Cancers* **2021**, *13*, 3095. [CrossRef] [PubMed]
53. Gallyamov, M.; Meyrick, D.; Barley, J.; Lenzo, N. Renal outcomes of radioligand therapy: Experience of ^{177}lutetium—prostate-specific membrane antigen ligand therapy in metastatic castrate-resistant prostate cancer. *Clin. Kidney J.* **2019**, *13*, 1049–1055. [CrossRef] [PubMed]
54. Ngoc, C.N.; Happel, C.; Davis, K.; Groener, D.; Mader, N.; Mandel, P.; Tselis, N.; Gruenwald, F.; Sabet, A. Renal Function after Radioligand Treatment with ^{177}Lu-PSMA-617. *J. Nucl. Med.* **2020**, *61* (Suppl. 1), 1279.
55. Yadav, M.P.; Ballal, S.; Tripathi, M.; Damle, N.A.; Sahoo, R.K.; Seth, A.; Tselis, N.; Gruenwald, F.; Sabet, A. (^{177})Lu-DKFZ-PSMA-617 therapy in metastatic castration resistant prostate cancer: Safety, efficacy, and quality of life assessment. *Eur. J. Nucl. Med. Mol. Imaging* **2017**, *44*, 81–91. [CrossRef] [PubMed]
56. Rahbar, K.; Schmidt, M.; Heinzel, A.; Eppard, E.; Bode, A.; Yordanova, A.; Claesener, M.; Ahmadzadehfar, H. Response and Tolerability of a Single Dose of ^{177}Lu-PSMA-617 in Patients with Metastatic Castration-Resistant Prostate Cancer: A Multicenter Retrospective Analysis. *J. Nucl. Med.* **2016**, *57*, 1334–1338. [CrossRef]

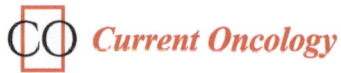

Article

Quality of Life Determinants in Patients with Metastatic Prostate Cancer: Insights from a Cross-Sectional Questionnaire-Based Study

Chetanya Mittal [1,†], Hardik Gupta [1,†], Chitrakshi Nagpal [2], Ranjit K. Sahoo [2], Aparna Sharma [3], Bharat B. Gangadharaiah [2], Ghazal Tansir [2], Sridhar Panaiyadiyan [4], Shamim A. Shamim [5], Seema Kaushal [6], Chandan J. Das [7], Kunhi P. Haresh [8], Amlesh Seth [9], Brusabhanu Nayak [9] and Atul Batra [2,*]

[1] All India Institute of Medical Sciences, New Delhi 110029, India; chetanyamittal35@aiims.edu (C.M.); hardikg2001@aiims.edu (H.G.)
[2] Department of Medical Oncology, Dr. B.R.A. Institute Rotary Cancer Hospital, All India Institute of Medical Sciences, New Delhi 110029, India; chitrakshinagpal11.jan20@aiims.edu (C.N.); drranjitmd@aiims.edu (R.K.S.); bharathbg01.jan21@aiims.edu (B.B.G.); ghzl_complique@yahoo.com (G.T.)
[3] Department of Medical Oncology, National Cancer Institute, All India Institute of Medical Sciences, New Delhi 110029, India; aparnasharma@aiims.edu
[4] Department of Urology, National Cancer Institute, All India Institute of Medical Sciences, New Delhi 110029, India; sridharsoul@gmail.com
[5] Department of Nuclear Medicine, All India Institute of Medical Sciences, New Delhi 110029, India; sashamim2002@aiims.edu
[6] Department of Pathology, All India Institute of Medical Sciences, New Delhi 110029, India; seema.dr@aiims.edu
[7] Department of Radiodiagnosis, All India Institute of Medical Sciences, New Delhi 110029, India; chandan.das@aiims.edu
[8] Department of Radiation Oncology, Dr. B.R.A. Institute Rotary Cancer Hospital, All India Institute of Medical Sciences, New Delhi 110029, India; drkpharesh@gmail.com
[9] Department of Urology, All India Institute of Medical Sciences, New Delhi 110029, India; amlesh.seth@aiims.edu (A.S.); brusabhanu@aiims.edu (B.N.)
* Correspondence: batraatul85@gmail.com; Tel.: +91-11-2957-5043
† These authors contributed equally to this work.

Citation: Mittal, C.; Gupta, H.; Nagpal, C.; Sahoo, R.K.; Sharma, A.; Gangadharaiah, B.B.; Tansir, G.; Panaiyadiyan, S.; Shamim, S.A.; Kaushal, S.; et al. Quality of Life Determinants in Patients with Metastatic Prostate Cancer: Insights from a Cross-Sectional Questionnaire-Based Study. *Curr. Oncol.* **2024**, *31*, 4940–4954. https://doi.org/10.3390/curroncol31090366

Received: 13 July 2024
Revised: 22 August 2024
Accepted: 25 August 2024
Published: 26 August 2024

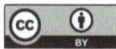

Copyright: © 2024 by the authors. Licensee MDPI, Basel, Switzerland. This article is an open access article distributed under the terms and conditions of the Creative Commons Attribution (CC BY) license (https://creativecommons.org/licenses/by/4.0/).

Abstract: Introduction: Prostate cancer is one of the most prevalent malignancies affecting men globally, with a significant impact on health-related quality of life (HRQOL). With the recent therapeutic advancements and improvements in survival, there is a need to understand the determinants of HRQOL in metastatic prostate cancer patients to optimize treatment strategies for quality of life as the number of survivors increases. The aim of this study was to identify clinical variables that affect HRQOL and its domains in patients with metastatic prostate cancer. Methods: We conducted a cross-sectional questionnaire-based study in patients diagnosed with metastatic prostate cancer at a tertiary cancer center in India. Baseline clinical features, treatment details, and completed Functional Assessment of Cancer Therapy—Prostate (FACT-P), composed of FACT-general (FACT-G) and prostate cancer-specific concerns subscale (PCS) and FACT-P Trial Outcome Index (FACT-P TOI) questionnaires, were collected. The mean total, as well as individual domain scores, were calculated. Additionally, these were stratified by the current treatment being received by patients. Linear regression was used to identify independent factors affecting HRQOL in these patients. Results: Of the 106 enrolled patients, 84 completed the FACT-P questionnaire and were included in the analysis. The median age was 66 years, and at the time of assessment, 3 patients (3.6%) were receiving androgen deprivation therapy only, 53 patients (63.1%) were on ADT + androgen receptor-targeted agents (ARTAs), and 18 patients (21.4%) patients received ADT + chemotherapy. The mean (±standard deviation) of the FACT-P TOI score was 70.33 (±15.16); the PCS subscale was the most affected followed by functional well-being. Patients on chemotherapy scored significantly higher on PCS but the composite scores were not significantly different. Univariable regression identified obesity (body mass index > 25 kg/m^2) and duration of first-line treatment as significant predictors of better HRQOL; however, obesity was the only independent predictor in multivariable analysis (β = 8.2; 95%

confidence interval, 1.2 to 15.0; $p = 0.022$). Obesity also independently predicted a better FACT-P and its physical well-being domain score and PCS. Conclusion: Prostate cancer patients experience impaired QoL, especially in the prostate cancer-specific and functional well-being domains. Lower BMI is an independent predictor of poor QoL, and this requires efforts to assess the impact of strategies to manage the nutritional status of patients with metastatic disease on QoL outcomes.

Keywords: prostate cancer; quality of life; health-related quality of life

1. Introduction

Prostate cancer is the second most common malignancy in men worldwide [1]. The prognosis of prostate cancer has improved significantly due to recent advancements in therapies [2]. With an increasing number of patients living with metastatic prostate cancer, efforts are needed to understand the impact of the disease and its treatment on various dimensions of quality of life [3].

Health-related QOL (HRQOL) is a multidimensional assessment of how disease and its treatment affect a patient's overall function and well-being [4]. Several validated HRQOL assessment tools are available for prostate cancer, of which the most common is the Functional Assessment of Chronic Illness Therapy-Prostate (FACT-P) questionnaire [5].

The FACT-P scale is a combination of the FACT-General (FACT-G) scale with four dimensions: physical well-being (PWB), social/family well-being (SWB), emotional well-being (EWB), and functional well-being (FWB), along with a 12-item prostate cancer-specific concerns subscale (PCS). It is a validated assessment tool for HRQOL with high content validity and internal consistency and is thus extensively used for QOL assessment in prostate cancer [6]. Higher scores indicate a better quality of life, and a change of 6 to 10 points is considered clinically meaningful [7,8]. Previous studies have shown mean baseline FACT-P scores (scored from 0 to 156) in patients with locally advanced/metastatic prostate cancer varying between 87.73 ± 19.88 and 116.62 ± 18.13 in the Indian and Western populations, respectively, suggesting that Indian patients with prostate cancer experience worse HRQOL than Western populations [9,10].

The prognostic association of baseline patient-reported HRQOL using the FACT-P scale has been extensively studied in localized prostate cancer [11]. An exploratory analysis of the CHAARTED trial revealed that low BMI is associated with significantly poor baseline HRQOL in patients with metastatic castration-sensitive prostate cancer, likely related to cancer-induced cachexia [12]. Apart from this, there have been very limited efforts to identify the status of patients with advanced disease, especially in the Indian setting, where HRQOL scores are comparatively lower than in the Western setting [9,10]. In this study, we aim to assess patient-reported HRQOL and identify prognostic factors that affect the quality of life in patients with metastatic prostate cancer [9,10].

2. Methodology
2.1. Study Design

The primary aim of this study was to identify the determinants of the HRQOL of patients with metastatic prostate cancer. We also sought to study the clinical variables affecting the various domains of HRQOL. It was a cross-sectional study conducted at the All India Institute of Medical Sciences (AIIMS), New Delhi, a tertiary cancer care center in India that caters to the populations of North India. Dr. B. R. A. Institute Rotary Cancer Hospital (IRCH), AIIMS, is the regional cancer center where approximately 15,000 patients with a new cancer diagnosis are treated annually [13].

This study was planned as a pilot study with a sample size of convenience screening and recruiting consecutive patients over 18 years of age with a histologically confirmed diagnosis of primary metastatic prostate cancer who were receiving systemic treatment at our center for a predetermined duration between September 2021 and June 2022. Patients with an expected life expectancy of <12 weeks, as determined by the treating oncologist, were excluded. All patients in this study had de novo metastatic prostate cancer, and none of them had been treated for local disease in the past (Figure 1). Demographic data were collected from all the participants, which included age, urban or rural residence (as reported by the patients), education status (categorized as illiterate—someone who cannot read and write [14]; the ones who were literate were categorized into those who have completed primary, middle, or high school or those who have a graduation or post-graduation degree), presence of comorbidities (comorbidities expected to be in a frequency of greater than 1% in our patient population were pre-specified and included in the case record form—diabetes mellitus, hypertension, hypothyroidism, CAD, CKD, stroke, and TIAs; the rest were classified as others), addictions, and accessibility to the hospital (calculated by measuring the distance from the patient's PIN code to the PIN code of the hospital using Google Maps, 2021).

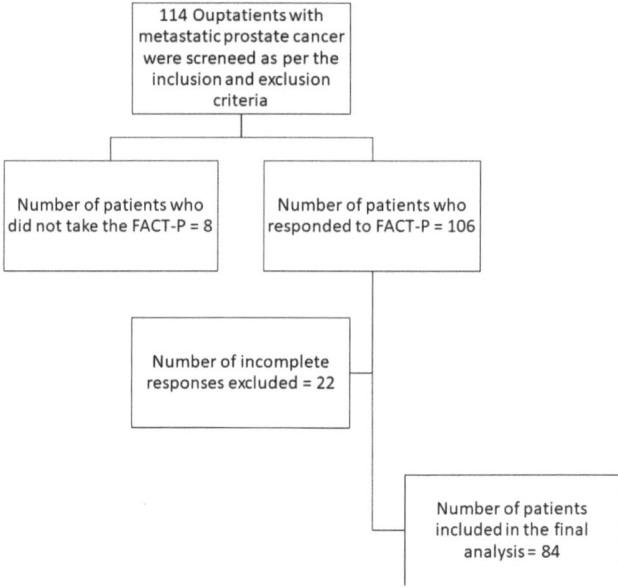

Figure 1. Enrollment of study participants and Health-Related Quality of Life Assessment. FACT-P, Functional Assessment of Cancer Therapy – Prostate.

Clinical data collected included the duration of disease, site of metastasis, anthropometry (body mass index defined as per South-Asian cutoffs—underweight (<18.5 kg/m^2), normal (18.5–22.9 kg/m^2), overweight (23.0–24.9 kg/m^2), and obese (≥ 25 kg/m^2) [15], Eastern Cooperative Oncology Group (ECOG) performance status, and risk-stratification of metastatic disease (high-risk disease defined as ≥ 2 of the following: visceral metastasis, Gleason score ≥ 8, ≥ 3 bone lesions) [16], and burden of disease (high-volume disease defined as presence of visceral metastasis and/or ≥ 4 bone metastases, including at least one outside the vertebral bodies and pelvis) [17]. Laboratory values included serum prostate-specific antigen (PSA) at the time of assessment and the Gleason score of the prostate biopsy specimens. Treatment details collected included the type of androgen deprivation therapy received (ADT), the number of lines and types of treatment received, and their duration. The assessment of these baseline factors was stratified on the basis of the current therapy being received by the patient at the cross-sectional time point of assessment.

The institutional ethics committee approved the study (reference number IEC-646/03.09.2021 RP-23/2021). Written informed consent was obtained from all patients before their participation

2.2. Assessment of HRQOL

We utilized the FACT-P measure to determine the HRQOL, which has been concluded to be the most appropriate patient-reported outcome measure for patients with metastatic prostate cancer by the PIONEER (Prostate Cancer DIagnOsis and TreatmeNt Enhancement through the Power of Big Data in EuRope) consortium [6]. All participants were assessed using this questionnaire at a single time point (in Hindi or English according to the patient's comprehension) [18]. The license for the English and Hindi versions for clinical providers was obtained in the institution's name from the Functional Assessment of Chronic Illness Therapy (FACIT) System Organization in the name of the institution vide agreement dated 9 August 2021.

Self-administration of the measure was the preferred mode of administering the questionnaire. Patients with difficulty comprehending the questions received assistance from our research staff, limited to explaining the literal meaning of the question in further, simpler terms without interfering with the responses. The FACT-P scale consists of the FACT-G and PCS subscales. The FACT-G (version 4) is a 27-item questionnaire comprising four dimensions (PWB, SWB, EWB, and FWB). Each domain has seven items and is scored out of 28, except EWB (6 items, scored out of 24) [7]. All items are answered on a Likert scale ranging from 0 to 4, with 0 representing "not at all" and 4 representing "very much." The subscale comprises 12 items encompassing bowel and bladder function, sexual activity, and pain, and is scored out of 48. The combination of the scales provides a global HRQOL score and domain-specific scores [19]. A modified version of FACT-P, called the FACT-P trial outcome index (FACT-P TOI), includes only the physical and functional domain scores and the PCS subscale. It takes less time to fill, is more sensitive than the FACT-P score, and is thus extensively used as an end-point in clinical trials [20]. The FACT-P is scored from 0 to 156, the FACT-G from 0 to 108, and the FACT-P TOI from 0 to 104. A higher score is indicative of a better quality of life.

A response rate of at least 50% in each subscale and 80% overall was required to include incompletely filled questionnaires. If less than 50% of individual items were skipped, subscale scores were prorated using the average of the other answers in the scale. This imputation method is standard across The Functional Assessment of Chronic Illness Therapy (FACIT) measurement system [20]. Patients with less than 50% of the forms filled out were excluded from the study.

2.3. Statistics

Descriptive statistics were used to present demographics and baseline clinical parameters. Categorical data were described as percentages, and continuous variables were described as mean ($\pm$ standard deviation). The means of the FACT-P, FACT-P TOI, and FACT-G scores were calculated as the composite scores and domain-wise subscores of the FACT-P tool and demonstrated as box and whiskers plots. Potential predictive factors associated with better or worse FACT-P TOI, FACT-P, and FACT-G scores were identified using linear regression analysis. Univariable linear regression analysis was performed on all the baseline demographic and clinical factors reported with the linear regression coefficient, beta, and its 95% confidence interval. Those with a p-value of <0.05 or previously studied prognostic factors were included in the multivariable analysis. The significant p-value used was specified as <0.05 a priori. Statistical analysis was performed using R version 4.3.2 (RStudio, R Foundation for Statistical Computing, Vienna, Austria).

3. Results

3.1. Baseline Characteristics

A total of 106 patients with metastatic prostate cancer were screened during the study period, and they consented to complete the questionnaire. A total of 84 patients who completed a FACT-P measure with an overall response rate of >80% were included in the final analysis. A total of 3 patients (3.6%) were receiving androgen deprivation therapy only; 53 patients (63.1%) were on ADT + androgen receptor-targeted agents

(ARTAs)—90.6% abiraterone and 9.4% enzalutamide. A total of 18 patients (21.4%) received ADT + chemotherapy—docetaxel—94% and cabazitaxel—5.6%. The median age of the participants was 66 (59–71) years; one-third belonged to a rural area (35%), and around 10% were illiterate. About half of the patients (48%) had one or more comorbid medical conditions (35% hypertension and 15% diabetes mellitus), and 46% of patients were obese. The median duration from diagnosis of metastatic prostate cancer to the assessment of HRQOL was 11 months (IQR, 4–38), with a higher median duration—25 months in chemotherapy patients versus 10 months in those receiving ADT/ADT + ARTA therapy, 65% had high-risk disease, and 62% of them had high-volume disease. Almost equal numbers had castration-sensitive and resistant diseases, respectively. Most of our patients had received androgen deprivation therapy; 69% underwent bilateral orchiectomy; and the remaining received medical castration. Forty-one percent of our patients received more than one line of treatment. Abiraterone was the choice of first-line therapy in 72% of patients, with others having received docetaxel (23%), enzalutamide (2.7%), and fosfestrol (2.7%). The median duration of first-line treatment was one year (IQR, 5–21 months). As of 31 December 2023, 45 (54%) patients in our cohort were alive (Table 1).

Table 1. Baseline Characteristics; [1]M: N Missing (% Missing), IQR, interquartile range; ADT, androgen deprivation therapy; TIAs, transient ischemic attacks; AIDS, acquired immunodeficiency syndrome; Ca Bladder, carcinoma bladder; BMI, body mass index; ECOG, Eastern Cooperative Oncology Group, PSA, prostate-specific antigen; ADT, androgen deprivation therapy; ¶ High-volume disease was defined as per the protocol of the CHAARTED trial by Sweeney et al., 2015 [17].

Characteristic	[1]M	Overall, N = 84
Age, Median (IQR)		66 (59–71)
Area, n (%)		
Rural		29 (35)
Urban		55 (65)
Education, n (%)		
Illiterate		8 (9.5)
Schooling		47 (56)
Graduate and above		29 (35)
Duration of Disease (Months), Median (IQR)	10 (12)	11 (4–38)
Comorbidities, n (%)		
Diabetes Mellitus, n (%)		15 (18)
Hypertension, n (%)		29 (35)
Hypothyroidism, n (%)		2 (2.4)
Coronary Artery Disease, n (%)		5 (6.0)
Chronic Kidney Disease, n (%)		1 (1.2)
Stroke and TIAs, n (%)		2 (2.4)
Other (AIDS, Hepatitis B, Ca Bladder, Hernia), n (%)		4 (4.8)
Number of Comorbidities, n (%)		
None		44 (52)
1 Comorbidity		29 (35)
>1 Comorbidity		11 (13)
Tobacco (Smokeless), n (%)		49 (58)
Smoking, n (%)		30 (36)
Alcohol, n (%)		25 (30)

Table 1. Cont.

Characteristic	¹M	Overall, N = 84
Type of Metastasis, n (%)	5 (6.0)	
Bony metastasis		22 (28)
Visceral metastasis		9 (11)
Bony and Visceral metastasis		48 (61)
Accessibility to AIIMS (kilometers), Median (IQR)	2 (2.4)	70 (21–400)
BMI, n (%)		
Underweight (< 18.5)		6 (7.1)
Normal (18.5–22.9)		25 (30)
Overweight (23–24.9)		14 (17)
Obese (> 25)		39 (46)
ECOG Status, n (%)	4 (4.8)	
ECOG (0–1)		47 (59)
ECOG (2–3)		33 (41)
PSA (ng/mL), Median (IQR)	3 (3.6)	7 (1–71)
Gleason Score, n (%)	6 (7.1)	
6 and 7, Low and Medium Risk		19 (24)
8, High Risk		23 (29)
9 and 10, High Risk		36 (46)
Castration Sensitivity, n (%)	5 (6.0)	
Castration-Sensitive, CSPC		39 (49)
Castration-Resistant, CRPC		40 (51)
Type of ADT, n (%)	6 (7.1)	
Medical		24 (31)
Surgical		54 (69)
Risk-Stratification, n (%)	5 (6.0)	
Low-risk		28 (35)
High-risk		51 (65)
Burden of Disease, n (%) ¶	5 (6.0)	
Low-volume		30 (38)
High-volume		49 (62)
Number of Treatment Lines, n (%)	5 (6.0)	
1 Line of Treatment		47 (59)
>1 Lines of Treatment		32 (41)
1st Line Treatment Received, n (%)	10 (12)	
ADT + Abiraterone		53 (72)
ADT + Docetaxel		17 (23)
ADT + Enzalutamide		2 (2.7)
ADT + Fosfosterol		2 (2.7)

Table 1. *Cont.*

Characteristic	[1]M	Overall, N = 84
Treatment at the Time of Assessment, n (%)	10 (12)	
ADT + Abiraterone		51 (69)
ADT + Docetaxel		17 (23)
ADT + Enzalutamide		5 (6.8)
ADT + Cabazitaxel		1 (1.4)
Duration of 1st Line Treatment (Months), Median (IQR)	13 (15)	12 (5–21)
Current Status, n (%)		
Alive		45 (54)
Dead		39 (46)

3.2. Quality of Life

The mean composite FACT-P, FACT-P TOI, and FACT-G scores and their respective standard deviations (SD) were 110.27 (20.18), 70.33 (15.16), and 79.25 (15.02), respectively. The domain-wise mean scores and SD for the subscales of physical well-being (PWB), social/family well-being (SWB), emotional well-being (EWB), functional well-being (FWB), and prostate cancer-specific subscale (PCS) were 20.41 (5.69), 21.24 (5.46), 18.70 (4.39), 18.90 (5.60), and 31.02 (7.10), respectively. Patients on chemotherapy had a significantly higher PCS ($p = 0.03$); however, the distributions were not significantly different for the composite scores across these subgroups (Figure 2 and Table 2).

Table 2. Domain-wise HRQOL; ADT, androgen deprivation therapy; ARTA, androgen receptor-targeted agent.

Characteristic	Overall, N = 84	ADT + ARTA, N = 56	ADT + Chemotherapy, N = 18	Unknown/Missing, N = 10	*p*-Value [1]
Physical Well-Being (0–28)					0.93
Mean (SD)	20.41 (5.69)	20.37 (5.64)	20.31 (5.75)	20.82 (6.48)	
Social/Family Well-Being (0–28)					0.76
Mean (SD)	21.24 (5.46)	20.98 (5.46)	21.29 (6.63)	22.60 (2.74)	
Emotional Well-Being (0–24)					0.29
Mean (SD)	18.70 (4.39)	18.10 (4.70)	19.78 (3.90)	20.10 (2.64)	
Functional Well-Being (0–28)					0.71
Mean (SD)	18.90 (5.60)	19.14 (5.77)	18.43 (5.69)	18.40 (4.88)	
Prostate Cancer Subscale (0–48)					**0.031**
Mean (SD)	31.02 (7.10)	30.15 (7.09)	34.82 (6.36)	29.06 (6.57)	
FACT-P TOI (Trial Outcome Index) (0–104)					0.56
Mean (SD)	70.33 (15.16)	69.66 (15.49)	73.56 (14.33)	68.28 (15.43)	
FACT-G (General Cancer) (0–108)					0.73
Mean (SD)	79.25 (15.02)	78.59 (15.27)	79.81 (15.23)	81.92 (14.33)	
FACT-P (Prostate Cancer) (0–156)					0.53
Mean (SD)	110.27 (20.18)	108.74 (20.46)	114.62 (20.02)	110.98 (19.63)	

[1] Kruskal–Wallis rank sum test. Bold values denote statistical significance at the $p < 0.05$ level.

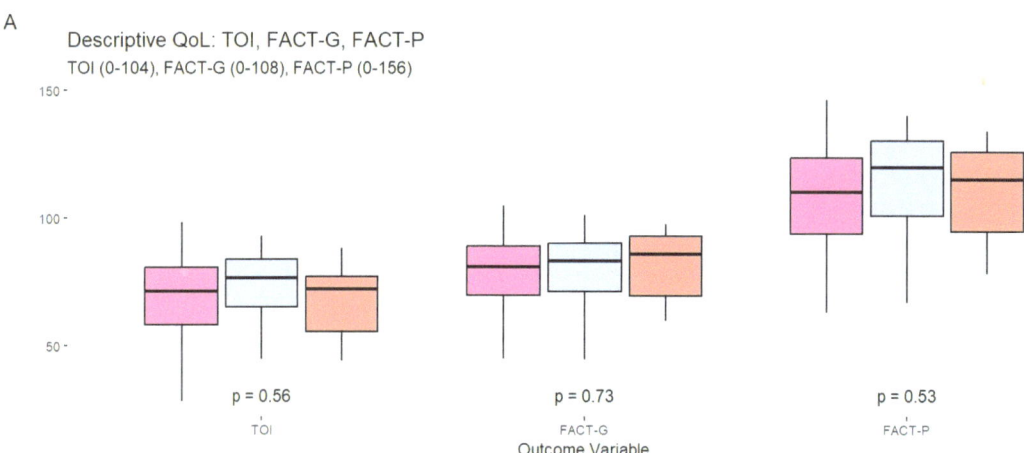
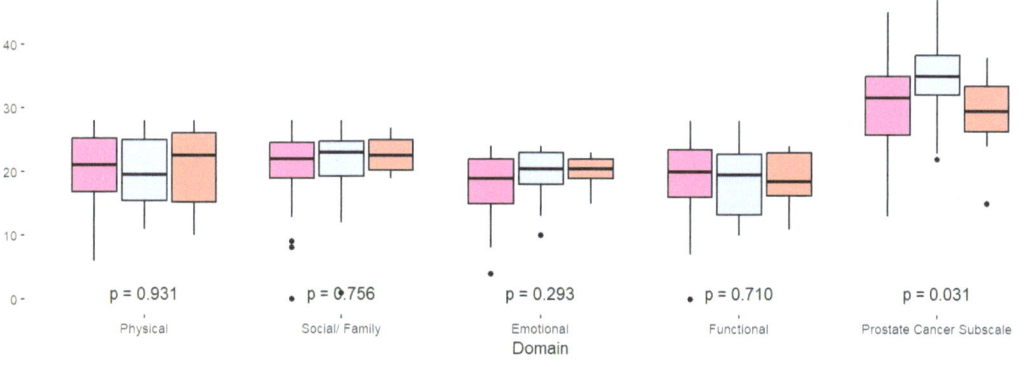

Figure 2. Composite outcome scores (**A**) and domain-wise score constituting FACT-P (**B**) stratified by the current treatment received; FACT-P: Functional Assessment of Cancer Therapy-Prostate; FACT-G: Functional Assessment of Cancer Therapy-General; TOI: Trial Outcome Index; ADT: androgen deprivation therapy; ARTA: androgen receptor-targeted agent.

3.3. Factors Affecting HRQoL

In univariable regression analysis, the FACT-P TOI was significantly better in patients with a longer duration of first-line treatment received ($\beta = 0.28$; 95% confidence interval [CI], 0.04 to 0.52; $p = 0.02$) and those with a higher body mass index (BMI) ($\beta = 6.80$; 95% CI, 0.30 to 13.0; $p = 0.04$) (Table 3). On multivariable analysis, BMI > 25 was the only factor associated with a better QOL ($\beta = 8.20$; 95% CI, 1.20 to 15.0; $p = 0.02$). Additionally, obesity (BMI > 25) was also an independent predictor of a higher FACT-P score ($\beta = 11.0$; 95% CI, 1.60 to 21.0; $p = 0.02$). BMI > 25 also correlated positively with the composite FACT-G score ($\beta = 6.50$; 95% CI, 0.05 to 13.0; $p = 0.05$), while higher PSA levels were negatively affecting the total FACT-G score ($\beta = -0.01$; 95% CI, -0.02 to 0.00; $p = 0.03$). On multivariable analysis, serum PSA levels independently predicted a worse FACT-G score, and obesity had a trend towards significance ($\beta = 7.20$; 95% CI, -0.10 to 14.0; $p = 0.054$) on multivariable analysis (Table 4).

Table 3. Univariable Regression Analysis; FACT-P: Functional Assessment of Cancer Therapy—Prostate; FACT-G: Functional Assessment of Cancer Therapy—General; TOI: Trial Outcome Index; ADT, androgen deprivation therapy; ARTA, androgen receptor-targeted agent; ECOG, Eastern Cooperative Oncology Group; PSA, prostate-specific antigen; BMI, body mass index.

Characteristic	TOI		FACT-G		FACT-P	
	Beta (95% CI) [1]	p-Value	Beta (95% CI) [1]	p-Value	Beta (95% CI) [1]	p-Value
Age	−0.14 (−0.51 to 0.23)	0.44	−0.05 (−0.42 to 0.32)	0.78	−0.17 (−0.67 to 0.32)	0.49
Area		0.72		0.95		0.82
Rural	—		—		—	
Urban	1.3 (−5.7 to 8.2)		−0.21 (−7.1 to 6.7)		−1.0 (−10 to 8.2)	
Accessibility to AIIMS with respect to Median Distance		0.13		0.92		0.60
Lesser/Equal	—		—		—	
Greater	−5.1 (−12 to 1.6)		−0.33 (−7.0 to 6.3)		−2.3 (−11 to 6.6)	
Education		0.97		0.67		0.93
Illiterate	—		—		—	
Schooling	0.36 (−11 to 12)		2.6 (−8.9 to 14)		1.2 (−14 to 17)	
Graduate and above	1.2 (−11 to 13)		4.9 (−7.1 to 17)		2.6 (−14 to 19)	
Duration of Disease with respect to Median Duration		0.88		0.63		0.61
Lesser/Equal	—		—		—	
Greater	0.55 (−6.6 to 7.8)		1.7 (−5.4 to 8.9)		2.4 (−7.1 to 12)	
Number of Comorbidities		0.63		0.81		0.87
None	—		—		—	
1 Comorbidity	0.65 (−6.6 to 7.9)		2.3 (−4.9 to 9.5)		1.2 (−8.5 to 11)	
>1 Comorbidity	−4.4 (−15 to 5.8)		0.33 (−9.8 to 10)		−2.7 (−16 to 11)	
Tobacco (Smokeless)	−2.6 (−9.3 to 4.1)	0.44	−0.68 (−7.3 to 6.0)	0.84	−0.66 (−9.6 to 8.3)	0.88
Alcohol	0.54 (−6.7 to 7.8)	0.88	2.4 (−4.7 to 9.6)	0.50	0.93 (−8.7 to 11)	0.85
Type of Metastasis		0.23		0.48		0.32
Bony metastasis	—		—		—	
Visceral metastasis	−10 (−22 to 1.5)		−7.2 (−19 to 4.7)		−12 (−28 to 3.7)	
Bony and Visceral metastasis	−3.2 (−11 to 4.4)		−1.4 (−9.1 to 6.3)		−3.7 (−14 to 6.5)	
Obese: BMI > 25	6.8 (0.31 to 13)	**0.040**	6.5 (0.05 to 13)	**0.048**	9.6 (1.0 to 18)	**0.028**
ECOG		0.072		0.44		0.36
ECOG (0–1)	—		—		—	
ECOG (2–3)	−6.2 (−13 to 0.57)		−2.7 (−9.5 to 4.1)		−4.2 (−13 to 4.9)	
PSA	−0.01 (−0.01 to 0.00)	0.16	−0.01 (−0.02 to 0.00)	**0.029**	−0.01 (−0.02 to 0.00)	0.062
Gleason Score Category		0.96		0.44		0.79
6 and 7, Low and Medium Risk	—		—		—	
8, High Risk	−0.36 (−9.8 to 9.1)		−4.0 (−13 to 5.3)		−2.9 (−16 to 9.8)	
9 and 10, High Risk	0.75 (−7.9 to 9.4)		1.1 (−7.5 to 9.7)		0.78 (−11 to 12)	
Castration Sensitivity		0.15		0.40		0.30
Castration-Sensitive, CSPC	—		—		—	
Castration-Resistant, CRPC	−5.0 (−12 to 1.9)		−2.9 (−9.7 to 3.9)		−4.9 (−14 to 4.3)	

Table 3. Cont.

Characteristic	TOI		FACT-G		FACT-P	
	Beta (95% CI) [1]	p-Value	Beta (95% CI) [1]	p-Value	Beta (95% CI) [1]	p-Value
Type of ADT Received		0.53		0.67		0.85
Medical	—		—		—	
Surgical	−2.4 (−10 to 5.2)		1.6 (−5.9 to 9.1)		0.95 (−9.1 to 11)	
Burden of Disease		0.37		0.24		0.24
Low-volume	—		—		—	
High-volume	−3.2 (−10 to 3.9)		−4.2 (−11 to 2.8)		−5.6 (−15 to 3.9)	
Number of Treatment Lines Received		0.60		0.72		0.73
1 Line of Treatment	—		—		—	
>1 Lines of Treatment	−1.9 (−8.9 to 5.2)		−1.3 (−8.2 to 5.7)		−1.7 (−11 to 7.8)	
1st Line Treatment Received		0.053		0.055		0.065
Abiraterone	—		—		—	
Docetaxel	−9.7 (−18 to −1.6)		−9.8 (−18 to −1.7)		−12 (−23 to −1.1)	
Enzalutamide	5.5 (−16 to 27)		3.5 (−18 to 25)		7.3 (−21 to 36)	
Fosfosterol	12 (−9.0 to 33)		12 (−8.8 to 33)		18 (−10 to 47)	
Duration of First-Line Treatment Received	0.28 (0.04 to 0.52)	**0.020**	0.19 (−0.06 to 0.43)	0.13	0.31 (−0.02 to 0.63)	0.063
Current Treatment Received		0.35		0.77		0.29
ADT + ARTA	—		—		—	
ADT + Chemotherapy	3.9 (−4.3 to 12)		1.2 (−7.0 to 9.5)		5.9 (−5.1 to 17)	

[1] CI = Confidence Interval. Bold values denote statistical significance at the $p < 0.05$ level.

Table 4. Multivariable Regression Analysis; ECOG, Eastern Cooperative Oncology Group; PSA, prostate-specific antigen; BMI, body mass index.

Characteristic	TOI		FACT-G		FACT-P	
	Beta (95% CI) [1]	p-Value	Beta (95% CI) [1]	p-Value	Beta (95% CI) [1]	p-Value
Age	−0.28 (−0.71 to 0.15)	0.20	−0.17 (−0.62 to 0.28)	0.45	−0.40 (−0.99 to 0.20)	0.19
Number of Comorbidities		0.35		0.96		0.69
None	—		—		—	
1 Comorbidity	−3.0 (−11 to 5.3)		−0.54 (−9.1 to 8.1)		−2.2 (−14 to 9.2)	
>1 Comorbidity	−7.9 (−19 to 3.5)		−1.7 (−14 to 10)		−6.5 (−22 to 9.1)	
Type of Metastasis		0.31		0.60		0.55
Bony metastasis	—		—		—	
Visceral metastasis	−10 (−23 to 3.1)		−5.8 (−19 to 7.8)		−9.5 (−27 to 8.4)	
Bony and Visceral metastasis	−2.0 (−10 to 6.1)		0.44 (−8.0 to 8.8)		−1.3 (−12 to 9.8)	
Obese: BMI > 25	8.2 (1.2 to 15)	**0.022**	7.2 (−0.12 to 14)	0.054	11 (1.6 to 21)	**0.023**
ECOG	−4.9 (−12 to 2.6)	0.19	−2.7 (−10 to 5.1)	0.49	−3.1 (−13 to 7.2)	0.55
PSA	−0.06 (−0.14 to 0.03)	0.19	−0.08 (−0.17 to 0.00)	0.061	−0.09 (−0.21 to 0.03)	0.12
1st Line Treatment Received		0.11		0.13		0.15
Abiraterone	—		—		—	
Docetaxel	−11 (−20 to −1.9)		−11 (−20 to −1.8)		−14 (−26 to −1.8)	
Enzalutamide	4.9 (−26 to 35)		2.8 (−29 to 35)		8.4 (−34 to 50)	
Fosfosterol	−3.7 (−28 to 20)		4.7 (−20 to 30)		1.0 (−32 to 34)	
Duration of First-Line Treatment Received	0.14 (−0.16 to 0.44)	0.35	0.04 (−0.27 to 0.35)	0.81	0.12 (−0.29 to 0.53)	0.56

[1] CI = Confidence Interval. Bold values denote statistical significance at the $p < 0.05$ level.

We also performed a domain-wise analysis with similar predictor variables. Obesity, duration of first-line treatment, and the current treatment received were significant predictors for the PCS subscale on univariable analysis; obesity and current treatment received were independently predictive on multivariable analysis (β = 4.20; 95% CI, 0.60 to 7.80; p = 0.02; β = 7.9; 95% CI, 3.0 to 13.0; p = 0.02). In the multivariable analysis, a higher ECOG PS score was associated with worse physical QOL (β = −3.3; 95% CI −6.20 to −0.50; p = 0.02), and obesity was significantly associated with a higher physical well-being domain score (β = 2.8; 95% CI, 0.1 to 5.5; p = 0.04). Higher PSA was found to impact emotional well-being (β (per 10 units change in PSA) = −0.029; 95% CI, −0.053 to −0.005; p = 0.02), and this association was consistent after adjusting for the other variables in multivariable analysis (β (per 10 units change in PSA) = −0.03; 95% CI, −0.06 to 0.00; p = 0.03) (Tables S1 and S2).

4. Discussion

We present cross-sectional HRQOL data from 84 patients with metastatic prostate cancer. We found that Indian patients with metastatic prostate cancer had a mean FACT-P QOL of 110.27 (SD ± 20.18). Weighing individual domains with the maximum scores, the worst affected domains included the prostate-specific subscale (including bowel and bladder function, sexual activity, and pain), followed by functional well-being. Further, patients with a higher BMI (>25 kg/m^2) had a better quality of life when adjusted for other baseline factors, including the prostate-specific subscale. There was no significant difference between the HRQOL outcomes between patients receiving ARTAs or chemotherapy at the time of assessment in our study cohort, except for the prostate-cancer-specific concerns subscale.

Indian population reference values are not available for the FACT-P questionnaire. However, compared with the United States reference values for the FACT-G scale, physical well-being is the most affected out of all domains in patients with metastatic prostate cancer, as shown in Figure S1 [21]. Surprisingly, our patients had higher scores for SWB [21.24 (5.6) versus 17.2 (6.9)], which may be due to the presence of a more cohesive social and family structure in the Indian setting, where the elderly often reside with their children in a joint family and are thus a source of social support [22]. Our outcome parameters were in close agreement with the baseline parameters reported by a Canadian study [23] with a FACT-P score of 111.3 (19.56) and similar means across domains. A study enrolling 280 patients from Europe, Australia, and North America reported a total FACT-P score of 105.1 ± 22.5 versus 110.27 ± 20.18 in our study [24]. This study enrolled patients with metastatic hormone-resistant prostate cancer, and this may explain the similar or lower HRQOL scores across FACT-G, FACT-P, and all its domains, as our study has almost an equal proportion of patients with CSPC and CRPC. Additionally, our patients had a better quality of life when compared with other metastatic solid organ tumors (lung, breast, cervical, and oral malignancies mainly), as depicted by the FACT-G scale [25].

We found that BMI was an independent predictor of quality of life scores. A lower BMI is the strongest predictor of a poor quality of life. The relationship between baseline BMI and HRQOL was explored in the CHAARTED study, and it was hypothesized that patients in the low BMI group had a poorer QOL because of the higher disease burden in these patients [12]. However, we found no significant difference in the disease burden between the two groups in our cohorts. The low BMI in our patients likely represents cancer-induced cachexia or weight loss due to disease activity. This causes significant impairment and a worse perception of the disease effect [26]. Patients with a high BMI have fat reserves, which may prevent cancer cachexia from manifesting [27]. Additionally, obese men are likely to have a higher estrogen level in their bodies due to peripheral conversion, which might be responsible for inhibiting tumor growth [27]. This relationship is similar to other cancers, such as breast cancer, where significant weight loss after diagnosis is an independent prognostic indicator [28]. However, it is noteworthy that obesity is associated with a higher recurrence rate, and the association is well-established in estrogen receptor-positive breast cancer [29]. Notably, sarcopenia and obesity may co-exist in men with androgen deprivation [30]. However, high BMI has previously been shown to have better outcomes, irrespective of the presence of sarcopenia [30]. However, it is relevant to note that due to the heterogeneous nature of our study population, this result may also reflect post-chemotherapy weight loss in the subset of patients on ADT + chemotherapy experiencing a worse HRQOL due to the effects of chemotherapy. We adjusted for this in the multivariable regression and noted worsening HRQOL with ADT + Docetaxel as 1st line therapy compared to ADT + Abiraterone ($\beta = -14$; 95% CI, -26 to -1.8), but the association was not significant ($p = 0.15$).

In addition to higher BMI, we found that serum PSA levels significantly predicted the FACT-G score but not the FACT-P scores. This reflects the variance of various composite scores for different predictor variables. Patients with a higher PSA had worse composite general scores. This is likely due to the higher disease burden, as is shown in the secondary analysis of the ALSYMPCA trial, where worsening of PSA overtime is associated with worse FACT-G scores [31]. The validation study for FACT-P also reported the statistically significant sensitivity of FACT-G to a change in PSA levels. However, they reported no statistically significant domain-wise changes, and we observed significant improvement in emotional well-being in patients with lower PSA levels [7]. This is expected as PSA anxiety is a prominent symptom for prostate cancer patients, with a prevalence of around 22%, and has been associated with poorer quality of life [32]. It is also interesting to note that while serum PSA levels are significantly associated with the FACT-G score, variables such as tumor load or type of metastasis do not seem to have an effect. Serum PSA levels are taken at the time of assessment; therefore, they represent the current status more accurately, and thus, they correlate better with HRQOL. In alia manu, the imaging studies (PET-CT) represent an earlier disease burden as they would have been conducted at an earlier time point and do not have a significant correlation with HRQOL.

Poorer ECOG performance status was associated with worse physical well-being, but not with the composite FACT-P score. ECOG is more directly representative of the physical status of the patient, minimizing its contribution to the composite score. This is somewhat in agreement with the FACT-P validation study, where, in addition to physical well-being, functional well-being, and the prostate cancer subscale, TOI and FACT-P had statistically significant sensitivity to changes in ECOG PS [7]. Performance status has previously been linked with worse physical symptoms using the National Comprehensive Cancer Network/Functional Assessment of Cancer Therapy—Prostate Symptom Index-Physical Scale (NFPSI-P) at baseline and after treatment [31]. ECOG PS has previously been identified as a strong prognostic factor in patients with metastatic prostate cancer [33]. This association of ECOG performance status with physical well-being and survival has also been shown in patients with metastatic lung cancer [34].

The striking absence of a lack of significant differences in HRQOL between the patients receiving chemotherapy and ARTAs may be hypothesized to reflect the advanced nature of metastatic prostate cancer, where the disease has more impact on the quality of life as opposed to the adverse effect profile of the patient's treatment. This may also reflect better disease control with chemotherapy. This is supported by the observation that patients on chemotherapy had a significantly better score on the prostate-cancer-specific concerns subscale ($\beta = 7.9$; 95% CI, 3.0 to 13.0; $p = 0.02$). Our results are in agreement with the results of the TAX 327 study, which suggests that docetaxel, despite its toxicity, has efficacious palliative effects as assessed by the FACT-P measure, with the greatest benefit for the PCS subscale [35].

The limitations of our study include the cross-sectional nature of a relatively small sample size, which represents only a screenshot of the data with no follow-up data after therapy. Additionally, the lack of population reference for the Indian subcontinent makes it difficult to accurately understand the magnitude of the deterioration of quality of life. A domain-wise analysis is difficult with FACT-P, where the contribution of domains depends on the number of items; weighted domain-wise subscores to calculate an adjusted FACT-P approach still remain to be validated [36]. The various indices have slight variations in the sensitivities to multiple dependent variables, and there is a possibility of type 1 statistical errors. Moreover, data and evidence are lacking as to what extent HRQOL can be improved by manipulation of the cachectic state by nutritional therapies or otherwise. Ours is one of the first studies in India to assess HRQOL in patients with prostate cancer and their demographic and cultural predictors individually.

5. Conclusions

The FACT-P measure is a useful patient-reported outcome measure assessing HRQOL in patients with metastatic prostate cancer in a tertiary care setting. However, there is a need to develop an independent population reference sample in India for FACT-G and FACT-P. We found that low BMI is an independent predictor of poor QoL. Thus, efforts are required to develop strategies to manage the nutritional status of patients with metastatic disease and to prospectively assess such interventions and their impact on HRQOL. Doublet therapy was the contemporary standard of care during the period of the study. Based on the change in institutional protocols, patients at our center have now been receiving triplet therapy, and it will also be of interest to us to study HRQOL in these patients. Future prospective studies that include a longitudinal follow-up of patients will provide more insight into how HRQOL changes as the disease progresses and with therapy and will help expand the use of the FACT-P questionnaire in our setting.

Supplementary Materials: The following supporting information can be downloaded at: https://www.mdpi.com/article/10.3390/curroncol31090366/s1, Figure S1: Domain-wise scores constituting FACT-P compared with United States population reference values.; Table S1: Domain-wise univariable regression analysis; Table S2: Domain-wise multivariable regression analysis.

Author Contributions: Conception and design: C.M., H.G., R.K.S., and A.B.; provision of study materials or patients: R.K.S., A.S. (Aparna Sharma), S.P., S.A.S., S.K., C.J.D., K.P.H., A.S. (Amlesh Seth), B.N., and A.B.; collection and assembly of data: C.M., H.G., C.N., A.S., B.B.G., and G.T.; data analysis and interpretation: C.M., H.G., C.N., and A.B.; manuscript writing: C.M., H.G., C.N., R.K.S. A.S. (Aparna Sharma), B.B.G., G.T., S.P., S.A.S., S.K., C.J.D., K.P.H., A.S. (Amlesh Seth), B.N., and A.B. All authors have read and agreed to the published version of the manuscript.

Funding: This research received no external funding.

Institutional Review Board Statement: All procedures performed in studies involving human participants were in accordance with the ethical standards of the institutional ethics committee and with the 1964 Helsinki Declaration and its later amendments or comparable ethical standards. The institutional ethics committee approved the study (reference number IEC-646/03.09.2021, RP-23/2021). Written informed consent was obtained from all patients before their participation.

Informed Consent Statement: Written and informed consent was obtained from each participant prior to recruitment in the study.

Data Availability Statement: The datasets used and/or analyzed during the current study are available from the corresponding author upon reasonable request.

Conflicts of Interest: The authors declare that they have no competing interests.

References

1. Ferlay, J.; Ervik, M.; Lam, F.; Colombet, M.; Mery, L.; Piñeros, M.; Znaor, A.; Soerjomataram, I.; Bray, F. *Global Cancer Observatory: Cancer Today*; International Agency for Research on Cancer: Lyon, France, 2020; Available online: https://gco.iarc.fr/today (accessed on 28 January 2024).
2. Sayegh, N.; Swami, U.; Agarwal, N. Recent Advances in the Management of Metastatic Prostate Cancer. *JCO Oncol. Pract.* **2022**, *18*, 45–55. [CrossRef] [PubMed]
3. Leaning, D.; Kaur, G.; Morgans, A.K.; Ghouse, R.; Mirante, O.; Chowdhury, S. Treatment landscape and burden of disease in metastatic castration-resistant prostate cancer: Systematic and structured literature reviews. *Front. Oncol.* **2023**, *13*, 1240864. [CrossRef]
4. Megari, K. Quality of life in chronic disease patients. *Health Psychol. Res.* **2013**, *1*, e27. [CrossRef]

5. Chu, D.; Popovic, M.; Chow, E.; Cella, D.; Beaumont, J.L.; Lam, H.; Nguyen, J.; Giovanni, J.D.; Pulenzas, N.; Bedard, G.; et al. Development, characteristics and validity of the EORTC QLQ-PR25 and the FACT-P for assessment of quality of life in prostate cancer patients. *J. Comp. Eff. Res.* **2014**, *3*, 523–531. [CrossRef]
6. Ratti, M.M.; Gandaglia, G.; Sisca, E.S.; Derevianko, A.; Alleva, E.; Beyer, K.; Moss, C.; Barletta, F.; Scuderi, S.; Omar, M.I.; et al. A Systematic Review to Evaluate Patient-Reported Outcome Measures (PROMs) for Metastatic Prostate Cancer According to the COnsensus-Based Standard for the Selection of Health Measurement INstruments (COSMIN) Methodology. *Cancers* **2022**, *14*, 5120. [CrossRef] [PubMed]
7. Esper, P.; Mo, F.; Chodak, G.; Sinner, M.; Cella, D.; Pienta, K.J. Measuring quality of life in men with prostate cancer using the Functional Assessment of Cancer Therapy-prostate instrument. *Urology* **1997**, *50*, 920–928. [CrossRef]
8. Cella, D.; Nichol, M.B.; Eton, D.; Nelson, J.B.; Mulani, P. Estimating Clinically Meaningful Changes for the Functional Assessment of Cancer Therapy—Prostate: Results from a Clinical Trial of Patients with Metastatic Hormone-Refractory Prostate Cancer. *Value Health* **2009**, *12*, 124–129. [CrossRef]
9. Sharma, A.; Garg, G.; Sadasukhi, N.; Sadasukhi, T.C.; Gupta, H.L.; Gupta, M.; Malik, S.; Patel, K.; Sinha, R.J. A prospective longitudinal study to evaluate bone health, implication of FRAX tool and impact on quality of life (FACT-P) in advanced prostate cancer patients. *Am. J. Clin. Exp. Urol.* **2021**, *9*, 211–220. [PubMed]
10. Sullivan, P.W.; Nelson, J.B.; Mulani, P.M.; Sleep, D. Quality of life as a potential predictor for morbidity and mortality in patients with metastatic hormone-refractory prostate cancer. *Qual. Life Res. Int. J. Qual. Life Asp. Treat. Care Rehabil.* **2006**, *15*, 1297–1306. [CrossRef]
11. Roy, S.; Morgan, S.C.; Spratt, D.E.; MacRae, R.M.; Grimes, S.; Malone, J.; Mukherjee, D.; Malone, S. Association of Baseline Patient-reported Health-related Quality of Life Metrics with Outcome in Localised Prostate Cancer. *Clin. Oncol.* **2022**, *34*, e61–e68. [CrossRef]
12. Morgans, A.K.; Chen, Y.; Jarrard, D.F.; Carducci, M.; Liu, G.; Eisenberger, M.; Plimack, E.R.; Bryce, A.; Garcia, J.A.; Dreicer, R.; et al. Association between baseline body mass index and survival in men with metastatic hormone-sensitive prostate cancer: ECOG-ACRIN CHAARTED E3805. *Prostate* **2022**, *82*, 1176–1185. [CrossRef]
13. 66th Annual Report, 2021–2022. All India Institute of Medical Sciences, New Delhi—110029. Available online: https://www.aiims.edu/images/pdf/annual_reports/english.pdf (accessed on 3 March 2024).
14. India 2020: Reference Annual. Profile—Literacy—Know India: National Portal of India. Publications Division, Ministry of Information and Broadcasting, Government of India, 2020. Available online: https://pmindiaun.gov.in/public_files/assets/pdf/India_2020_REFERENCEANNUAL.pdf (accessed on 2 March 2024).
15. Misra, A.; Chowbey, P.; Makkar, B.M.; Vikram, N.K.; Wasir, J.S.; Chadha, D.; Joshi, S.R.; Sadikot, S.; Gupta, R.; Gulati, S.; et al. Consensus statement for diagnosis of obesity, abdominal obesity and the metabolic syndrome for Asian Indians and recommendations for physical activity, medical and surgical management. *J. Assoc. Physicians India.* **2009**, *57*, 163–170.
16. Hussain, M.; Tombal, B.; Saad, F.; Fizazi, K.; Sternberg, C.N.; Crawford, E.D.; Kopyltso, E.; Kalebasty, A.R.; Bögemann, M.; Ye, D.; et al. Darolutamide Plus Androgen-Deprivation Therapy and Docetaxel in Metastatic Hormone-Sensitive Prostate Cancer by Disease Volume and Risk Subgroups in the Phase III ARASENS Trial. *J. Clin. Oncol.* **2023**, *41*, 3595–3607. [CrossRef]
17. Sweeney, C.J.; Chen, Y.H.; Carducci, M.; Liu, G.; Jarrard, D.F.; Eisenberger, M.; Wong, Y.-N.; Hahn, N.; Kohli, M.; Cooney, M.M.; et al. Chemohormonal Therapy in Metastatic Hormone-Sensitive Prostate Cancer. *N. Engl. J. Med.* **2015**, *373*, 737–746. [CrossRef] [PubMed]
18. Singh, D. Quality of life in cancer patients receiving palliative care. *Indian. J. Palliat. Care* **2010**, *16*, 36. [CrossRef] [PubMed]
19. Kretschmer, A.; van den Bergh, R.C.N.; Martini, A.; Marra, G.; Valerio, M.; Tsaur, I.; Heidegger, I.; Kasivisvanathan, V.; Kesch, C.; Preisser, F.; et al. Assessment of Health-Related Quality of Life in Patients with Advanced Prostate Cancer—Current State and Future Perspectives. *Cancers* **2021**, *14*, 147. [CrossRef] [PubMed]
20. Webster, K.; Cella, D.; Yost, K. The Functional Assessment of Chronic Illness Therapy (FACIT) Measurement System: Properties, applications, and interpretation. *Health Qual. Life Outcomes* **2003**, *1*, 79. [CrossRef] [PubMed]
21. Cella, D.; Ganguli, A.; Turnbull, J.; Rohay, J.; Morlock, R. US Population Reference Values for Health-Related Quality of Life Questionnaires Based on Demographics of Patients with Prostate Cancer. *Adv. Ther.* **2022**, *39*, 3696–3710. [CrossRef]
22. Han, J.; Yang, D.L.; Liu, J.H.; Li, B.H.; Kan, Y.; Ma, S.; Mao, L.J. Family-centered psychological support helps improve illness cognition and quality of life in patients with advanced prostate cancer. *Zhonghua Nan Ke Xue Natl. J. Androl.* **2020**, *26*, 505–512.
23. Gotto, G.; Drachenberg, D.E.; Chin, J.; Casey, R.; Fradet, V.; Sabbagh, R.; Shayegan, B.; Rendon, R.A.; Danielson, B.; Camacho, F.; et al. Real-world evidence in patient-reported outcomes (PROs) of metastatic castrate-resistant prostate cancer (mCRPC) patients treated with abiraterone acetate + prednisone (AA+P) across Canada: Final results of COSMiC. *Can. Urol. Assoc. J.* **2020**, *14*. Available online: https://cuaj.ca/index.php/journal/article/view/6388 (accessed on 29 January 2024). [CrossRef]
24. Wu, E.Q.; Mulani, P.; Farrell, M.H.; Sleep, D. Mapping FACT-P and EORTC QLQ-C30 to Patient Health Status Measured by EQ-5D in Metastatic Hormone-Refractory Prostate Cancer Patients. *Value Health* **2007**, *10*, 408–414. [CrossRef]
25. Jacob, J.; Palat, G.; Verghese, N.; Chandran, P.; Rapelli, V.; Kumari, S.; Malhotra, C.; Teo, I.; Finkelstein, E. Health-related quality of life and its socio-economic and cultural predictors among advanced cancer patients: Evidence from the APPROACH cross-sectional survey in Hyderabad-India. *BMC Palliat. Care* **2019**, *18*, 94. [CrossRef] [PubMed]
26. Vaughan, V.C.; Martin, P.; Lewandowski, P.A. Cancer cachexia: Impact, mechanisms and emerging treatments. *J. Cachexia Sarcopenia Muscle* **2013**, *4*, 95–109. [CrossRef]

27. Montgomery, B.; Nelson, P.S.; Vessella, R.; Kalhorn, T.; Hess, D.; Corey, E. Estradiol suppresses tissue androgens and prostate cancer growth in castration resistant prostate cancer. *BMC Cancer* **2010**, *10*, 244. [CrossRef] [PubMed]
28. Cespedes Feliciano, E.M.; Kroenke, C.H.; Bradshaw, P.T.; Chen, W.Y.; Prado, C.M.; Weltzien, E.K.; Castillo, A.L.; Caan, B.J. Postdiagnosis Weight Change and Survival Following a Diagnosis of Early-Stage Breast Cancer. *Cancer Epidemiol. Biomark. Prev.* **2017**, *26*, 44–50. [CrossRef] [PubMed]
29. Jiralerspong, S.; Goodwin, P.J. Obesity and Breast Cancer Prognosis: Evidence, Challenges, and Opportunities. *J. Clin. Oncol.* **2016**, *34*, 4203–4216. [CrossRef]
30. Xu, M.C.; Huelster, H.L.; Hatcher, J.B.; Avulova, S.; Stocks, B.T.; Glaser, Z.A.; Moses, K.A.; Silver, H.J. Obesity is Associated with Longer Survival Independent of Sarcopenia and Myosteatosis in Metastatic and/or Castrate-Resistant Prostate Cancer. *J. Urol.* **2021**, *205*, 800–805. [CrossRef]
31. Beaumont, J.L.; Butt, Z.; Li, R.; Cella, D. Meaningful differences and validity for the NCCN/FACT-P Symptom Index: An analysis of the ALSYMPCA data. *Cancer* **2019**, *125*, 1877–1885. [CrossRef]
32. James, C.; Brunckhorst, O.; Eymech, O.; Stewart, R.; Dasgupta, P.; Ahmed, K. Fear of cancer recurrence and PSA anxiety in patients with prostate cancer: A systematic review. *Support. Care Cancer* **2022**, *30*, 5577–5589. [CrossRef] [PubMed]
33. Assayag, J.; Kim, C.; Chu, H.; Webster, J. The prognostic value of Eastern Cooperative Oncology Group performance status on overall survival among patients with metastatic prostate cancer: A systematic review and meta-analysis. *Front. Oncol.* **2023**, *13*, 1194718. [CrossRef]
34. Jeon, H.; Eo, W.; Shim, B.; Kim, S.; Lee, S. Prognostic Value of Functional Assessment of Cancer Therapy-General (FACT-G) in Advanced Non-Small-Cell Lung Cancer Treated with Korean Medicine. *Evid. Based Complement. Altern. Med.* **2020**, *2020*, 2845401. [CrossRef] [PubMed]
35. Tannock, I.F.; de Wit, R.; Berry, W.R.; Horti, J.; Pluzanska, A.; Chi, K.N.; Oudard, S.; Théodore, C.; James, N.D.; Turesson, I.; et al. Docetaxel plus Prednisone or Mitoxantrone plus Prednisone for Advanced Prostate Cancer. *N. Engl. J. Med.* **2004**, *351*, 1502–1512. [CrossRef] [PubMed]
36. Stone, P.C.; Murphy, R.F.; Matar, H.E.; Almerie, M.Q. Quality of life in patients with prostate cancer: Development and application of a hybrid assessment method. *Prostate Cancer Prostatic Dis.* **2009**, *12*, 72–77. [CrossRef] [PubMed]

Disclaimer/Publisher's Note: The statements, opinions and data contained in all publications are solely those of the individual author(s) and contributor(s) and not of MDPI and/or the editor(s). MDPI and/or the editor(s) disclaim responsibility for any injury to people or property resulting from any ideas, methods, instructions or products referred to in the content.

MDPI AG
Grosspeteranlage 5
4052 Basel
Switzerland
Tel.: +41 61 683 77 34

Current Oncology Editorial Office
E-mail: curroncol@mdpi.com
www.mdpi.com/journal/curroncol

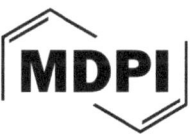

Disclaimer/Publisher's Note: The title and front matter of this reprint are at the discretion of the Guest Editor. The publisher is not responsible for their content or any associated concerns. The statements, opinions and data contained in all individual articles are solely those of the individual Editor and contributors and not of MDPI. MDPI disclaims responsibility for any injury to people or property resulting from any ideas, methods, instructions or products referred to in the content.

www.ingramcontent.com/pod-product-compliance
Lightning Source LLC
LaVergne TN
LVHW072325090526
838202LV00019B/2356